Primary Care Procedures in Women's Health

Sandra M. Sulik · Cathryn B. Heath
Editors

Primary Care Procedures in Women's Health

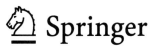 Springer

Editors

Sandra M. Sulik, MD, MS
Associate Professor, Family Medicine
St. Joseph's Family Medicine Residency
SUNY Upstate Medical Center
Department of Family Medicine
Syracuse, NY
USA

Cathryn B. Heath, MD
Clinical Associate Professor
of Family Medicine
UMDNJ
Department of Family Medicine
New Brunswick, NJ
USA

ISBN 978-0-387-76598-3   e-ISBN 978-0-387-76604-1
DOI 10.1007/978-0-387-76604-1
Springer New York Dordrecht Heidelberg London

Library of Congress Control Number: 2010927498

Printed on acid-free paper

Springer is part of Springer Science+Business Media (www.springer.com)

To my mom, who has provided constant faithful support, and to my family, Jeff, Maryann, Julie, Read, Tammy, Abbie, Joe, Lydia, and Lisa, who have always believed in me. Specials thanks to Ferne for her photo help, to my nurses and to my many patients who graciously allowed pictures to be taken during their procedures. My thanks to Cathy and Liz Corra for their support and energy throughout this process. Thanks to all our contributing authors for making the time to write their chapters and share their expertise and wisdom.

SMS

To my family, colleagues, staff, and patients: How lucky to be surrounded by such wonderful people! Special thanks to my husband John, Sandy, and Liz, all of whom have provided strength, encouragement, wisdom, and patience. To Brendan, Austin, and Claire – thanks for putting up with Mom's "homework."

CBH

Preface

Despite the common perception that medicine is becoming specialty driven, there are many reasons for primary care providers to offer women's health procedures in an office setting. Women feel more comfortable having procedures done by providers whom they already know and trust. Continuity of care is still valued by patients, who trust their primary care providers to work with them as collaborators in the decision-making process. Women have found that their options for care have become limited, not by their own decision, but by the lack of training of their provider. In rural areas, the barriers of time, expense, and travel often prevent many women from obtaining necessary care; yet many of the procedures that these women are requesting are relatively easy to learn. Positive experiences are shared by women who then refer friends and family by word of mouth.

This book has been designed to assist not only the clinician performing the procedures covered, but also the office staff with setting up the equipment tray prior to performing the procedure and with preparing office documents and coding information needed to complete the procedure. Most procedures covered can be done with a minimum investment in equipment and require minimal training. Some of the procedures are best done after a training course has been completed; however, even in these cases, this book will serve as a solid aid and review to the practitioner in performing the procedures within the office setting. It can also be used as a quick reference guide to refamiliarize the practitioner with the steps to a given procedure.

Each chapter outlines one women's health procedure and contains an overview of background information, indications, contraindications, complications, equipment needed, procedure steps, an office note, patient instructions, and a patient handout. Typical case studies and case study outcomes serve as illustrations of typical women found in practices who have needed each procedure. The "tricks and helpful hints" section draws on the years of experience of providers who have performed each procedure many times and have overcome common difficulties often encountered by newcomers to the procedure. A set-up picture of equipment is included to assist office staff in gathering the appropriate materials prior to starting the procedure. Algorithms assisting the provider with the steps to take at decision points of each procedure are also included to serve as a quick guide. References and additional resources are listed for further education, learning, and equipment needs. Illustrations, images, and photos further enrich the chapters.

We have elected to start our procedure book with the most common of procedures found in women's health – these include pelvic examinations and Pap smear collection – and its content extends to some of the more complicated office procedures, such as laser surgery and LEEP. There are sections on basic women's health procedures, contraceptive procedures, diagnostic procedures, therapeutic procedures, and cosmetic procedures. The chapters are authored by family physicians experienced with the procedure covered. Also included are specific chapters on coding and billing, authored by a physician who oversees a 35-physican practice and has had additional training in coding and billing. A separate chapter is included on the medicolegal aspects of performing women's health procedures in an office setting. This chapter outlines the necessary legal and regulatory considerations that must be addressed before adding many of these procedures to an office practice.

Many procedures have become a "lost art." For example, as fewer patients choose diaphragms as a method of contraception, fewer clinicians are being trained in fitting and inserting them. A number of these common women's health procedures are not routinely taught in residency or training programs, and, hence, many practitioners do not offer them in their offices. Some are trained during residency but have not performed the procedure for some time and need a review prior to performing the procedure. This book will serve as a quick refresher for those procedures for which the clinician may have had previous training but may not have performed for a while.

The old standard of "see one, teach one, do one" gets more difficult as procedures become more complex and require more training before they can be performed. A number of excellent procedures courses are offered by the American Academy of Family Physicians, American College of Obstetrics and Gynecology, and the American Society of Cervical Pathology and Colposcopy. Suppliers of medical equipment also offer training courses. Often, a training package is offered as part of the purchase of more expensive pieces of equipment. Finding a local experienced physician to precept and mentor a less experienced physician in the initial few procedures is another way to become skilled in performing most of these procedures after a training course has been taken. Proctoring or precepted experience is crucial, especially for complex procedures, not only to reduce medicolegal liability but also to ensure patient safety.

Having the patient schedule a separate appointment to have a procedure performed allows the patient time to read the information provided about the upcoming procedure, ask appropriate questions, and prepare herself for the actual procedure. This allows for the proper amount of time to be scheduled for the procedure to be done; for the inexperienced clinician, additional time should be scheduled. Scheduling new procedures at the end of an office session allows more time for the clinician. As the practitioner's confidence grows, scheduling times can be adjusted. Scheduling an office session dedicated to just procedures can also be helpful.

A well-trained staff is the provider's best asset. A lunchtime training session can be very helpful for teaching the staff proper equipment set-up, proper sterile technique for set-up and assisting with the procedure, and how best to assist with the procedure itself. Appropriate equipment set-ups can greatly ease the procedure.

Proper Occupational Safety and Health Administration (OSHA) guidelines must also be followed. For most women's health procedures, it is wise to have an assistant in the room with the provider, to assist as well as to comfort and to chaperone the patient. All procedures should be done with a consent signed by the patient.

It is important to understand the appropriate billing of your services in order to be properly compensated for your work. Both CPT® codes developed by the American Medical Association and the ICD9 (International Classification of Diseases, 9th Revision, Center for Disease Control and Prevention) codes are provided as suggested codes for each procedure. There may be other more appropriate codes; therefore, each procedure should be coded based on the procedures done or services rendered. Some minor procedures, such as cervical polyp removal, do not have a specific CPT® code. In those circumstances, the CPT® manual recommends that the clinician code the appropriate-level office visit. As covered in our billing and coding chapter, certain insurance plans reimburse differently for some of the contraception devices, and insurance reimbursement varies across the county. It is important that the provider be aware of these differences as he/she offers certain procedures in the office. Prior authorization is sometimes necessary as well. Some devices (levonorgestrel intrauterine system or etonorgestrel implantables) may need to be ordered through the patient's insurance company and delivered to the office before insertion.

It is our hope that this book will act as a manual for women's health procedures for all providers, including family physicians, gynecologists, general internists, residents, nurse practitioners, nurse midwives, and physician's assistants. There are presently no other texts specifically written for providers and staff of women's health services. It is our hope that this procedures text will allow the practitioner to be competent, efficient, and comfortable in performing each procedure in the office on a regular basis.

Syracuse, NY   Sandra M. Sulik, MD, MS
New Brunswick, NJ   Cathryn B. Heath, MD

Contents

Contributors

Rhina Acevedo, MD
Assistant Professor, Department of Family Medicine, University of Medicine and Dentistry of New Jersey, New Brunswick, NJ, USA

Donald J. Brideau, Jr., MD, MMM
President, Springfield Family Medicine and Cosmetic Laser and Skin Services, Alexandria, VA, USA
Assistant Clinical Professor, Georgetown University Medical School and George Washington School of Medicine and Health Science, Alexandria, VA, USA

Dawn Brink-Cymerman, MD
Assistant Professor, Department of Family Medicine, SUNY Upstate Medical Center, St. Joseph's Hospital Family Medicine Residency, Syracuse, NY, USA

John Ladislav Bucek, MD, FAAFP
Program Director, Somerset Family Medicine Residency Program, Somerset Medical Center, Somerville, NJ, USA

DeAnn Cummings, MD
Assistant Professor, Department of Family Medicine, SUNY Upstate Medical Center, St. Joseph's Hospital Family Medicine Residency, Syracuse, NY, USA

Janice E. Daugherty, MD
Associate Professor, Director of Predoctoral Education, Department of Family Medicine, Brody School of Medicine, East Carolina University, Greenville, NC, USA

Sharon D. Gertzman, DO
Medical Director, Serenity Medical Spa, Pennington, NJ, USA

Cathryn B. Heath, MD
Clinical Associate Professor of Family Medicine, Department of Family Medicine, Robert Wood Johnson Medical School, University of Medicine and Dentistry of New Jersey, New Brunswick, NJ, USA

Joel A. Kase, DO, MPH
Division Chief for Public Health, Department of Family Medicine
University of New England, College of Osteopathic Medicine,
Biddeford, ME, USA

Catherine I. Keating, MD
Family Health Network of Central New York, Cortland, New York, USA
Department of Family Medicine, St. Joseph's Hospital Health Center,
Syracuse, NY, USA

David E. Kolva, MD
Clinical Associate Professor, Department of Family Medicine,
SUNY Upstate Medical Center, Clinical Faculty,
St. Joseph's Hospital Family Medicine Residency, Syracuse, NY

Jeffrey P. Levine, MD, MPH
Professor, Director, Women's Health Programs, Department of Family Medicine,
Robert Wood Johnson Medical School, University of Medicine
and Dentistry of New Jersey, New Brunswick, NJ, USA

Jennifer N. McCaul, MD
Assistant Professor, Department of Family Medicine, St. Joseph's Hospital
Family Medicine Residency, Syracuse, NY, USA

Barbara Jo McGarry, MD
Clinical Assistant Professor, Department of Family Medicine,
Robert Wood Johnson Medical School, University of Medicine
and Dentistry of New Jersey, New Brunswick, NJ, USA

Kristen McNamara, MD
Assistant Professor, Department of Family Medicine,
St. Joseph's Hospital Family Medicine Residency, Syracuse, NY, USA

Elizabeth H. McNany, MD
Assistant Professor, Department of Family Medicine, St. Joseph's Hospital
Family Medicine Residency, Syracuse, NY, USA
Department of Medical Education, St. Joseph's Hospital, Syracuse, NY, USA

Kathleen M. O'Hanlon, MD
Professor, Department of Family Practice, Joan C. Edwards Marshall University
School of Medicine, Huntington, WV, USA

Matthew L. Picone, MD, MSEd
Assistant Professor, Department of Family Medicine, SUNY Upstate Medical
Center, St. Joseph's Hospital Family Medicine Residency, Syracuse, NY, USA

Beverly A. Poelstra, MD, FAAP
Clinical Associate Professor of Pediatrics, Department of Pediatrics,
Division of Pediatric Emergency Medicine, The Bristol-Myers Squibb Children's
Hospital of Robert Wood Johnson University Hospital, University of Medicine
and Dentistry of New Jersey, New Brunswick, NJ, USA

Sandra M. Sulik, MD, MS
Associate Professor, Department of Family Medicine, Upstate Medical Center,
St. Joseph's Family Medicine Residency, Syracuse, NY, USA

Laurie Turenne-Kolpan, MD
Faculty Physician, Department of Family Practice, Hunterdon Medical Center,
Flemington, NJ, USA

Justine Wu, MD, MPH
Clinical Assistant Professor, Department of Family Medicine, Robert Wood
Johnson Medical School, University of Medicine and Dentistry of New Jersey,
New Brunswick, NJ, USA

Chapter 1
Introduction: The Case for Procedures in Primary Care

Cathryn B. Heath and Sandra M. Sulik

Case Studies

Dr. Jerri Neilsen had a problem. She needed to do a procedure that she had never performed on anyone. There were no specialists available to do it. The nearest specialist was a continent away. What did she do? According to her first-hand account in *Ice Bound: A Doctor's Incredible Battle for Survival at the South Pole*, she received instructions by computer and by satellite telephone on how to do a Fine Needle Aspiration (FNA). She and her assistant, who was an Emergency Medical Technician (EMT), practiced the aspiration technique on some fruit, and then both she and her assistant did an FNA – on Dr. Jerri Neilsen [1].

One of the authors and editors of this book (CBH) was taking care of one of her patients in New Jersey, a state with more specialist physicians per capita than any state in the United States. A woman requested an Intrauterine Device (IUD) placement, a procedure that the author had not done in several years. She told the patient that she had not done this procedure in quite some time and offered to send her to another physician. The patient's response was that she preferred her own primary care physician do the procedure, and the patient suggested that the author "just read the book and then go ahead." The procedure was successful, and was the first of many IUD placements within this physician's practice in New Jersey.

A patient came in to see one of the other authors and editors of this book (SMS) with symptoms of pressure in her vagina which worsened upon standing. With many health problems, the patient was considered at high risk for major morbidity and mortality from surgery. She came to the author's office for a pessary fitting, as there were few physicians in town who fit pessaries. SMS successfully treated the woman's symptoms with a pessary, which avoided major surgery and relieved her urinary incontinence. The grateful woman used the pessary successfully for many years.

C.B. Heath (✉)
Department of Family Medicine, Robert Wood Johnson Medical School, University of Medicine and Dentistry of New Jersey, New Brunswick, NJ 08901, USA
e-mail: cheath1965@aol.com

S.M. Sulik and C.B. Heath (eds.), *Primary Care Procedures in Women's Health*, DOI 10.1007/978-0-387-76604-1_1, © Springer Science+Business Media, LLC 2010

Location of Practice

These cases exemplify the necessity for women's health procedures being done by primary care physicians such as family physicians and obstetricians/gynecologists, and by primary care practitioners such as midwives, nurse practitioners, and physician's assistants. Although obviously an extreme case, Dr. Neilsen's case typified a situation in which a woman has difficulty finding a physician to do a basic procedure, a concern common with many women who reside in rural areas. Currently, a significant health care disparity exists for women who reside in rural areas, with over 20% of the population of the United States residing in rural areas and only 9% of the US physician population caring for patients in these areas [2].

The scope of practice of rural physicians has by necessity been broad, with rural physicians being much more likely to do procedures not done by their suburban and urban counterparts. Male physicians are more likely to do procedures than women physicians in urban and suburban settings; however, in rural settings, women physicians are equally as likely as male physicians to perform procedures [3]. In a study of Canadian physicians, younger male physicians were more likely than middle-aged to older physicians to do procedures, except for women's health procedures, which were more likely to be done by women physicians [4]. In a survey of Wisconsin family physicians, Eliason and colleagues noted that 40% of family physicians reported doing skin surgery, flexible sigmoidoscopy, breast cyst aspiration, joint arthrocentesis, and Norplant® (Population Council, New York, NY, and Washington, DC) insertion. Female physicians performed more women's health procedures than other procedures in any setting [5].

In many instances, access to a specialist for routine procedures is difficult, and, thus, many generalist providers are doing procedures that in more suburban and urban regions are considered reserved for specialists. In a study of colonoscopy in rural communities, family physicians performed colonoscopies on patients with symptoms as well as on patients for screening. Family physicians successfully reached the cecum in 96% of the cases, with an average time of 15.9 min, finding neoplastic polyps in 22% of the patients and cancer in 2.5% of the patients [6].

Continuity of Care: "The Medical Home"

Patients prefer seeing the same provider and consider seeing the same provider every time they have a health problem as very important [7]. Patients prefer, in many cases, to have procedures done by a practitioner whom they know and trust. For instance, in a study conducted at an inner city clinic, 70% of patients thought it appropriate for their family physicians to do medical abortions. Forty-seven percent thought it appropriate for their family physicians to do first-trimester surgical abortions. Of the women who would personally consider an abortion, 73% preferred to have it done by their family physician, 22% preferred to go to a free-standing abortion clinic, and 5% had no preference [8]. In a survey done by the Kaiser Family Foundation, 54% of obstetricians/gynecologists stated that they would be very or somewhat likely to prescribe mifepristone for medication abortions. Fifty percent of family physicians, nurse practitioners, and physician's assistants reported interest in prescribing mifepristone. At the time of the survey, only 5% of family physicians currently performed surgical abortions [9].

Many patients expect their generalist providers to perform common procedures, especially those done in an outpatient setting. Most patients appreciate continuity and find that receiving care (including procedures) from one provider improved the physician–patient relationship [10, 11].

Procedure Training

A number of procedures have become a lost art, making it difficult for patients to access providers who feel comfortable performing these procedures. Physicians in the past have relied on learning procedures in medical school or residency; yet newer, more advanced procedures can only be offered in a postgraduate setting for most practicing physicians. In Canada, 91% of physicians reported learning procedures in medical school or in a family medicine residency, whereas only 12.6% learned procedures in clinical practice settings, followed by 6.4% who reported learning procedures in formal skills training. Those in rural practice learned a relatively greater proportion of procedural skills through formal skills training [12]. While the general guidelines for women's health procedure skills within a family medicine residency [13] have mandatory procedures (Endometrial Biopsy, Pap Smears, Wet Mount, KOH Prep), some less common procedures are no longer considered mandatory but are "recommended" (Breast Cyst Aspiration, Diaphragm Fitting, IUD Insertion and Removal). Bartholin Cyst or Abscess Treatment and Colposcopy are considered "elective."

Unfortunately, if physicians tend to do only procedures that they learned in residency, women who prefer uncommon contraceptives may have fewer options than previously. In a study by Cheng of final year residents in all family practice and obstetrics/gynecology training programs in Maryland, 50% of family practice residents had never inserted an IUD and 77% had never removed one; 30% of family practice residents had never fitted a diaphragm; 97% had no experience with elective termination; 43% had never inserted a subdermal contraceptive. In the same study, 20% of *obstetrics/gynecology residents* had never inserted an IUD, 16% had never inserted subdermal implants, 20% had never fitted a diaphragm, and 36% had no experience with elective termination [14]. This lack of experience may subvert the physician's confidence about incorporating procedures into his/her office setting. Sempowski and colleagues did a cross-sectional survey of Canadian family physicians' provision of minor office procedures and found that of the 108 family physicians and general practitioners in Kingston, Ontario, only 35.4% reported performing endometrial biopsies. The most common reason for not performing a specific procedure was the "lack of up-to-date skills" [15].

Insurance Coverage

The good news is that many insurance plans across the United States are covering contraceptive procedures more commonly than ever before. In a study of insurance coverage for contraceptives, 86% of the plans covered the five leading prescription methods: diaphragm, 3-month injectables, IUD, and oral contraceptives. Insurance companies in states with mandated coverage were significantly more likely (87–92%) to cover the five leading prescription methods of contraceptives than states without mandates [16].

Patient (and Provider) Satisfaction

Doing procedures in the office leads to *both* patient and physician satisfaction *and* to strengthening the physician–patient bond. In addition, it can improve practice income. Offering cash-only cosmetic procedures has become popular among primary care providers, and offering these procedures may improve the cash flow in one's office. Some primary care providers do cosmetic surgery in their office, which can be rewarding and offer respite from the insurance company reimbursement issues so common in primary care today.

Conclusion

Whatever the rationale, women's health procedures are in demand, especially in a primary care setting, and are rewarding for both physician and patient alike. No matter where the location of the practice or what type of patient or provider may be involved, generalist providers can offer these procedures as part of their daily practice. All of these procedures are easy to learn, most require minimal equipment, and they offer services that improve women's health and the range of options for the care that all patients wish to receive from their provider.

References

1. Nielsen J, Vollers MA. *Ice bound: a doctor's incredible battle for survival at the south pole.* New York: Hyperion, 2001.
2. Jolly P, Hudley DM (eds). *AAMC data book: statistical information related to medical education.* Washington, DC: Association of American Medical Colleges, 1998.
3. Hutten-Czapski P, Pitblado R, Slade S. Short report: scope of family practice in rural and urban settings. *Can Fam Physician* 2004;50:1548–1550.

4. Chaytors RG, Szafran O, Crutcher RA. Rural-urban and gender differences in procedures performed by family practice residency graduates. *Fam Med* 2001;33:766–771.
5. Eliason BC, Lofton SA, Mark DH. Influence of demographics and profitability on physician selection of family practice procedures. *J Fam Pract* 1995;40(3):223–224.
6. Edwards JK, Norris TE. Colonoscopy in rural communities: can family physicians perform the procedure with safe and efficaceous results? *J Am Board Fam Pract* 2004;17:353–358.
7. Baker R, Mainous AG, Gray DP, Love MM. Exploration of the relationship between continuity, trust in regular doctors and patient satisfaction with consultations with family doctors. *Scand J Prim Health Care* 2003;21(1):27–32.
8. Rubin SE, Godfrey E, Gold M. Patient attitudes toward early abortion services in the family medicine clinic. *J Am Board Fam Med* 2008;21(2):162–164.
9. Koenig JD, Tapias MP, Hoff T. Are US health professionals likely to prescribe mifepristone or methotrexate? *J Am Med Womens Assoc* 2000;55:155–160.
10. Norris TE, Cullison SW, Fihn SD. Teaching procedural skills. *J Gen Intern Med* 1997;12(S2):S64–S70.
11. Haggerty JL, Pineault R, Beaulieu MD, Brunelle Y, Gauthier J, Goulet F, Rodriguez J. Practice features associated with patient-reported accessibility, continuity, and coordination of primary health care. *Ann Fam Med* 2008;6:116–123.
12. Crutcher RA, Szafran O, Woloschuk W, Chaytors RG, Topps DA, Humphries PW, Norton PG. Where Canadian family physicians learn procedural skills. *Fam Med* 2005;37(7):491–495.
13. Edwards FD, Frey KA. The future of residency education: implementing a competency-based educational model. *Fam Med* 2007;39(2):116–125.
14. Cheng D. Family planning training in Maryland family practice and obstetrics/gynecology residency programs. *J Am Med Womens Assoc* 1999;54:208–210.
15. Sempowski IP, Rungi AA, Seguin R. A cross sectional survey of urban Canadian family physicians' provision of minor office procedures. *BMC Fam Pract* 2006;7:18.
16. Sonfield A, Gold R, Frost JJ, Darroch JE. U.S. insurance coverage of contraceptive and the impact of contraceptive coverage mandates. *Perspect Sex Reprod Health* 2004;36(2):72–79.

Chapter 2
Coding, Billing, and Reimbursement for Procedures

Cathryn B. Heath

Introduction

Coding, billing, and reimbursement are an integral part of the procedures performed in today's modern medical office. Gone are the days when one could learn a procedure and then just expect payment for services rendered. Performing the actual procedure is only part of the process. At times, billing and coding can be even more complicated and time-consuming than actually performing the procedure itself. However, once learned, procedure billing can become as routine as office visit billing. Appropriate billing with concomitant reimbursement is very satisfying and can gradually change the emphasis and tenor of a clinician's practice. It is crucial that, before instituting a new office procedure, the clinician and the billing staff review the proper billing and coding to ensure that payment will occur.

Procedure Coding

As seen in the various procedure chapters in this book, included within each chapter are appropriate codes that must be compatible with the procedures discussed and shown. If a clinician is seeing a patient for diagnoses other than just the procedure, each diagnosis and procedure need to be coded separately. For instance, if a patient is being seen for a gynecologic exam and requests that her Intrauterine Device (IUD) be removed, the clinician would code the appropriate health maintenance code for the exam, use a -25 modifier, and then code for the IUD removal [1]. If the patient prefers to return another day for the IUD removal, one would only code for the actual procedure on the IUD removal visit.

C.B. Heath (✉)
Department of Family Medicine, Robert Wood Johnson Medical School, University of Medicine and Dentistry of New Jersey, New Brunswick, NJ 08901, USA

S.M. Sulik and C.B. Heath (eds.), *Primary Care Procedures in Women's Health*,
DOI 10.1007/978-0-387-76604-1_2, © Springer Science+Business Media, LLC 2010

Many procedures have global codes. Thus, if a procedure such as a Bartholin's gland excision requires a second visit for a recheck, the recheck is considered part of the original global procedure code and would not be billed as a second office visit. Similarly, if there are sutures being removed for a procedure done in the office, the suture removal should be covered in the global fee. There are some exceptions to the rule: for example, one can bill separately for a visit to review and discuss treatment options of colposcopy pathology.

Coding compatibility with the procedure is essential to ensure payment. Checking with the Local Medical Review Processes (LMRP) in the state of the practice is essential, as this will lead the practitioner and his/her office staff to use the appropriate diagnosis codes as per the Centers for Medicare and Medicaid Services (CMS). Medicare's website (http://www.cms.hhs.gov) is an excellent place to start [2]. There are stipulations for which ICD 9 (International Classification of Diseases, 9th Revision, Center for Disease Control and Prevention) codes will be covered by private payers and CMS for a specific procedure. Thus, a code that sounds appropriate in one state may be covered while another code will not be covered. Reviewing the state's LMRP will decrease the number of rejected claims and improve the efficiency of the billing process. Inadvertent coding discrepancies also may be found by office staff who are assigned to check rejected claims. It is imperative to have someone in your financial office who is prepared to review rejected claims, particularly for procedures, and who can pursue the reasons for rejection. As billing improves, rejected claims decrease in number.

Coding also can be improved and facilitated by using specific coding software, some of which may even be accessed by either an electronic medical record or a handheld electronic device. There are many coding and billing software packages available in the market that will help promote effective coding [3].

Documentation of Procedures

All procedures need appropriate notes written by the clinician. Size and location of excised lesions should be documented, as reimbursement is determined by size, location, number of lesions removed, and the pathology of the lesion (benign versus malignant). Billing should be submitted based not only on the size of the lesion but also on the size of the margins. For instance, if a 1 cm lesion is removed using a margin of 0.2 cm on each side, the size would be considered 1.4 cm [4]. Follow-up should be clearly stated in order to document whether a subsequent visit should be considered part of the procedure.

Coding and billing for skin procedures is further complicated by the specific pathologic diagnosis of the lesion itself. For instance, coding for removal of a benign versus malignant lesion may be difficult until the biopsy results have returned to the office, which may be anywhere from 10 to 14 days after the date the actual procedure is performed. However, removal of a malignancy is generally reimbursed at an average of two to three times the amount of the removal of a benign lesion. Thus, in some instances in which the CPT® (AMA, Chicago, IL) code may be dramatically changed by the pathology results, it may be advisable to hold billing the particular procedure until the pathology report returns and is reviewed.

One can also attempt to bill for an unsuccessful procedure, though the likelihood of being reimbursed is obviously much less [5]. Some insurances do pay for an attempted procedure, while others do not. Attempted procedures that are unsuccessful should have a modifier -52 attached to show that the actual procedure was not completed. The payer will need to know the extent of what was done; attaching a copy of the office note to the claim will usually suffice.

Health Maintenance Organization Billing

Medical procedures are highly scrutinized by Health Maintenance Organizations (HMOs) due to the expense of the procedure itself. Some HMOs require prior authorization for procedures, which may include submitting prior office notes, labs, or radiology reports to substantiate the need for the actual procedure [6]. This varies nationally by region and by the policy negotiated by the patient's employer. This is particularly pertinent in regard to payment for a contraception procedure, which is often considered a separate benefit purchased by some employers and not by others. In all cases, contacting the patient's insurance company to check coverage for the particular procedure is a proactive measure that will save time and money. If there is a concern that the insurance will not cover the procedure, consider having the patient sign a document (Advance Beneficiary Notice or ABN) stating that she will be willing to pay for the procedure if it is considered a noncovered service by her insurance company.

Most insurance companies will consider the procedures listed in this book as billable procedures over and above any negotiated capitation rates. However, if the clinician is practicing in a primary care office, he or she should know specifically which procedures are considered billable. If the specific procedure is not listed in the insurance company's billable list, the insurance company may deny payment, citing the procedure as part of standard care and covered by the capitation rate. The list of billable procedures may not be standardized, even by insurance vendors. It is vital to obtain the region's billable procedure list from each one of the insurance companies that are accepted by an office. If a given procedure is not present on the billable list, the clinician may need to negotiate with the insurance company for inclusion of that particular procedure. Typically, this might involve a discussion with a medical director within the insurance company and a presentation of the number of such procedures performed so as to judge the competence of the clinician. Credentialing with the insurance company prior to initiation of a procedure will improve the likelihood of payment.

Durable Medical Goods

Durable goods, such as IUDs, may be stocked by an office if they are used on a frequent basis. Another alternative to stocking durable goods is to have the patient contact the supply company directly and for the patient to pay directly for the durable good. For example, at times, it is necessary for the practitioner to write a prescription for the actual IUD; in other cases, it can be ordered online. The IUD is then sent to the office in the patient's name: when it is sent, the patient is called so that insertion can be scheduled. Some insurance companies will only reimburse for the cost of the insertion, but will not cover the cost of the actual IUD. Other insurance companies may cover both procedure and durable goods. It is always important to have the patient sign an ABN stating that she is willing to pay for the procedure and the durable good prior to performing the procedure. Alternatively, some offices require that the patient provide payment prior to the procedure.

Charity Care Procedures

Charity care services also may be available for procedures such as IUD insertion. The Arch Foundation was established as a not-for-profit institution to help low income women who have no insurance coverage for the levonorgestrel Intrauterine System. The copper IUD manufacturer has a similar program for low income women who are interested in an IUD. In each program, the clinician has to agree to put the IUD in at no cost to the patient.

Cosmetic Surgery Billing

Most cosmetic surgery is not covered by insurance companies and is considered an "out of pocket" expense. Most clinicians who provide cosmetic surgery will stipulate that the patient pay prior to the actual procedure being performed. It is best to do a consultation prior to the actual procedure and to clearly provide the price of each procedure both verbally and in writing. Payment is then made prior to the actual procedure.

Summary

Appropriate coding and billing improves women's access to important health procedures, as practitioners are more likely to continue doing procedures for which they can be paid. Due to the coding specificity, tracking payment and improving the process of payment are relatively easy tasks for any clinician's practice. Familiarizing oneself and one's billing staff with coding for procedures by type of procedure and by type of payment by specific insurance company will increase the likelihood of payment, thus rewarding the clinician for providing services that are requested by the patient or necessary for good clinical care.

References

1. Hughes C. Multiple procedures at the same visit. *Family Practice Management* July/Aug 2007, vol 14(7).
2. Moore KJ. Navigating the medicare web site. *Family Practice Management* Nov/Dec 2004, vol 11(10), p 31.
3. Morrison KM. Coding and billing software for palm-top computers. *Family Practice Management* May 2002, vol 9(5), p 33.
4. Moore KJ. CPT code update 2003. *Family Practice Management* Jan 2003, vol 10(1), p 14.
5. Hughes C. Discontinued procedures. *Family Practice Management* Oct 2006, vol 13(9).
6. Reichman M. Managed care administrative tasks: cutting the red tape. *Family Practice Management* Oct 2006, vol 13(9), p 32.

Additional Resources

Web Sites

The physicians' guide to handheld computer software: www.fphandheld.com
http://www.archfoundation.com/
The Arch Foundation: http://www.archfoundation.com

Chapter 3
Legal Aspects of Office-Based Women's Health Procedures

David E. Kolva

Introduction

As primary care practitioners face increasing liability risk in this litigious society, careful planning and timely consultation with a competent legal advisor is critically important to reduce exposure to lawsuits or conduct sanctions. Since the regulation of medical practice is largely an individual state activity and since laws vary widely by locality, this chapter is not intended to provide personal legal advice. When a practice makes decisions about new policies or procedures, it should be clearly recorded in a practice policy and procedure manual. A user-friendly manual, in print or electronic form, will standardize policy and procedure throughout a medical practice and facilitate training of new employees.

Office Physical Plant Concerns

Local zoning laws regulate use of the office building premises for provision of medical services. If an existing practice location is in complete compliance with local zoning law requirements, none of the procedures described in this book should require additional special permits or variances since they fall into the category of usual medical diagnostic and therapeutic services for licensed physicians.

If cosmetic laser or electrosurgery services are being added to a practice, an electrician should be consulted in order to evaluate electrical service requirements. Equipment manufacturers will provide the detailed specifications to ensure safe operation.

D.E. Kolva, M.D.
Department of Family Medicine, SUNY Upstate Medical University, Syracuse, NY, USA

Family Medicine Residency Program, St. Joseph's Hospital Health Center,
301 Prospect Avenue, Syracuse, NY 13203, USA

S.M. Sulik and C.B. Heath (eds.), *Primary Care Procedures in Women's Health*,
DOI 10.1007/978-0-387-76604-1_3, © Springer Science+Business Media, LLC 2010

The decision as to whether to purchase or to lease new equipment has important tax implications. Consultation with an accountant is mandatory before any large practice expense. For example, the cost of a new colposcopy suite may easily surpass $15,000. The cost of necessary electrical, plumbing, and storage improvements on physical plants should be budgeted carefully. One must remember to review office/business property insurance policy to include the new equipment and leasehold improvements.

OSHA Concerns

In 2001, the federal Occupational Safety and Health Administration (OSHA) substantially revised the 1991 compliance standards for employers in order to prevent employees' exposure to bloodborne pathogens [1]. A practice must have an Exposure Control Plan to reflect these standards, and it must be reviewed and updated at least once a year. The employer is responsible for staff training and compliance as well as for proper documentation of these activities. Practitioners and assistants who perform these women's health procedures should have serological documented immunity to Hepatitis B. The practice must have a written protocol that clearly outlines proper handling, storage, and disposal of "sharps" (needles and blades), toxic chemicals (acetic acid, Lugol's and Monsel's solutions), and regulated medical waste. Personal protective equipment and emergency eyewash stations must be provided by the employer.

The practice must create engineering controls that allow for the proper ventilation of waste nitrous oxide gas from certain cryosurgical instruments if this equipment is used for cryosurgery of cervical or vulvar lesions. Similarly, a smoke evacuation system should be available for electrosurgical procedures to minimize aerosolized tissue inhalation.

Promotion of Services

If the practitioner is providing outpatient women's health procedures for patients outside of the practice's enrolled panel on a referral basis from other practitioners, then state and federal "anti-kickback" laws prevail. These laws, commonly known as Stark I and II rules, prohibit self-referrals, fee-splitting arrangements, and other types of activity between business entities [2]. An attorney knowledgeable in this technical area of the law must be consulted before promoting or advertising services to patients outside of a group practice.

Individual states regulate the scope and content of advertisement of physician's services. Fraudulent or misleading advertisement is considered professional misconduct in most states and may negate malpractice insurance coverage for these services if results are guaranteed or falsely solicited.[1]

Credentialing Concerns

While surgery performed in facilities licensed under state Public Health Laws (such as hospitals or ambulatory surgery centers) is subject to regulatory standards established under such law, procedures performed by primary care practitioners in private offices are not subjected to the same standards. The practitioner's authority to perform office-based procedures is derived from the license to practice medicine issued by the states. States are increasingly establishing clinical guidelines for office-based surgery [3]. The practitioner should become familiar with his or her state's guidelines for definitions of standards of care and quality. These guidelines can serve as a good resource template for creating office policy concerning staff education and training for individual procedures.

One of the most important rules of risk management is that the practitioner must be able to prove competency in the performance of these outpatient procedures. Procedure-specific competence should include education, training, experience, and evaluations of performance. Proof of competence should include documentation of procedures performed during postgraduate residency programs and/or proof of satisfactory completion of approved didactic courses offered as Continuing Medical Education (CME). For Example, the American Academy of Family Physicians offers a CME syllabus in Colposcopy and outlines methods to facilitate credentialing [4]. A practice should have a system to record the ongoing number of procedures performed by each practitioner and have a formal "re-evaluation of competency" policy in place.

The practitioner must research the terms of coverage of the practice's professional malpractice policy to make sure that the planned procedures are covered under the existing policy. Unlicensed personnel should not be assigned duties or responsibilities that require professional licensure [3]. The practice should have a formal "in-service" instruction program for office assistants involved in these procedures and document successful completion in the personnel record. This program should also address the knowledge needs of telephone-triage or advice nurses who are most likely to receive telephone calls for postoperative care concerns from patients.

---

[1] All professional liability policies have "intentional acts exclusions" where coverage may be reserved or denied. Some companies provide a more exhaustive list of acts that would trigger denial of coverage.

Informed Consent

Informed consent is a process of communication with a competent patient about the planned procedure in sufficient detail to allow a decision regarding whether or not to proceed with the intervention [5]. The key legal components of informed consent have evolved over the last 50 years in the United States. Not only is this process an ethical obligation, it is now a legal duty of professional conduct as described in statutes and case law in all 50 states. Informed consent is also a key component of the "shared decision making" process that is replacing the "paternalistic" practice of medicine [6].

For the procedures described in this book, informed consent must include the following components:

1. Information on the patient's pathology or current medical condition.
2. Other scientifically valid treatment options.
3. Rationale for the chosen procedure.
4. Anticipated beneficial outcomes of the procedure.
5. Potential harmful complications or consequences of the procedure.
6. Consequences of *not* having the procedure [Informed Refusal].

There can be no deliberate or willful misrepresentation of facts in these discussions with patients. In addition, the discussion must be in language that is understandable to the patient in terms of education level and language of preference. Certified medical interpreters should be provided for patients whose language of preference is discordant with the practitioner. Many studies have shown a higher medicolegal risk when using family members as "ad hoc" interpreters [7].

The Americans with Disabilities Act requires the provider of medical services to provide appropriate means for hearing impaired patients to function in the medical environment. Because informed consent discussions are of the highest importance, only medically certified interpreters should be hired by the practice to serve in this function with hearing impaired patients. The cost of this service must be absorbed by the practice and may not be billed to the patient.

The informed consent discussion should be performed by the practitioner in the office setting. This discussion should be recorded in the patient's medical record, with care to mention the use of any drawings or audiovisual aids [8]. Many practices have preprinted informational brochures that are part of the informed consent discussion. The patient's signature authorizes the procedure *only at the successful conclusion of the informed consent process*. If the patient refuses to have the intervention after this discussion, this refusal should be documented, with a discussion of the repercussions fully acknowledged by the patient.

The increasingly popular usage of Electronic Medical Records (EMR) has allowed groups to create standardized electronic consent systems and forms. The use of these new standardized systems has improved the documentation accuracy of the informed consent process [9].

Rights of Minors

While primary care physicians provide the majority of health care to adolescents, there is significant evidence that both physicians and adolescents are uninformed of adolescent's legal rights to confidential reproductive health care [10]. The Guttmacher Institute sponsors an online reference source that is updated monthly to provide information on key issues affecting these rights, indexed by each individual state [11]. The practitioner *and* the office staff must be knowledgeable about their own state's law concerning consent and confidentiality when treating minors. In general, the law recognizes special conditions in which the minor child may consent to diagnostic and treatment activities without parental approval or knowledge, in matters concerning: Sexually Transmitted Infections (STIs), contraception, and reproductive (pregnancy) health, including abortion [12]. When the practitioner consents to performance of these women's health procedures on minors, there are practical clinical concerns that may arise in the office with regards to billing, scheduling, telephone calls, and medical records privacy. The practice's policy and procedure manual should anticipate these potential breaches and detail the proper method of handling each issue. If a practice participates in the federal Title X Family Planning Program or in the State Children Health Insurance Program (SCHIP), it must be knowledgeable about the confidentiality and consent rules for these programs. The major specialty organizations have all published policy statements regarding health care for adolescents [13]. These comprehensive guides should be required reading by practitioners who perform these gynecological procedures.

Use of Chaperones

There is no *uniform* national legal requirement mandating the use of a chaperone during female pelvic examinations or procedures. Even though all medicolegal risk managers recommend the routine use of chaperones, there is wide variation in this practice between physicians in the United States [14] and their European counterparts [15]. The American Medical Association has addressed this deficiency by publishing a Policy Compendium stating that, from the standpoint of ethics and prudence, the protocol of having chaperones available on a consistent basis for patient examinations is recommended [16].

In April 2006, the Federation of State Medical Boards adopted a policy that defines physician sexual misconduct and provides recommendations for physician education [17]. When reviewing the definitions of sexual impropriety and sexual violation in this publication, it is clear that most false accusations or misunderstandings can be avoided with the proper use of a *medically trained* chaperone *always* when performing these women's health procedures. The practice policy and procedure manual should state this clearly. It is also a good investment to avoid the emotionally wrenching experience of a false sexual misconduct charge. For most of the procedures described in this book, a chaperone is the beneficial "second pair" of hands to assist the operator in the completion of the procedure. Most experts recommend that the chaperone be the same sex as the patient; thus, a male physician should have a female chaperone for a female patient.

Patient Preprocedure Preparation Concerns

Solutions to prevent health care errors were unveiled in May 2007 by the World Health Organization's (WHO) Collaborating Centre for Patient Safety Solutions. Two of the solutions deal with office-based procedures: patient identification and performance of correct procedure at correct body site. A practice should adopt the "Universal Protocol for Preventing Wrong Site, Wrong Procedure, Wrong Person Surgery" as standard office policy [18]. It is the responsibility of the practitioner to verify the adequacy of the informed consent process and to double-check the patient's identity and planned procedure. The office should have an adequate privacy area to allow for patient disrobing and gowning.

Procedure-Specific Legal Concerns

Cervical Cytology and Pap Smears

An office should have an established policy for the review of all laboratory reports before the reports are filed into the medical record [19]. The primary care provider must review and acknowledge *all* Pap smear cytology reports. An office notification system must be fool-proof and have built-in reminders for follow-up of patients with abnormal Pap smear results until diagnostic resolution. Patient risk factors contributing to inadequate follow-up include low-income ethnic minority and low health literacy [20]. Clinical errors occurring that led to Pap smear litigation include failure to notify patients of their abnormal test result, missing or inconsistent follow-up patterns, failure to investigate persistent bleeding following a Pap smear, and failure to biopsy an abnormal cervix given a normal Pap smear result [21]. Thankfully, the increased utilization of EMR with built in laboratory results management programs will improve the follow-up process [22]. The practitioner *must* be knowledgeable about the positive and negative predictive value of the Pap smear results in order to give adequate informed consent.

Pessary

New self-positioning pessaries are effective, easy to use, and have few complications [23]. The most serious complications from pessary use are attributable to neglected devices in patients lost to follow-up [24]. These rare complications include urosepsis, impaction, vesicovaginal fistulae, and incarceration of cervix and small bowel.

Contraceptives

When the practitioner discusses the contraceptive needs of the patient, the six key components of the previously discussed informed consent process must be addressed. Elements of the patient's current medical condition that are important in choosing the proper contraceptive method include:

- Age
- Emotional maturity
- Health literacy
- Parity
- Number of sexual partners
- Cardiac risk profile (including hypertension and diabetes)
- Migraines
- Coagulopathy
- History of cancers
- History of pelvic inflammatory disease or STIs
- HIV and Hepatitis B status
- Tobacco use, street drug, or alcohol use
- Access to medical care follow-up
- Family history
- Latex allergy

The practitioner must also have published information available to compare the relative effectiveness rates of each method [25]. This information should be included in table form on the practice's informed consent forms.

Diaphragms

"Items that come in contact with mucous membranes or nonintact skin are defined by the CDC as semicritical. These medical devices should be free of all microorganisms, although small numbers of bacterial spores may be present." Diaphragm fitting rings are considered to be "semicritical" items for disinfection following use [26]. The manufacturer's recommendations for cleaning and disinfecting must be followed, and this procedure must be part of the practice's OSHA blood borne pathogens exposure control plan.

Effectiveness of the diaphragm for pregnancy prevention is very dependent upon proper inspection of the device prior to use, correct initial fitting on a suitable patient, proper insertion, duration of use postcoitus, and storage of the device [27]. Patient education during the fitting/insertion office visit is critical. The most significant complication of diaphragm use is toxic shock syndrome.

Intrauterine Devices

The thought process of a generation of physicians was forever changed by the Dalkon Shield litigation history during the 1970s. It was the largest "defective product" tort case in history and has reduced Intrauterine Device (IUD) usage in the United States to the lowest level of any industrialized nation in the world [28]. The new approved IUDs for use in the United States have eliminated the design flaws that plagued the Dalkon Shield. Proper patient selection and postinsertion education and follow-up are important factors to reduce complications and to enhance effectiveness [29]. Contraindications and adverse effects should be included on the informed consent forms. Documentation of absence of pregnancy before insertion is legally critical. The most serious complication of the IUD insertion procedure is uterine perforation, with a reported rate of 1 per 1,000 insertions for copper IUDs [30] and 2.2 per 1,000 insertions for hormone-releasing IUDs (LNG IUS) [31]. Recently, published practice guidelines by the American College of Obstetricians and Gynecologists have concluded that IUDs "offer safe, effective, long-term contraception and should be considered for all women who seek reliable, reversible contraception" [32]. It is hoped that the publication of evidence-based patient selection criteria and conclusions regarding pelvic inflammatory disease can improve the usage of these devices and reduce the unwarranted fear of litigation over modern IUDs [33].

Colposcopy and Loop Electrocautery Excision Procedure

The process of informed consent is of the utmost importance when discussing abnormal Pap smear results with patients and determining who should undergo further procedures. Some patients consider an abnormal Pap smear to automatically indicate cancer and wonder why they are not being managed more aggressively. Even the majority of college educated women do not know the role of Human Papilloma Virus (HPV) in cervical neoplasia [34]. An overlooked communication problem is the confusion among the abbreviations "HPV" and "HIV" (Human Immunodeficiency Virus) and "HSV" (Herpes Simplex Virus) when talking with patients. Caution is required!

Recent publications contain excellent consensus statements that summarize the 2006 American Society for Colposcopy and Cervical Pathology Guidelines for evidence-based management of abnormal cervical cytology [35, 36]. These protocol algorithms should be referenced in informed consent discussions and documentation. The highest medicolegal risk in the performance of a colposcopy is an inadequate examination with inappropriate follow-up. An office notification system must be fool-proof and have built-in reminders for follow-up of patients with abnormal colposcopic findings until diagnostic resolution. A telephone call to a patient before a scheduled recheck appointment has been shown to improve compliance with follow-up. Mail reminders have *not* been found to be helpful to improve compliance, but these are legally important for documentation purposes.

Even though colposcopy is regarded as a core procedural technique for family physicians, the skill and comfort level of the individual practitioner must be assessed with a verifiable credentialing process and ongoing quality assurance process. The practice should tabulate the clinical and pathologic situations in which referral to a gynecology specialist is required since "failure to diagnose cancer" is still a leading cause of malpractice actions against primary care practitioners [37].

Loop Electrosurgical Excision Procedure of the cervix has been shown to be an effective office technique in the treatment of CIN 2 and CIN 3 [38]. The informed consent discussion must include the reason for selection of the cervix ablation procedure, including risks of incomplete excision, cervical stenosis, and incompetent cervix in subsequent pregnancy [39]. A practice must have an adequate reminder system for postprocedure follow-up of pathology reports and patient recall.

Endometrial Biopsy

In an effort to reduce the number of operative Dilatation and Curettage (D&C) procedures in the diagnostic evaluation of dysfunctional uterine bleeding, several excellent outpatient endometrial biopsy instruments were developed. One randomized controlled study showed that when endometrial biopsy was coupled with transvaginal ultrasound, saline sonohysterography, and/or hysteroscopy in patients with low-risk for endometrial cancer, the combined results had accuracy rates comparable to formal D&C [40]. During an informed consent discussion with patients with unexplained uterine bleeding, the risk assessment for uterine cancer must be categorized on the basis of age, menopause status, nulliparity, body–mass index, insulin resistance syndromes (such as polycystic ovary syndrome), family history, hormone replacement therapy, and tamoxifen use. Documentation of absence of pregnancy before endometrial biopsy is legally critical. A nondiagnostic tissue sample in patients with persistent bleeding requires referral for operative D&C. Again, one must remember that failure to diagnose cancer is still a leading cause of malpractice actions against primary care practitioners. The main complication of endometrial biopsy is uterine perforation, although the reported rates are extremely rare.

Elective Termination of Pregnancy in the United States

There is probably no other medical procedure that provokes as much worldwide divisive emotional and ethical debate as the elective termination of pregnancy. Since the United States Supreme Court upheld the constitutionality of the federal Partial-Birth Abortion Ban Act of 2003 in April 2007 [*Gonzales v. Carhart*], it is imperative for women's healthcare practitioners to know their own state's laws and terminology regarding the elective termination of pregnancy. Two excellent internet sites contain up-to-date information on the status of state laws governing elective termination of pregnancy: the Guttmacher Institute [41] and the National Abortion Federation. These sites contain information on Medicaid abortion funding, mandatory counseling and waiting periods, parental involvement in a minor's abortions, and mandatory reporting to state health department requirements.

Pregnancy termination and miscarriage treatment use overlapping sets of skills and procedures [42]. It is critical for the practitioner to perform a thorough history, physical examination, and determination of gestational age for all pregnant patients. All of the elements of the informed consent process need to be well documented. The risk of the planned procedure on future fertility must be discussed and documented. Postprocedure contraception needs also should be answered. The practitioner's office staff and after-hours call groups should be comfortable providing advice and care for any postprocedure complications to avoid any charge of patient abandonment.

The utility of mifepristone and misoprostol regimens as nonsurgical methods of abortion continues to gain acceptance as the regimens allow for participation by a broader range of providers [43]. The manufacturers of mifepristone require that all practitioners who administer the medication undergo training in patient selection, informed consent, and postprocedure care.

Cosmetic Laser Surgery, Dermabrasion, Chemical Peels, and Botox Injections (Esthetic or Cosmetic Medicine)

There has been a virtual explosion of growth in demand for esthetic procedures by patients as various technologies have evolved over the last 25 years. Once the exclusive domain of the plastic surgeon in the operating room, now even nonphysician practitioners in day-spas are performing these procedures. As economic pressures from reduced reimbursements continue to mount on primary care providers, the addition of these types of procedures is increasingly tempting.

Various specialty organizations have attempted to set guidelines to govern the training, education, and standard of practice for these procedures [44]. The general conclusions of most organizations' guidelines can be generalized into topics already covered in this chapter: proper patient selection, accurate diagnosis of condition, full informed consent including realistic expectations, documentation of operator's training and experience, safe operation of equipment in the proper environment, and comprehensive patient postprocedure follow-up. The practitioner must be able to diagnose patients with Body Dysmorphic Disorder, who comprise 7–15% of patients presenting for cosmetic procedures [45]. These patients typically do not benefit from cosmetic procedures. Practitioners must consult with their professional liability insurance company to purchase cosmetic surgery riders.

Summary

In general, procedures can enhance office income and provide valuable services to one's own patients. Proper training for each procedure offered must be accomplished by the clinicians who will offer these services. A dedicated procedure room or cart with the needed equipment and supplies should be established prior to offering these procedures. Both OSHA regulations and local and state standards of care must be explored and incorporated into the office policies and procedures training manual. Training of office staff to provide patient education, responses to triage questions, and assistance during the procedure is crucial to a smooth and safe experience for the patient. Written patient information and standardized permits that include known complications should be available. Use of the EMR if available can enhance patient tracking for follow-up.

References

1. http://www.osha.gov/dcsp/osp/index.html Accessed May 28, 2007.
2. Satiani B. Exceptions to the Stark law: practical considerations for surgeons. *Plast Reconstr Surg* 2006;117(3):1012–1022, discussion 1023.
3. Clinical guidelines for Office-Based Surgery. Committee on quality assurance in office-based surgery. A report to: New York State Public Health Council and New York State Department of Health, July 2000. Accessed May 29, 2007 at www.health.state.ny.us/nysdoh/obs/purpose.html.
4. American Academy of Family Physicians. Position paper: colposcopy. http://www.aafp.org/online/en/home/policy/policies/c/colposcopypositionpaper.html#Parsys0006.
5. American Medical Association Standards: Office of the General Counsel: informed consent. Updated May 07, 2007. http://www.ama-assn.org/ama/pub/category/4608.html Accessed September 29, 2007.
6. Woolf SH, Krist A. The liability of giving patients a choice: shared decision making and prostate cancer. Editorial. *Am Fam Physician* 2005;71(10):1915–1922.
7. Betancourt JR, Jacobs EA. Language barriers to informed consent and confidentiality: the impact on women's health. *J Am Med Womens Assoc* 2000;55(5):294–295.
8. Issa MM, Setzer E, Charaf C, Webb AL, Derico R, Kimberl IJ, Fink AS. Informed versus uninformed consent for prostate surgery: the value of electronic consents. *J Urol* 2006;176(2):694–699.
9. Moseley TH, Wiggins MN, O'Sullivan P. Effects of presentation method on the understanding of informed consent. *Br J Ophthalmol* 2006;90(8):990–993.

10. Lieberman D, Feierman J. Legal issues in the reproductive health care of adolescents. *J Am Med Womens Assoc* 1999;54(3):109–114.
11. Guttmacher Institute. State policies in brief. http://www.guttmacher.org/ Accessed September 28, 2007.
12. Ford C, English A, Sigman G. Confidential health care for adolescents: position paper of the Society for Adolescent Medicine. *J Adolesc Health* 2004;35(2):160–167.
13. Diaz A, Neal WP, Nucci AT, Ludmer P, Bitterman J, Edwards S. Legal and ethical issues facing adolescent health care professionals. *Mt Sinai J Med* 2004;71(3):181–185.
14. Rockwell P, Steyer TE, Ruffin MT IV. Chaperone use by family physicians during the collection of a Pap smear. *Ann Fam Med* 2003;1:218–220.
15. Rymer J, Durbaba S, Rosenthal J, Jones RH. Use of chaperones by obstetricians and gynaecologists: a cross-sectional survey. *J Obstet Gynaecol* 2007;27(1):8–11.
16. AMA Policy E-8.21 on Use of chaperones during physical exams, adopted June 1998, www.ama-assn.org/ama/pub/category/2503.html under Code of Ethics.
17. Federation of State Medical Boards Policy Statement. Addressing sexual boundaries: guidelines for state medical boards. Adopted April 2006. http://www.fsmb.org/grpol_policydocs.html Accessed May 29, 2007.
18. http://www.jointcommission.org/PatientSafety/UniversalProtocol. Accessed May 28, 2007.
19. White B. Four principles for better test-result tracking. *Fam Pract Manag* 2002;9(7):41–44.
20. Engelstad LP, Stewart LS, Nguyen BH, Bedeian KL, Rubin MM, Pasick RJ, Hiatt RA. Abnormal Pap smear follow-up in a high-risk population. *Cancer Epidemiol Biomarkers Prev* 2001;10:1015–1020.
21. Frable WJ. Litigation in gynecologic cytology. *Pathol Case Rev* 2005;10(3):106–114.
22. Murff HJ, Gandhi TK, Karson AK, Mort EA, Poon EG, Wang SJ, Fairchild DG, Bates DW. Primary care physician attitudes concerning follow-up of abnormal test results and ambulatory decision support systems. *Int J Med Inform* 2003;71(2–3):137–149.
23. Farrell SA, Baydock S, Amir B, Fanning C. Effectiveness of a new self-positioning pessary for the management of urinary incontinence in women. *Am J Obstet Gynecol* 2007;196:474.e1–474.e8.
24. Trowbridge ER, Fenner DE. Conservative management of pelvic organ prolapse. *Clin Obstet Gynecol* 2005;48(3):668–681.
25. Trussell J. Contraceptive failure in the United States. *Contraception* 2004;70:89–96.
26. Rutala WA, Weber DJ. Disinfection and sterilization in health care facilities: what clinicians need to know. *Clin Infect Dis* 2004;39:702–709.
27. Allen RE. Diaphragm fitting. *Am Fam Physician* 2004;69:97–100.
28. Hubacher D. The checkered history and bright future of intrauterine contraception in the United States. *Perspect Sex Reprod Health* 2002;34(2):98.
29. Johnson BA. Insertion and removal of intrauterine devices. *Am Fam Physician* 2005;71(1):95–102.
30. FFPRHC guidance (January 2004). The copper intrauterine device as long-term contraception. *J Fam Plann Reprod Health Care* 2004;30(1):29–41.
31. Van Houdenhoven K, van Klam KJAF, van Grootheest AC, Salemans T, Dunselman G. Uterine perforation in women using a levonorgestrel-releasing intrauterine system. *Contraception* 2006;73:257–260.
32. Intrauterine device. ACOG practice bulletin no. 59. American College of Obstetricians and Gynecologists. *Obstet Gynecol* 2005;105:223–232.
33. Stanwood NL, Garrett JM, Konrad TR. Obstetric-gynecologists and the intrauterine device: a survey of attitudes and practice. *Obstet Gynecol* 2002;99:275–280.
34. Le T, Hicks W, Menard C, Boyd D, Hewson T, Hopkins L, Kee Fung MF. Human papillomavirus testing knowledge and attitudes among women attending colposcopy clinic with ASCUS/LGSIL pap smears. *J Obstet Gynaecol Can* 2004;26(9):788–792.
35. Kyrgiou M, Tsoumpou I, Vrekoussis T, Martin-Hirsch P, Arbyn M, Prendiville W, Mitrou S, Koliopoulos G, Dalkalitsis N, Stamatopoulos P, Paraskevaidis E. The up-to-date evidence on

colposcopy practice and treatment of cervical intraepithelial neoplasia: the Cochrane colposcopy and cervical cytopathology collaborative group (C5 group) approach. *Cancer Treat Rev* 2006;32(7):516–523.

36. Wright TC, Massad LS, Dunton CJ, Spitzer M, Wilkinson EJ, Solomon D. The 2006 consensus guidelines for the management of women with abnormal cervical cancer screening tests. *Am J Ob Gyn* 2007;197(4):346–355.

37. Callaway P. Does a family physician who offers colposcopy and LEEP need to refer patients to a gynecologist? *J Fam Pract* 2000;49:534–536.

38. Lyman DJ, Morris B. LEEP in the family practice setting. *J Am Board Fam Pract* 2003;16(3):204–208.

39. Mathevet P, Chemali E, Roy M, Dargent D. Long-term outcome of a randomized study comparing three techniques of conization: cold knife, laser and LEEP. *Eur J Obstet Gynecol Reprod Biol* 2003;106(2):214–218.

40. Tahir MM, Bigrigg MA, Browning JJ, Brookes ST, Smith PA. A randomized controlled trial comparing transvaginal ultrasound, outpatient hysteroscopy and endometrial biopsy with inpatient hysteroscopy and curettage. *Br J Obstet Gynaecol* 1999;106(12):1259–1264.

41. The National Abortion Federation: www.prochoice.org Guttmacher Institute. State policies in brief as of September 1, 2007: an overview of abortion laws. http://www.guttmacher.org Accessed September 29, 2007.

42. Johnson TRB, Harris LH, Dalton VK, Howell JD. Language matters: legislation, medical practice, and the classification of abortion procedures. *Obstet Gynecol* 2005;105(1):201–204.

43. Grimes DA, Creinin MD. Induced abortion: a review for internists. *Ann Intern Med* 2004;140(8):620–626.

44. Alam A, Dover JS, Arndt KA. Use of cutaneous lasers and light sources: appropriate training and delegation. *Skin Therapy Lett* 2007;12(5):5–9.

45. Crerand CE, Franklin ME, Sarwer DB. Body dysmorphic disorder and cosmetic surgery. *Plast Reconstr Surg* 2006;118(7):167e–180e.

Additional Resources

Web Sites

The Guttmacher Institute: http://www.guttmacher.org/
The National Abortion Federation: www.prochoice.org

Chapter 4
Empathic Pelvic Examination

Rhina Acevedo

Introduction

The pelvic examination is an important and basic procedure for women's healthcare providers. It is an integral part of the evaluation of common gynecologic and abdominal complaints including pelvic pain, vaginal discharge, vaginal bleeding, and irregular menses. Pelvic examinations are also part of the annual routine women's health examination [1]. The American College of Obstetrics and Gynecology recommends a routine biennial gynecologic examination beginning at age 21 [2]. If a woman has had three normal examinations on a yearly basis, the interval between examinations may increase to every 1–3 years after age 30, at the discretion of the woman and her clinician [3].

Women with a past history of abnormal Pap smears, women with a history of breast or ovarian cancer, women at risk for sexually transmitted infections, and women who cannot remember to have pelvic examinations unless they have them every year are candidates to continue yearly screening. There is currently no evidence to continue yearly pelvic examinations after the age of 65, but consideration needs to be made for personal history (including recent change in sexual partner and multiple partners), family history, expected longevity, and frequency of prior Pap smears [2]. The American Cancer Society recommends discontinuing Pap smears after the age of 70 after three consecutive normal Pap smears and no abnormal Pap smears within the last 10 years [3]. The United States Preventative Services Task Forces found insufficient evidence to do routine screening examinations past the age of 65. Medicare presently does not pay for yearly routine screening pelvic examinations.

Although the Pap smear has been a mainstay for evaluation of cancer of the cervix, there is no recommended screening for ovarian cancer. A large prospective

R. Acevedo

Department of Family Medicine, University of Medicine and Dentistry of New Jersey,
New Brunswick, NJ, USA
e-mail: Racevedo97@gmail.com

S.M. Sulik and C.B. Heath (eds.), *Primary Care Procedures in Women's Health*, 27
DOI 10.1007/978-0-387-76604-1_4, © Springer Science+Business Media, LLC 2010

trial is presently underway to assess a variety of screening measures for ovarian cancer. Patients with a personal history of ovarian cancer are candidates for yearly examinations and serum laboratory CA 125 levels [4, 5].

See Algorithm 4-1 for the decision tree on the necessity of performing a pelvic exam.

Case Study

A 21-year-old G0P0 woman presents to your office for her first annual gynecological evaluation. She has become sexually active in the last 2 years. She denies any current complaints. She reports that her menses are regular. She is not currently using any contraceptive method. She is very nervous about her gynecologic examination.

Diagnosis (Algorithm 4-1)

Routine annual women's health examination.

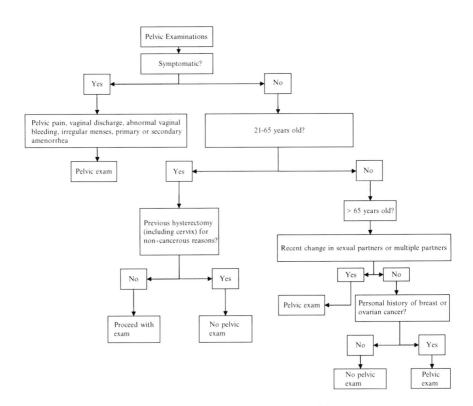

Algorithm 4-1 Decision tree on the necessity of performing a pelvic exam

Indications (Algorithm 4-1)

- Routine annual women's health exam
- Lower abdominal or pelvic pain
- Menstrual irregularities including:
    ○ Primary amenorrhea (no menses by age 16)
    ○ Secondary amenorrhea
    ○ Menorrhagia (heavy bleeding)
    ○ Menometrorrhagia (irregular heavy bleeding)
- Vaginal discharge
- Postcoital bleeding
- Dyspareunia
- Dysmenorrhea
- Pregnancy
- Vaginal bleeding in pregnancy
- Postmenopausal bleeding
- Sexual assault
- Vaginal warts

Contraindications

- Patient refusal
- Placenta previa (contraindication to digital vaginal exam)

Equipment (Fig. 4-1a)

- Appropriately sized gown
- Sheet
- Light source
- Nonsterile nonlatex gloves
- Lubricating gel
- Scopettes® (Birchwood Labs, Eden Prairie, MN)
- Speculum: comes in different sizes and forms, from metal to plastic, Pedersen and Graves
- If clinically appropriate:
    – Pap smear (Fig. 4-1b)
        (a) For fixed glass slide specimens – glass slide, wooden cervical spatula, and endocervical brush; or endocervical broom, cell fixation spray
        (b) For liquid Pap – plastic spatula and endocervical brush or endocervical broom, liquid Pap smear jar

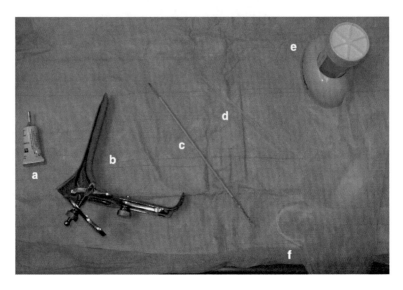

Fig. 4-1 Set-up for pelvic examination: (a) Surgilube® water-based lubricant (E. Fougera & Co, Melville, NY); (b) speculum; (c) endocervial brush; (d) spatula; (e) liquid-based cytology Pap jar with base; (f) nonsterile nonlatex gloves

- Wet mount
  (a) Cotton swab, small test tube, saline, pH paper, glass slide
- Additional cultures – for gonorrhea and chlamydia cultures, HPV and Group b Strep

Procedure

1. Take history before the patient changes into the gown. Using the appropriate language and/or drawings, describe the pelvic examination to the patient. Answer any questions the patient may have regarding the upcoming procedure. Let the patient know that although the exam may be uncomfortable, it should not be painful and that every effort will be made to minimize her discomfort.
2. Offer a chaperone: ask if the patient wishes to have another person present in the room at the time of the examination. Chaperones may be a requirement in some states and generally should be the same sex as the patient.
3. Step out of the room so that the patient may change into a gown, instructing her to take off her clothing, including underwear and bra.
4. Ask the patient to lie down on the table. Do the rest of the examination, leaving the pelvic examination for last. Have her lie down on the table, placing the stirrups in the appropriate positions, extending and externally rotating the stirrups.
5. Ask the patient to place her feet in the stirrups and to slide down so that her perineum reaches the edge of the examination table. Be sure to use the drape or sheet across her abdomen and pelvic area.
6. Put on nonsterile gloves on both hands.
7. Ask the patient to relax her legs, and let her knees fall to the sides as much as possible (Fig. 4-2). Describe to the patient each part of the procedure that you are about to perform.

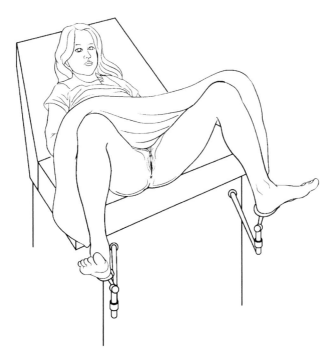

Fig. 4-2 Dorsal lithotomy position and pelvic exam position

8. Examine the labia for the presence of any lesions (warts, ulcerations, abnormal moles). Also examine the patient for the presence of a cystocele or rectocele.

9. If you are using a self-lit speculum, place the light source in the appropriate segment of the handle. If you are using a gooseneck lamp as a light source, position to provide appropriate lighting for visualization inside the vagina without burning the patient's thigh.

10. Apply warm water and/or warm lubricant gel to the blades of the speculum. Introduce the tip of the speculum at a 45-90 degree angle to the introitus, and apply downward and posterior pressure until approximately ¾ of the speculum's blades have been introduced.

11. Rotate the speculum so that the blades are at a perpendicular position in relation to the vaginal canal, and open the blades (Fig. 4-3a).

12. Reposition as needed in order to bring the cervix into full visualization between the blades of the speculum.

13. Inspect the vaginal walls for the presence of any lesions (i.e., warts and ulcers). Also note for presence or lack of moisture or rugae indicating atrophy.

14. Clean any cervical mucus from the cervix with the Scopette® prior to obtaining either Pap smear or gonorrhea and chlamydia DNA probes.

15. Obtain clinically appropriate vaginal/cervical/endocervical samples and Pap smear, if indicated (Fig. 4-3a,b). Obtain culture specimens prior to obtaining Pap smear specimens. Many times, the use of the endocervical brush to obtain an

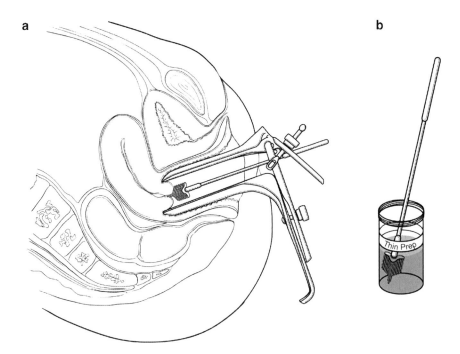

Fig. 4-3 (a) Speculum examination. (b) Liquid Pap smear

endocervical sample can produce some bleeding, which could affect the evaluation of other samples such as a wet mount or gonorrhea/chlamydia DNA probes.

16. Withdraw the speculum from the vaginal canal, being careful not to release the cervix quickly (do not "pop" the cervix).
17. Perform a bimanual examination by introducing the index and middle finger of the dominant hand into the vaginal canal. The examiner then places the non-dominant hand over the patient's lower abdomen. With the finger located inside the vagina, locate the cervix and apply upwards pressure to the body of the uterus. Sweep the external hand down the midline of the lower abdomen to palpate the size of the uterus in order to measure uterine size.
18. Move internally placed fingers laterally to the adnexae on each side, applying upwards pressure while applying downward pressure on the external hand to locate the ovaries.
19. If indicated, perform a rectovaginal examination, withdrawing the internal vaginal fingers, changing gloves and relubricating, and then placing one finger inside the vaginal canal and one finger of the same hand into the rectum. Palpate the rectovaginal wall for thickening or herniations, and ovarian enlargement or pain.
20. If the woman is over 50, do a stool guaiac evaluation from the finger used for the rectal examination.
21. Help the woman into a seated position by sliding back up the table first, and then removing feet from the stirrups. Offer tissues for cleaning lubricant and sanitary pads for any bleeding. Allow her to change prior to going over any results. Let her know when she can expect to be contacted about her results.

Complications and Risks

Although there is a small risk of trauma to the adjacent tissue, it is usually not necessary to obtain a consent form for the performance of a pelvic examination.

Tricks and Helpful Hints

- Specula come in various sizes and configurations:
  - Pedersen: more narrow and useful in patients who are not sexually active, nulliparous, or postmenopausal
  - Graves: wider blades, which are more useful in multiparous women or women with redundant vaginal walls
  - Smaller-sized specula are more appropriate for women who have never been sexually active.
  - Larger specula may be useful in patients with a cystocele or rectocele. It may be necessary to use vaginal wall retractors (see Chap. 5).
  - It is best to start with the smallest speculum that will allow full visualization of the cervix and to change to a larger size if needed.

- Have the patient take a deep breath to relax the perineal muscles while you are inserting the speculum.
- If you are having difficulty finding the cervix, withdraw the speculum from the vaginal canal and perform a digital examination to identify the presence and location of the cervix. Alternatively, withdraw the speculum approximately half way down the vagina, being careful not to pinch the patient as the blades close slightly. Apply downward pressure on the entire speculum toward the rectum. Open speculum blades partially to view the vaginal tissue. If more tissue is found superiorly, aim the speculum tip downward. Conversely, if more tissue is found inferiorly, aim the speculum tip upward.
- Inserting the speculum slowly allows the woman's tissues to accommodate to the blades. This is especially important with women who are postmenopausal or nulliparous, or women with vaginal infections.
- Be aware of your patient's cultural needs. Different ethnic groups may hold to different belief and health practices than the clinician. When appropriate, ask the patient about any other health beliefs or health maintenance practices in which she may participate. Be respectful, listen with an open mind, and welcome the opportunity to learn about these differences. Being judgmental may be detrimental toward building trust between the patient and clinician. If the clinician is concerned that a belief may be harmful, present the reservations in an open dialog and negotiate a solution that is acceptable to all.
- Some women may find it more comfortable to have a "stirrup-free" pelvic examination. To use this technique, have the woman slide herself down to the edge of the exam table, placing her feet on the corners of the withdrawn extension of the table. She then externally rotates her knees. This technique was found to decrease both physical discomfort and the sense of vulnerability [6].
- If the male partner insists on being present, make sure that there is some time during the examination that the clinician and patient are alone. Be sure to ask the patient if she has been harmed in any way. Posting discrete notices about safe houses for abuse in discrete places (usually restrooms) may be helpful.

Procedure Note

(Provider to fill in blanks/circle applicable choice when given multiple choices and customize as necessary.)

Patient placed in a dorsal lithotomy position. External genitalia examined without lesions or abnormalities. Speculum inserted without difficulty; cervix visualized; Pap smear (done/not done due to _____). Bimanual examination performed with uterus noted to be in _____ (anteverted, retroverted) position. Approximately _____ cm in size. Adnexae without masses or tenderness. Rectal examination (performed, not performed) with no noted lesions.

Coding

CPT® Codes (Current Procedural Terminology, AMA, Chicago, IL)
89.26   Gynecological examination
V70.0   Well woman examination

Postprocedure Patient Instructions

Patient may experience some vaginal spotting; she is to be instructed to call if it does not resolve spontaneously within 2 days. She should be told to call the office with heavy vaginal bleeding (>1 pad per hour), vaginal discharge, or pain. She needs to be told how to expect the results of any Pap smears or cultures and how soon to expect the results.

Case Study Outcome

A breast and pelvic examination were performed. A Pap smear was obtained and sent to the laboratory. Contraception options were discussed with the patient and prescribed. One week later, results revealed normal cytology and cultures. Patient was advised to return to the office in 1 year.

Postprocedure Patient Handout

(Provider to customize as necessary.)

You have had a pelvic examination today and may experience some vaginal spotting for 1 or 2 days, which will resolve spontaneously. Please call the office if you have heavy bleeding, vaginal discharge, or abdominal or pelvic pain. You will be notified of the results of your Pap smear and/or cultures within the next 2 weeks. If you have not heard from this office by then, please call us.

References

1. Saslow D, Runowicz CD, Solomon D, Moscicki AB, Smith RA, Eyre HJ, Cohen C. American Cancer Society guideline for the early detection of cervical neoplasia and cancer. *CA Cancer J Clin* 2002;52(6):342–362.
2. ACOG Practice Bulletin #109 "Cervical cytology screening." *Obstet Gynecol.* 2009.
3. Smith RA, Cokkinides V, von Eschenbach AC, Levin B, Cohen C, Runowicz CD, Sener S, Saslow D, Eyre HJ. American Cancer Society Guideline for the early detection of cervical neoplasia and cancer. *CA Cancer J Clin* 2002;52(1):8–22.
4. Bohm-Velez M, Fleischer AC, Andreotti RF, Fishman EK, Horrow MM, Hricak H, Thurmond A, Zelop C. Expert panel on women's imaging. *Ovarian cancer screening*. [online publication]. Reston, VA: American College of Radiology (ACR), 2005.
5. Chu CS, Rubin SC. Screening for ovarian cancer in the general population. *Best Pract Res Clin Obstet Gynaecol* 2006;20(2);307–320.
6. Seehusen DA, Johnson DR, Earwood JS, Sethuraman SN, Cornali J, Gillespie K, Doria M, Farnell E IV, Lanham J. Improving women's experience during speculum examinations at routine gynaecological visits: randomised clinical trial. *BMJ* 2006;333(7560):171.

Additional Resources

Articles

Edelman A, Anderson J, Lai S, Braner DA, Tegtmeyer K. Pelvic examination. In Videos in clinical medicine. *N Engl J Med* 2007;356(26):e26.

Web Sites

http://www.familydoctor.org/138.xml.
http://www.guideline.gov.

Chapter 5
Difficult Exams: Cystocele, Rectocele, Stenotic Cervix/Cervical Dilatation, Nonsexually Active Women, Elderly Women

Rhina Acevedo

Introduction

There are various anatomical conditions that can affect the performance of the pelvic exam and may lead to modifications of your pelvic examination techniques. These conditions include examinations of women who are not sexually active, women with cystoceles or rectoceles, women with atrophic vaginitis, and women with cervical stenosis.

Women who have never been sexually active may have greater anxiety about their first pelvic examination; these patients would benefit from more time, explanation, and support during their examinations. Using the smallest speculum will also improve their comfort during the exam, as well as using lubricant liberally. Indications for examination of women who have never been sexually active are limited to those with pelvic pain, discharge, or women above the age of 21 as per ACOG guidelines [1]. Most examinations are possible; however, if examination becomes too painful, the provider should discontinue the examination and consider referral for an examination under anesthesia or, alternatively, using a pelvic ultrasound. For non-emergent situations (i.e., Pap smear), a woman without prior sexual contact may benefit from first using tampons during her menses prior to her first pelvic examination as tampon use may have the woman experience the physical sensation of having something placed inside her vagina.

There are other acquired and congenital changes of the pelvic structures that may also add difficulty to the performance of the pelvic exam. These include cystoceles and rectoceles, atrophic vaginitis, and cervical stenosis.

Cystoceles and rectoceles result from weakened pelvic support structures. This weakness can be attributed to such factors as childbirth, pelvic trauma, and the aging process. Cystoceles occur when the pubovesicle cervical fascia is

R. Acevedo (✉)
Department of Family Medicine, University of Medicine and Dentistry of New Jersey, New Brunswick, NJ 08820, USA
e-mail: Racevedo97@gmail.com

S.M. Sulik and C.B. Heath (eds.), *Primary Care Procedures in Women's Health*, DOI 10.1007/978-0-387-76604-1_5, © Springer Science+Business Media, LLC 2010

weakened and allows the descent of the bladder into the vaginal canal. Patients often have a sensation of fullness or pressure, stress incontinence, urinary urgency, or a feeling of incomplete voiding. A rectocele is produced when the weakened pelvic structure allows the rectum to bulge into the vaginal canal. The patient may report the presence of a sensation of heaviness in the vagina, constipation, and may need to splint the vagina with her fingers in order to evacuate stool during a bowel movement [2]. A cystocele is best observed with the patient in the dorsal lithotomy position. With the posterior wall of the vagina depressed (manually or with the use of a retractor), the patient is then asked to valsalva or cough to visualize the degree of cystocele that is present [2]. A cystocele that presents only on valsalva or upright posture is considered grade 1. A grade 2 cystocele occurs when the cystocele is present at the introitus. Grade 3 is a cystocele that protrudes halfway beyond the introitus; and, if it occurs with an everted vaginal cuff or cervix, it is called a "procidentia," complete pelvic floor collapse, or grade 4 cystocele. Alternatively, the Pelvic Organ Prolapse Quantification (POPQ) measures nine sites in centimeters between the vagina and perineal body to the hymen [3].

Cervical stenosis can be either acquired or congenital. It commonly occurs in the region of the internal os. Acquired cervical stenosis can result from radiation therapy, previous infection, cancer, atrophic changes, and surgical interventions. Cone biopsy and cautery of the cervix, electrocautery, and cryocoagulation can all lead to cervical stenosis [4]. Presenting symptoms vary depending on the patient's hormonal status (pre- or postmenopausal) and degree of obstruction present. Premenopausal women with cervical stenosis may present with complaints of dysmenorrhea, pelvic pain, abnormal uterine bleeding, amenorrhea, and infertility. Postmenopausal women are predominantly asymptomatic, but eventually may develop hydrometra (collection of clear fluid in the uterine cavity), hematometra (collection of blood in the uterine cavity), or pyometra (collection of exudate within the uterine cavity). The diagnosis of cervical stenosis is based on the inability to pass a 1–2 mm cervical dilator through the cervical os into the endocervical canal. The treatment for complete cervical stenosis is cervical dilatation (can be performed under ultrasound guidance). It is important to rule out the presence of endometrial carcinoma and endocervical carcinoma in patients with complete cervical stenosis [4, 5].

Vaginal atrophy is the result of estrogen deficiency. This commonly occurs in postmenopausal women, but it may also occur in premenopausal women who have a relative estrogen deficiency. Premenopausal atrophy due to estrogen deficiency can occur in the immediate postpartum period, during lactation, or with use of low-dose estrogen contraceptives, progesterone-only contraceptives, and estrogen blockers such as Danazol (Sanofi-Synthelabo, Bridgewater, NJ) (Danocrine®) and tamoxifen. Patients with atrophic vaginitis may present with complaints of vaginal itching, vaginal soreness, spotting, urinary incontinence, dysuria, or dyspareunia [6]. On exam, the vaginal tissues appear pale and dry, and have decreased distensibility and decreased vaginal rugae. The tissue may be friable and have areas of stenosis [3]. Patients may also have adhesions of the vaginal wall, either externally or internally.

Case Study

A 65-year-old woman, G5P5005, presents to your office for her annual well woman examination and Pap smear. The patient has had no vaginal bleeding since her last menses 12 years ago. She also reports some vaginal dryness and itching. As you introduce the speculum into the vaginal canal, the patient reports discomfort. As you examine the vagina, you notice that her vaginal walls are devoid of rugae and appear thin. When attempting to obtain an endocervical sample, it is impossible to insert the brush into the tightly closed cervical os.

Diagnosis (Algorithms 5-1, 5-2)

- Atrophic vaginitis
- Cervical stenosis

Differential Diagnosis (Algorithms 5-1, 5-2)

- Female sexual dysfunction
- Infectious vaginitis
- Vaginal neoplasia (most commonly squamous cell)
- Status postcervical cone or cryotherapy (differential for cervical stenosis)

Indications (Algorithms 5-1, 5-2)

- Routine women's health examination
- Lower abdominal and/or pelvic pain
- Irregular menses
- Postcoital bleeding
- Dyspareunia
- Pregnancy
- Postmenopausal bleeding
- Sexual assault

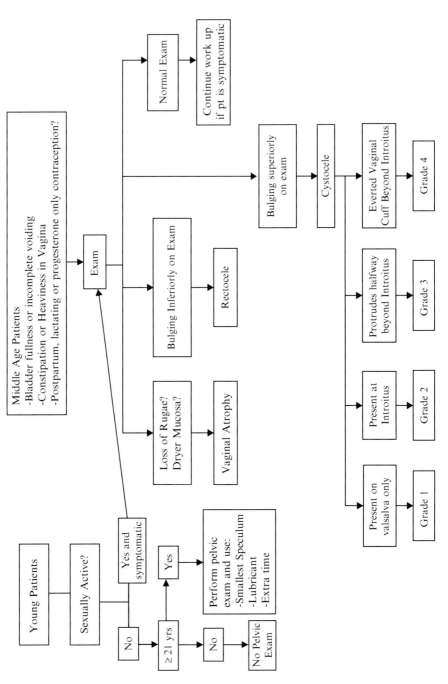

Algorithm 5-1 Decision tree for pelvic examinations of adolescent and middle age women

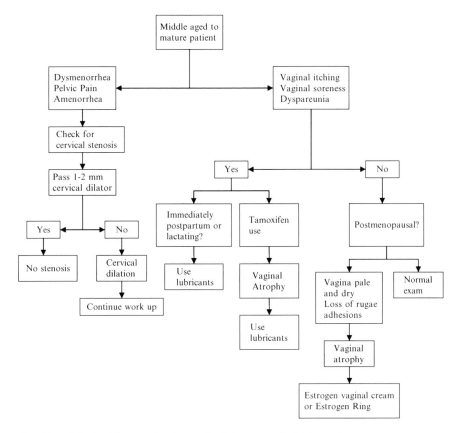

Algorithm 5-2 Decision tree for abnormal pelvic exams of middle-aged to mature women

Contraindications

- Patient refusal
- Placenta previa (contraindication to digital vaginal examination)

Equipment (Fig. 5-1)

- Gown (appropriately sized for patient)
- Sheet
- Light source
- Vaginal cotton swabs (Scopettes®, Birchwood Labs, Eden Prairie, MN)
- Non-sterile gloves (latex free if patient allergic)
- Lubricating gel

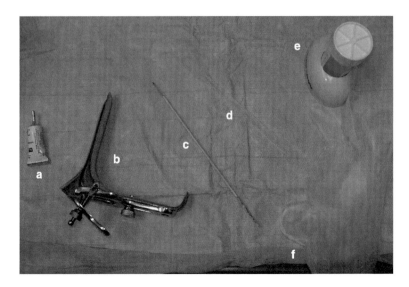

Fig. 5-1 Set-up for pelvic examination: (a) Surgilube® water-based lubricant (E. Fougera & Co, Melville, NY); (b) speculum; (c) endocervial brush; (d) spatula; (e) liquid-based cytology Pap jar with base; (f) non-sterile non-latex gloves

- Speculum (Fig. 5-2): Metal or plastic – Various sizes and shapes available, including Graves ("duck-billed") or Pederson ("straight"); each speculum comes in small (pediatric), medium, large, and extra large sizes.
- Vaginal wall retractors: may be separate from speculum or incorporated into speculum
- Wet mount specimen
  - Cotton swab
  - KOH
  - Small test tube with saline
  - pH paper
  - Glass slide with cover
  - Microscope

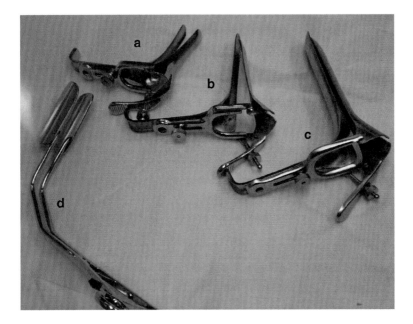

Fig. 5-2 Small Pederson speculum (**a**), medium Pederson speculum (**b**), large Graves speculum (**c**), with separate vaginal wall retractor/spreader (**d**)

- Additional cultures as necessary
  - Gonorrhea and chlamydia
  - HPV (Human Papilloma Virus)
  - HSV (Herpes Virus)
- Pap smear equipment
  - Glass slide method
    - (a) One glass slide
    - (b) Fixation spray or jar with alcohol
    - (c) Wooden cervical spatula and endocervical brush OR
    - (d) Cervical broom
  - Liquid cell medium
    - (a) Plastic cervical spatula and endocervical brush OR
    - (b) Cervical broom

Procedure

Proceed with the steps described in Chap. 4 in the Procedures section, with the following variations:

1. Examine the labia for the presence of any lesions (warts, ulcerations).
2. Separate the labia and inspect the introitus for any masses or bulges.
3. Ask the patient to valsalva and watch the area for any bulges on the superior (cystocele) (Fig. 5-3) or inferior (rectocele) (Fig. 5-4) aspect of the vaginal canal.
4. Place the index finger into the vaginal canal and apply downward pressure to displace the introitus, which will allow the examiner to visualize a cystocele or rectocele.
5. Position the light source in order to optimize visualization of the vaginal canal.
6. Apply a small amount of warm lubricant gel to the blades of the speculum or wet the metal speculum with warm water. Use the smallest speculum available that will permit visualization of the vaginal walls and cervix.
7. Introduce the tip of the speculum at an angle to the vaginal canal entry and apply slow downward and posterior pressure until approximately ¾ of the speculum blades have been introduced. Allow time to have the patient's vaginal tissue accommodate to the procedure.
8. Rotate the speculum so that the blades are perpendicular to the vaginal canal and open the blades. Reposition as needed in order to bring the cervix into full visualization between the blades of the speculum.

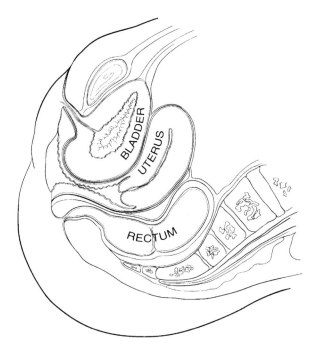

Fig. 5-3 Visualization of cystocele with patient in dorsal lithotomy position

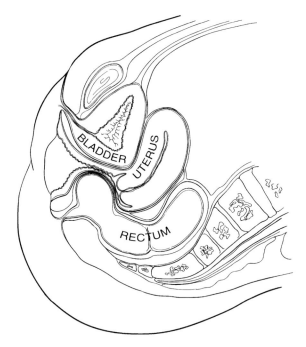

Fig. 5-4   Rectocele with patient in dorsal lithotomy position

9. Inspect the vaginal walls for the presence of any lesions. Also note the presence or absence of rugae and vaginal moisture.
10. Obtain clinically appropriate vaginal/cervical/endocervical samples.
11. Carefully withdraw the speculum from the vaginal canal.
12. Perform a bimanual examination. For women with a small introitus, one finger may be all that is necessary for the intra-vaginal portion of the bimanual examination.
13. Perform a recto-vaginal examination, with the middle finger being introduced into the rectum and the index finger into the vagina if necessary.

Complications and Risks

There is a small risk of trauma to the adjacent tissue.

Tricks and Helpful Hints

- Do not assume that postmenopausal women are not sexually active.
- Use a well-lubricated speculum when performing an examination of a woman with possible atrophic vaginitis. Consider using a Pedersen instead of a Graves speculum.

- A speculum with a wider blade (such as a medium or large-sized Graves) will provide better support of superior and posterior structures and will allow for better visualization of the cervix.
- For vaginal walls that persistently protrude into the field of vision, consider the following:
  - Use vaginal wall retractors with the speculum (must use medium or large Graves with retractors).
  - If vaginal wall retractors are unavailable, make a retractor out of a clean latex glove by cutting the thumb portion from the glove and then cutting the tip off the thumb portion of the glove (Fig. 5-5). Introduce the speculum blades into the rubber cylinder created (Fig. 5-6), and lubricate both the speculum and the cylinder prior to introducing it into the vagina.
  - Use a condom in the same fashion as the latex glove.
- For cervical stenosis:
  - Use an endometrial cell sampler to relieve mild cervical strictures. Then retry using the endocervical brush or broom.
  - Use cervical dilators.
  - Use intra-vaginal estrogen cream, one applicatorful, to vagina nightly for 2–4 weeks and then obtain the specimen.
  - Use laminaria.
  - Use misoprostel 200 mg orally or intra-vaginally 4 h prior to the exam.
- In women who have never been sexually active, the clinician may opt to insert only one finger intra-vaginally during the bimanual examination.
- In extreme cases of tenderness or pain with examination, discontinue the exam and consider doing under general anesthesia.

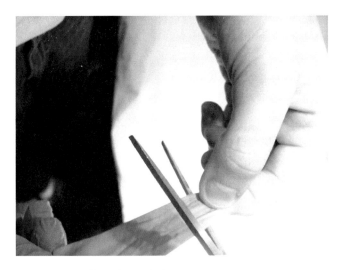

Fig. 5-5 Cutting latex glove finger for vaginal retractor

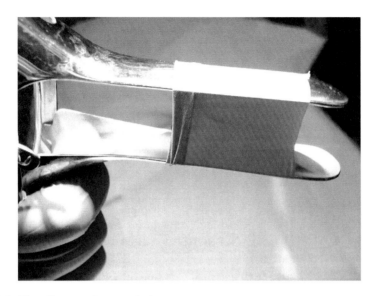

Fig. 5-6   Glove finger used as a vaginal retractor

- In extreme cases of tenderness or pain, consider gently questioning women about previous sexual abuse. In some cases, pelvic examinations may need to be done after desensitization programs or under general anesthesia.
- Be sure to question women alone about their needs for a chaperone. Chaperones in general should be health professionals, but they can be family members or partners if that is the preference of the patient. However, be sure to discuss this in private with the patient prior to agreeing to any non-professional chaperone, as abusive partners may insist on being present.

Procedure Note

(Provider to fill in blanks/circle applicable choice when given multiple choices and customize as necessary.)

> Patient was placed in the dorsal lithotomy position. Upon examination, _____ (cystocele, rectocele, vaginal atrophy, cervical stenosis) was noted. Careful speculum examination (with, without) vaginal retractors occurred; cervix was visualized, and Pap smear was obtained. Patient tolerated procedure well and a note will be mailed to her with her results.

Coding

CPT® Codes (Current Procedural Terminology, AMA, Chicago, IL)

89.26	Gynecological examination
V70.0	Well woman examination

ICD 9-CM-Diagnostic Codes (International Classification of Diseases, 9th Revision, Clinical Modification, Center for Disease Control and Prevention)

618.01	Cystocele, midline NOS
618.02	Cystocele, lateral, paravaginal
618.04	Rectocele
622.4	Stricture/stenosis of cervix (acquired)
627.3	Postmenopausal atrophic vaginitis

Postprocedure Patient Instructions

The patient should be advised of any findings on exam and how she will be notified of the results. She should also be advised that she may experience some scant vaginal spotting which is usually self limited. If the patient begins to experience significant vaginal symptoms of heavy bleeding, discharge or pelvic pain, she should return to the office for evaluation.

Case Study Outcomes

Vaginal examination revealed the presence of a cystocele and atrophic vaginitis. Patient was treated with estrogen vaginal cream. Upon re-evaluation 1 month later, the patient reported significant improvement of symptoms.

Postprocedure Patient Handout

(Provider to fill in blanks/circle applicable choice when given multiple choices and customize as necessary.)

You have just had a pelvic examination. This examination showed that you have (provider to circle diagnosis):

- A cystocele is a protrusion of the bladder into the vagina that happens due to the relaxation of the pelvic structures. Many women who have cystoceles have no symptoms at all. Some women notice urgency of urination, stress incontinence (losing urine with laughing, coughing or sneezing), or a sense that their bladder is just not emptying. Some women also experience only a vague sense of fullness of the bladder. If these symptoms are becoming bothersome to you, please make an appointment to discuss treatment options, such as pessary fitting or surgery.
- A rectocele occurs when the rectal mucosa protrudes into the vaginal wall. Many women with rectoceles have no symptoms, but some experience symptoms of heaviness in the vagina, constipation, or the need to provide support to their vagina to have a bowel movement. If these symptoms are becoming bothersome to you, please make an appointment to discuss treatment options, such as pessary fitting or surgery.
- Vaginal atrophy occurs when there is a lack of estrogen lubricating the vaginal walls, either from medications such as tamoxifen or progesterone-only birth control, menopause, breastfeeding, or hysterectomy with removal of both ovaries. Most women have no symptoms, but some may experience painful intercourse, vaginal itching or soreness, burning on urination, urinary incontinence, or vaginal spotting. If these symptoms are becoming bothersome to you, please make an appointment to discuss treatment options, such as hormone replacement, if indicated.
- Cervical stenosis occurs when there is a lack of estrogen lubricating the cervix or when there is a surgical procedure or radiation that has caused the cervical opening to become small. Symptoms of cervical stenosis for women who still are getting their periods include: dysmenorrhea (painful periods), pelvic pain, abnormal uterine bleeding, amenorrhea (no period), or infertility. Postmenopausal women usually have no symptoms but can experience abdominal cramping or pain from collections of blood or fluid in the uterus. This is very rare. If you are experiencing any of these symptoms, please make an appointment with your provider to discuss treatment options.

References

1. ACOG Committee Opinion. Primary and preventive care: periodic assessments. *Obstet Gynecol* 2003;102(5 Pt 1):1117–1124.
2. Lentz GM. Anatomic defects of the abdominal wall and pelvic floor. In Stenchever MA, Droegemueller W, Herbst AL, Mishell DR Jr (eds) *Comprehensive gynecology, fourth edition.* St. Louis, MO: Mosby, 2007.
3. Steers WD, Barret DM, Wein AJ. Voiding dysfunction: diagnosis, classification and management. In Gillenwater JA, Greywater JA, Greyhack JT, Howards SS, Mitchell ME (eds) *Adult and pediatric urology.* Philadelphia: Lippincott Williams and Wilkins, 2002.
4. Williams R, Elam G. Gynecology. In Rakel R (ed) *Textbook of family practice, sixth edition.* Philadelphia: WB Saunders, 2002.
5. Katz VL, Benign gynecological lesions. In Stenchever MA, Droegemueller W, Herbst AL, Mishell DR Jr (eds) *Comprehensive gynecology, fourth edition.* St. Louis, MO: Mosby, 2007.
6. Bachmann GA, Nevadunsky NS. Diagnosis and treatment of Atrophic vaginitis. *Am Fam Physician* 2000;61:3090–3096.

Chapter 6
Sexual Assault Victim Examination

Beverly A. Poelstra

Introduction

Sexual assault is defined as a threat of or actual sexual contact with or without penetration without the willing consent of the victim, whether by threat of physical force, psychological pressure, or facilitation by the use of alcohol or drugs [1]. Rape is considered an act requiring forced penetration of the mouth, genitals, or anus by the offender where the force is either physical or psychological [2]. One in six American women is a victim of sexual assault. In 2004–2005, there were an average of 200,780 victims of rape, attempted rape, or sexual assault. Of these women, 44% were under the age of 18 [3]. The rate of rape and sexual assault has fallen by more than half, although a large percentage of cases still go unreported [4].

When a victim of rape presents to the Emergency Department or private office for examination, one of the most important issues is to take steps to preserve all forensic evidence to insure that there are few impediments to prosecution. It is important to be complete and thorough in the exam and evidence gathering, while at the same time being sensitive to the fact that the victim has likely already endured a lengthy process prior to arriving for her physical examination. To that end, the number of examiners and interviews should be kept to a minimum with as much history as possible being obtained from law enforcement personnel, social workers, and family members. This use of the team approach toward evaluation and treatment is effective in minimizing the trauma of the emergency department setting [5]. With that background, a more focused interview can be obtained from the victim using as many of the victim's own words as possible in recording the history. The interview process need not be duplicated, except as it pertains to specific evidence that needs to be collected for a

B.A. Poelstra (✉)
Department of Pediatrics, Division of Pediatric Emergency Medicine, University of Medicine and Dentistry of New Jersey, The Bristol-Myers Squibb Children's Hospital at Robert Wood Johnson University Hospital, New Brunswick, NJ, USA
e-mail: poelstbe@umdnj.edu

S.M. Sulik and C.B. Heath (eds.), *Primary Care Procedures in Women's Health*,
DOI 10.1007/978-0-387-76604-1_6, © Springer Science+Business Media, LLC 2010

more in-depth, directed physical exam or specimen collection. Offering to have a support person present (who is not suspected of the abuse) may be reassuring to victims of all ages [6].

It is helpful to have a second professional (nurse, aide) assist during the exam and evidence collection, not only to serve as a witness, but also to provide materials and label evidence promptly as it is collected. This will lessen the possibility of lost specimens and speed up the process by allowing the examiner to continue wearing gloves during the entire examination without having to change them for record-keeping. Specially trained nurses in the Sexual Assault Nurse Examiner (SANE) program help coordinate all the team members and minimize further trauma to the victim [7].

Case Study

A 22-year-old woman was at a party with her friends where alcohol was being served. She does remember drinking two beers within a time span of 3 h but did not take any drugs. She recalls dancing with several young men, but she now has a headache, her clothing is disheveled, and she is experiencing vaginal spotting. She suspects that she may have been the victim of unwanted sexual advances, but her memory is fuzzy for the event. She is presently on oral contraceptives, and her last menstrual period was 1 week ago.

Indications (Algorithm 6-1)

Suspected rape

Contraindications

Unwilling or uncooperative patient

Equipment

- Speculum: disposable
- Lubricant
- Light source

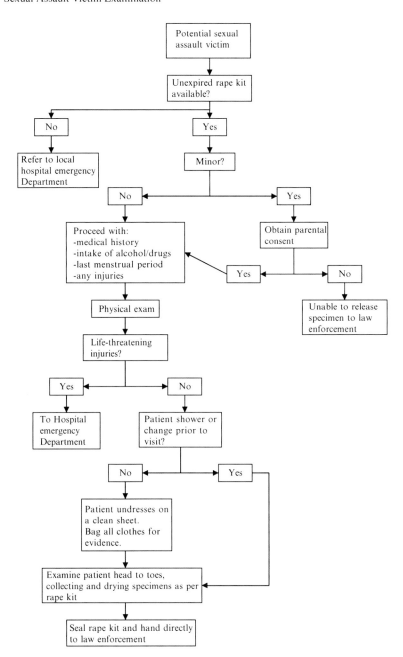

Algorithm 6-1   Decision tree for sexual assault victim

- Rape Kit: as determined by local law enforcement agencies. (This includes envelopes, swabs, and slides for evidence collection, as well as forms with routine questions and diagrams.)
- GC/Chlamydia test kit with swabs, depending on local custom.
- Venipuncture materials: needle, vacutainer collection tubes, alcohol prep, gloves, gauze
- Urine collection container with cleansing wipes
- Rapid pregnancy test kit
- Pencil for labeling specimens on glass slides
- Pen for recording findings and labeling envelopes
- Nonsterile exam gloves
- Clean sheet for patient to stand on while collecting clothing for evidence.
- Hospital gown for patient to wear during exam and clean sheet for cover-up.
- Water for dampening swabs to collect evidence
- Paper bags in various sizes to collect clothing
- Extra clothing for victim, preferably "street clothes" as opposed to hospital gown

Optional Equipment

- UV light (see Sect. "Tricks and Helpful Hints")
- Colposcope with video capabilities to record the evidence as collected

Procedure (Algorithm 6-1)

1. Consent must be obtained from the victim or a parent/legal guardian (in the case of a minor) in order to release the specimens to law enforcement authorities.
2. Medical history, noting:
    - Any complaints of injuries related to the alleged sexual abuse. The rape kit forms are very thorough in assessing and recording the circumstances of the sexual assault and which body parts of the victim came in contact with which body parts of the perpetrator.
    - The date and time of alcohol or drug intake, if applicable.
    - Last menstrual period (LMP), prior pregnancies, sexual partners, birth control.
    - Past medical history. List of current medications. Allergies.
3. Observe and record the general appearance and demeanor of the victim, noting any obvious injuries. Any potential life-threatening injuries should be attended to first.
4. Wearing nonsterile gloves lay out a clean white sheet on the floor.
5. Have the patient undress on the sheet, which will prevent any contamination of clothing and secure any fibers or evidence that may be on clothing, lodged in the patient's hair, or under her fingernails.

6. Have the patient completely disrobe while standing on the sheet and package each piece of clothing individually in a paper bag, which should then be sealed. If the victim has showered and changed clothing after the sexual assault has occurred, this step may be unnecessary. Provide patient with a hospital/office gown and a sheet.

7. A complete physical exam should be performed with special attention directed to the oral cavity, skin around and near the breasts, and the perineal area (Fig. 6-4).

8. Using the rape kit as a guide, proceed from head to toe gathering specimens as appropriate and placing them in the appropriate envelopes (Fig. 6-1).

9. Thoroughly dry all specimens prior to packaging to avoid the destruction of samples by mold growth (Fig. 6-2).

10. Obtain cervical swabs to be sent to the local laboratory for gonorrhea and chlamydia by the preferred local detection method.

11. In order to minimize further trauma to the patient, specimens of the victim's scalp hair and pubic hair (which must be plucked) can be obtained either at this step or at any follow up visit under less stressful circumstances.

12. Seal the rape kit with the special stickers provided and sign off each sticker with time and date and initials of the examiner. The kit must be handed directly to a law enforcement officer in order to preserve the chain of evidence (Fig. 6-4). Sign each page (usually 15–20 pages, not including duplicates) and

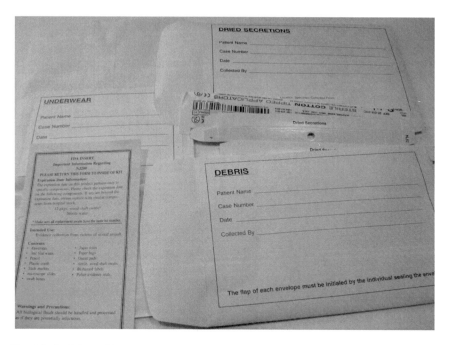

Fig. 6-1 Partial rape kit contents

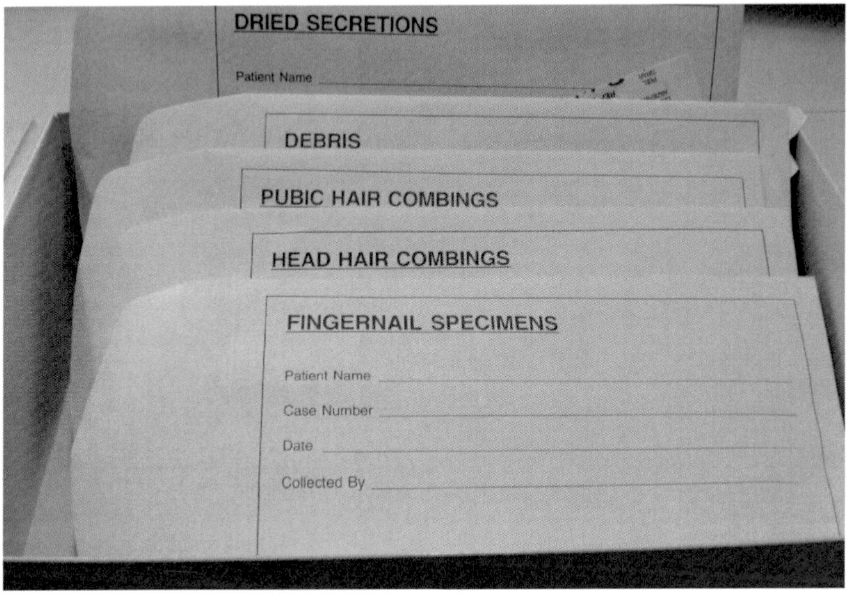

Fig. 6-2 Additional rape kit contents

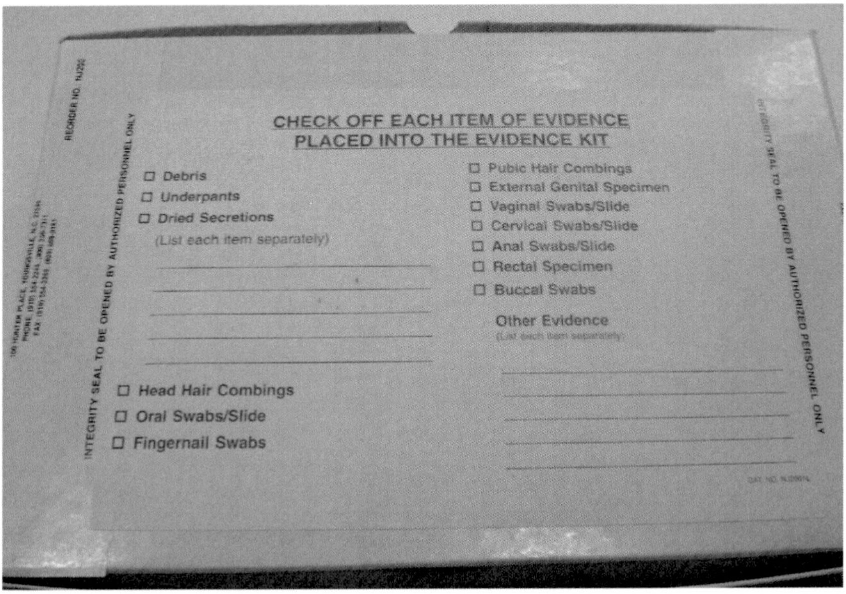

Fig. 6-3 Rape kit box with all necessary forms and packaging materials for samples collected. External portion of box with check-off list of sent contents

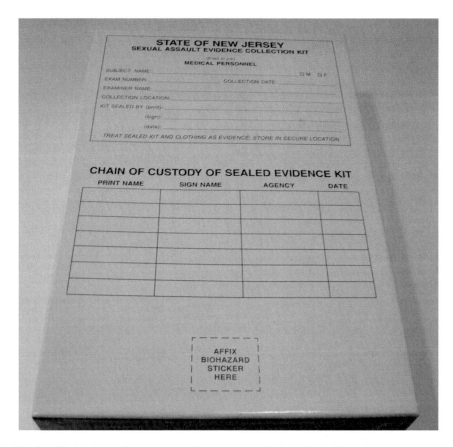

Fig. 6-4   Chain of custody sealed rape kit; front of rape kit box (State of New Jersey)

hand the originals to the officer, keeping copies for the chart and sexual abuse management (SAM) clinic.

13. Blood and urine specimens should be labeled and delivered to the lab. The prosecutor will obtain these results later.

14. Perform serum toxicology screens – alcohol, drug screen if indicated – noting time of alcohol ingestion obtained in history, if known. These specimens are sent to the local hospital laboratory. Specimens may also be sent for Hepatitis B, Hepatitis C, and HIV.

15. Results of the rapid pregnancy test and/or quantitative βHCG results should be obtained and recorded if the patient is a female of childbearing age.

16. Offer pregnancy prophylaxis, if indicated.

17. Sexually transmitted disease prophylaxis should be provided empirically based on local and current guidelines.

18. Arrange a follow up appointment to review labs, discuss emotions concerning the assault. Local support groups are often invaluable for handling the emotional aftermath.

Tricks and Helpful Hints

- UV light has been used in the past to highlight areas of semen on skin and in hair; however, studies have recently shown that this yields confusing results, as many common items (such as K-Y jelly and powder) will fluoresce. Local authorities may dictate whether this step is performed, but it is not recommended.
- It is *VERY IMPORTANT* to check the date on the seal of the rape kit before proceeding to determine that it has not expired. Otherwise, all evidence collected may be considered invalid and the case may not be able to be prosecuted.
- Many of the "date-rape" drugs do not have metabolites that can be detected on routine toxicology screens. However, some drugs may be possible to detect if special instructions are given to the laboratory. Check with local law enforcement as some specimens can be sent to the state lab for testing of metabolites. The length of time from drug ingestion to collection of the specimen also plays a role in the likelihood of detection [8].
- It is the patient's preference to decide on her own about pregnancy prophylaxis, even if that patient is a minor.
- Special handling and special consent may be needed for HIV serology.
- If the patient prefers, have a support person present during the exam.
- When an assessment is made, it is important to note that although the physical exam may be normal, this does not exclude the possibility that a sexual assault did indeed occur, and this should be discussed with the patient and with the authorities.
- In some areas of the country, clinicians use a colposcope to aid in recording details in the woman's examination, including bruising or bleeding consistent with trauma.

Procedure Note Provider to Customize as Needed

The rape kit provides a very elaborate and thorough form for recording various aspects of the history and physical exam. An additional note for the hospital or office record may make a reference to these documents and should summarize the major findings.

For example:

CC: 22 yo female c/o alleged sexual assault 12 h prior to admission. Patient consumed one beer at 1:00 am. Patient has voided and brushed her teeth, but has not showered, douched, or defecated since the event. She changed her clothes prior to going to police station. No other injuries. LMP 9/13/07 G1P0010 sexually active, one partner, on oral contraceptives. No significant past medical history. No other meds, no known allergies.

PE: Small abrasion of left labia minora with no active bleeding; exam otherwise normal. (See rape kit sheets.)

A/P: Alleged sexual assault. STD and pregnancy prophylaxis offered. Hepatitis, HIV, GC/ chlamydia pending. Patient to f/u with Sexual Abuse Management (SAM) Clinic.

Coding

CPT® Codes (Current Procedural Terminology, AMA, Chicago, IL)
E960.1   Rape; descriptor code used in conjunction with codes describing trauma.
V71.5   Observation following alleged rape or seduction. V codes are supplementary or secondary diagnosis codes to support other primary diagnosis and conditions.

Postprocedure Patient Instructions

Follow-up to be arranged with the local Sexual Abuse Management team or equivalent where counseling can be provided; follow up on infections and diseases can take place, and these can be treated if necessary. Appropriate follow up should also be made to manage any injuries that may have occurred during the sexual assault.

Case Study Outcome

The patient has been evaluated by the clinician in the emergency room for rape. She has elected to be treated for sexually transmitted infections. She decided to follow up with her primary care clinician and is planning on going to the next meeting of the support group for women who have been sexually abused.

Postprocedure Patient Handout

(Provider to customize as necessary.)

You have just been evaluated for sexual assault (rape). It is important to remember that what happened is not your fault. *No one* "deserves this" or was "asking for it." Rape is a crime. You have a right to report this to the police, and you have the right to be treated fairly during the justice process.

Many people experience a widely varying set of emotions, including rage, depression, anxiety, and fear. This is normal. In addition, it is very common for loved ones to have similar reactions. It is important not to "take the law into your own hands," as these actions will likely end in more hardship to you and to your loved ones. Allow the law to do its job. Law enforcers are specialists and are there to assist you in bringing the perpetrator to justice.

Some women prefer private counseling with a psychologist or mental health social worker. Many people find support groups quite helpful. These local support groups often have trained therapists and other women who have gone through similar circumstances. Talking with people who have also experienced rape often helps people understand their own feelings and emotions. There are also national groups to help support women through the crisis of rape:

- National Coalition Against Sexual Assault: telephone: 1-717-728-9764.
- Rape, Abuse and Incest National Network: telephone: 1-800-656-HOPE.

It is also important to follow up with the medical issues surrounding sexual assault. This can be done by a local Sexual Abuse Management team or at your primary care physician's office.

If you are on birth control and are taking it regularly, the likelihood of pregnancy is low. If you wish to be treated for prevention of pregnancy, you may be given a series of pills to take. It is important to take them as directed. If you are concerned about the possibility of infection, you may be treated for gonorrhea, chlamydia, and syphilis. If you are concerned about getting HIV, understand the risk of this is less than 1%. However, if you elect to be treated, be sure to take the medication as directed.

References

1. DeLahunta E, Baram DA. Sexual assault. *Obstet Gynecol* 1997;40:648.
2. Cantu M, Coppola M, Lindner AJ. Evaluation and management of the sexually assaulted woman. In Coppola M, Della Giurstina D (eds) *Emergency medicine clinics of North America: obstetric and gynecological emergencies*. Philadelphia: WB Saunders 2003;21:3.
3. Catalano SM. Criminal victimization 2005. Bureau of Justice Statistics Bulletin. 2006;NCJ 214644:3.
4. Statistics. Key facts. Rape, Abuse, & Incest National Network Website. 2005. Available at: http://www.rainn.org/statistics/index.html?PHPSESSID=20b163a7eabff1191d664c90a6f46 c02. Accessed October 28, 2007.
5. American Academy of Pediatrics Task Force on Adolescent Assault Victim Needs, Adolescent assault victim needs: a review of issues and a model protocol. *Pediatrics* 1996;98(5):991–999.
6. Kellogg N. Committee on Child Abuse and Neglect American Academy of Pediatrics. The evaluation of sexual abuse in children. *Pediatrics* 2005;116(2):506–512.
7. Taylor WK. Collecting evidence for sexual assault: The role of the sexual assault nurse examiner (SANE). *Int J Gynaecol Obstet* 2002;78:S91–S94.
8. Bechtel LK, Holstege CP. Criminal Poisoning: drug-facilitated sexual assault [Review]. *Emerg Med Clin North Am* 2005;25(2):499–525.

Additional Resources

Books

Crowley SR. *Sexual assault: the medical-legal examination*. Stamford (CT): Appleton & Lange, 1999.

Girardin BW, Faugno DK, Seneski PC, Slaughter L, Whelan M. *Color atlas of sexual assault*. St. Louis, MO: Mosby, 1997.

Lavelle J. Forensic evidence collection. In Giardino AP, Alexander R (eds): *Child maltreatment: a clinical guide and reference*, 3rd ed. St. Louis, MO: G.W. Medical Publishing, 2005.

Christian CW, Giardino AP. Forensic evidence collection. In Finkel MA, Giardino AP (eds) *Medical evaluation of child sexual abuse: a practical guide*, 2nd ed. Thousand Oaks, CA: Sage, 2002.

Sexual Assault Nurse Examiner (SANE): Development and Operation Guide, US Department of Justice, Office of Justice Programs, Office for Victims of Crimes, Washington, DC, 1999.

Article

Laraque D, DeMattia A, Low C. Forensic Child Abuse Evaluation: A Review. *Mt Sinai J Med* 2006;73(8):1138–1147.

Web Sites

Sexual Assault Resource Service (SARS): www.sane-sart.com.

Sexual Assault Nurse Examiner (SANE) Programs: www.ojp.usdoj.gov/ovc/publications/bulle-tins/sane_4_2001/welcome.htm.

Chapter 7
Pap Smear

DeAnn Cummings

Introduction

The Pap smear for cervical cancer screening was first introduced in the 1940s. Since then, the incidence of cervical cancer in the US has decreased from 14/100,000 to 7.8/100,000 in 1994 [1]. Despite this decline, cervical cancer continues to be the third most common gynecologic malignancy in the US and the second most common cancer in women worldwide. This underscores the need for continued vigilance.

Pathology of Pap smear specimens shows that 95–100% of squamous cell cancers and 75–95% of high-grade CIN lesions have detectable HPV-DNA [1]. This observation has led to new options for prevention, screening, and management of cervical cancer and its precursors. Vaccines against HPV types 16 and 18 have been introduced to reduce HPV infection. HPV DNA testing is now being utilized in the management of the abnormal Pap smear and cervical dysplasia.

HPV DNA testing is also under evaluation for primary screening of cervical cancer. HPV testing has a sensitivity of 82–96% and a specificity of 78–90% for the detection of high-grade cervical disease. While the sensitivity is improved over Pap smear testing, the specificity is decreased, which could lead to more unnecessary testing. The combination of Pap smear and HPV testing has been approved by the FDA for screening women over age 30 every 3 years. Combination screening improves the sensitivity but decreases the specificity [2].

Liquid-based cytology (ThinPrep®, SurePath™) as an alternative to the conventional Pap smear was introduced in 1996 to improve the sensitivity of the Pap smear (40–80%). Instead of applying the cervical specimen to a slide, the specimen (collected in the same fashion) is instead inserted into a vial of fluid which

DeAnn Cummings
Department of Family Medicine, St. Joseph's Hospital Health Center,
4104 Medical Center Drive, Fayetteville, NY 13066, USA
email: dcummin6@twcny.rr.com

S.M. Sulik and C.B. Heath (eds.), *Primary Care Procedures in Women's Health*,
DOI 10.1007/978-0-387-76604-1_7, © Springer Science+Business Media, LLC 2010

is later spun in the lab to remove excess material. With the SurePath™ method, the brush is detached and sent in the specimen container along with the sample. One meta-analysis found that liquid-based technology is as good or even better than a conventional Pap smear for detection of high-grade disease [3]. The United States Preventive Services Task Force found that liquid-based cytology is cost-effective only if used every 3 years [1]. However, another benefit of liquid-based cytology is the ability to obtain reflex HPV DNA testing from the same Pap test. Comparison between the two methods of liquid-based cytology shows that SurePath™ may have a higher specimen adequacy rate (therefore decreasing the number of unsatisfactory Pap smear results) [4]. Other studies have shown that the SurePath™ system may handle adverse limiting factors such as blood better than the ThinPrep® system [5].

A combination of Pap smear and speculoscopy is also available and approved by the FDA (PapSure®, Watson Diagnostics, Corona, CA). This involves using a chemiluminescent light to examine the cervix after application of acetic acid. A limited number of studies have shown improved sensitivity compared to Pap alone [6, 7].

New guidelines for the interpretation of the Pap smear results have been published and provide different options for following minor cytologic changes in younger women (<age 21), and postmenopausal and pregnant women [8]. New recommendations for management after colposcopy can be found in Chap. 22 on Colposcopy.

Case Study

A healthy 32-year-old G2P2 presents for her yearly physical exam. She has had consistent annual Pap smears over the past 10 years with no history of an abnormal result. She has had only one sexual partner.

Diagnosis (Algorithms 7-1, 7-2)

Normal exam

Differential Diagnosis (Algorithms 7-1, 7-2)

- Cervical dysplasia
- Human papilloma virus

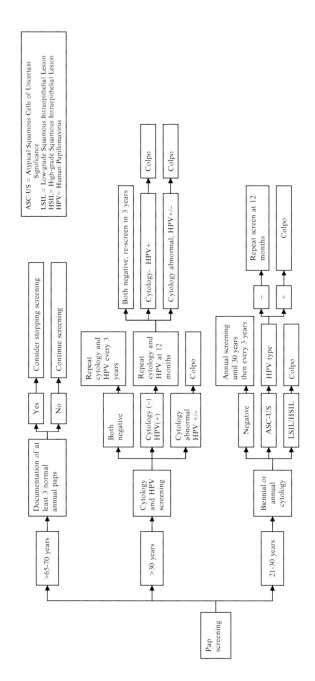

Algorithm 7-1 Algorithm for interpretation of Pap smear

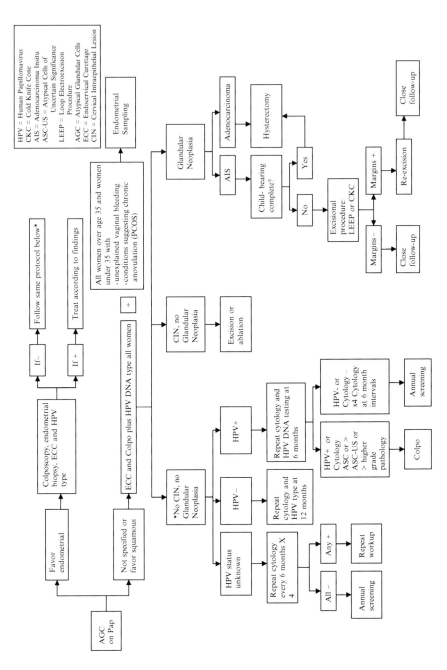

Algorithm 7-2 Algorithm for Atypical Glandular Cells (AGC)

Indications [1,2,9] (Algorithms 7-1, 7-2)

- Adolescents: Recommendations from the American College of Obstetricians and Gynecologists (ACOG) and from the American Cancer Society (ACS) state that screening should begin at age 21.
- Adult women 64 years of age or less: All guidelines recommend regular screening for cervical cancer. There is some debate about what interval is best:
  - ACOG
    (a) Biennial screening for all women <30
    (b) Women >30 who have had three recent, consecutive, normal Paps may be screened every 3 years
    (c) Alternative option: screen every 3 years with Pap + HPV test
  - ACS
    (a) For women <30, screen every year with conventional Pap or every 2 years with liquid-based cytology
    (b) Women >30 can be screened every 2–3 years
  - US Preventive Services Task Force (USPSTF)
    (a) No direct evidence that screening more often than every 3 years adds any additional benefit
- Women aged 65 or older:
  - ACOG: Must take into consideration a woman's past screening history, consecutive Pap smears, and risks for cervical cancer in making a decision to stop screening.
  - ACS: Discontinue screening after age 70.
  - USPSTF: No screening after age 65 if patient is at low risk for cervical cancer and has had recent adequate Pap screening. (D Recommendation – harms outweigh benefits)
- Women with history of total hysterectomy for benign disease:
  - ACOG: No screening unless history of CIN 2, CIN 3, or cancer. With history of CIN 2 or 3, get three normal yearly Paps, then stop.
  - USPSTF: Recommends against routine screening. (D Recommendation)

Contraindications

Uncooperative patient

Equipment (Fig. 7-1)

- Exam table equipped to place patient in lithotomy position
- Vaginal speculum (metal or plastic)

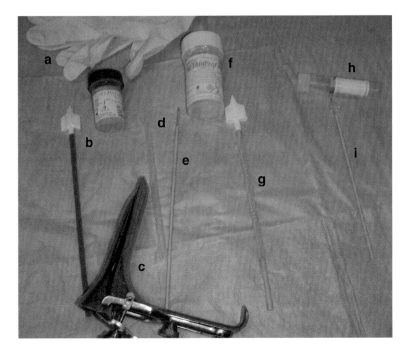

Fig. 7-1 Equipment set-up with Pap smear tools: (a) gloves; (b) SurePath™ [TriPath, Burlington, NC] Pap jar with detachable broom; (c) Graves speculum; (d) spatula; (e) endocervical brush; (f) ThinPrep® [Hologic, Bedford, MA] Pap jar with cervical broom; (g) cervical broom; (h) HPV specimen container; (i) HPV collection brush

- Light source
- Non-sterile gloves
- Large cotton swabs
- Pap broom (Cytobroom) or extended tip spatula plus endocervical brush
- Liquid transport medium or conventional Pap smear slide plus fixative
- HPV collection kit

Procedure

1. Place patient in dorsal lithotomy position.
2. Insert speculum to visualize entire transformation zone.
3. If STD testing indicated, perform after Pap smear.
4. Look for warts, lesions, erosions, or leukoplakia on the cervix.
5. Obtain Pap smear either with broom device or spatula plus endocervical brush:
   - Must obtain sample from both endocervix and ectocervix.
   - If using broom, rotate 360 degrees making sure that the long bristles in the center extend into the cervical os and rotate at least three times.
     - If using the spatula, take an ectocervical sample first by rotating the spatula around the ectocervix. Then insert the endocervical brush rotate 360 degrees.

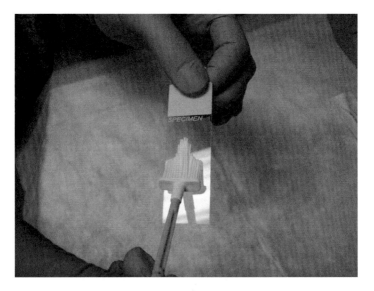

Fig. 7-2 Conventional Pap smear collection onto glass slide

6. Avoid using a swab on the cervix prior to Pap unless there is a large amount of blood or discharge.
7. For conventional Pap, smear specimen onto a prelabeled slide and apply fixative immediately. Both ectocervical and endocervical samples can go on the same slide (Fig. 7-2).
8. For liquid-based cytology, place collection device in liquid transport medium and vigorously twirl the device in the liquid (Fig. 7-3).
9. HPV testing can be done with the liquid transport medium, or a separate testing brush can be used. For the latter, insert the brush 2/3 of the way into the cervical os so that part of the brush is on the ectocervix and part is in the endocervix and rotate 360 degrees. Place brush into transportation device and break off the stem.
10. Upon removal of the speculum, observe the vaginal walls and vulva for any lesions.

Complications and Risks

False positive result with unnecessary additional tests.

Tricks and Helpful Hints

- Difficult to visualize cervix:
  - Move patient down on table so that her pelvis is just at the edge.
  - Have patient press down on her lower abdomen to raise cervix into view.

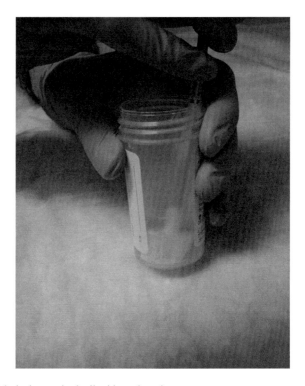

Fig. 7-3 Swish the broom in the liquid cytology jar

- – Try larger or longer speculum.
- – If using plastic speculum, try metal speculum.
- – If vaginal wall blocks view, try placing a condom with a small hole in the end over the blades of the speculum.
- Stenotic cervical os:
  - – Have patient use estrogen cream intravaginally for 3 weeks prior to Pap smear.
  - – Use endocervical brush.
- No endocervical cells on previous Paps: Use endocervical brush.
- Excessive cervical discharge or bleeding:
- Use large cotton swab in this instance to clear away exudate or blood.
- Consider using liquid-based cytology.
- If using conventional Pap slide, consider having the patient return for Pap at a later date.

Interpretation of Results [8,10] (Algorithms 7-1, 7-2)

- Unsatisfactory: Pap must be repeated.
- ASC-US (atypical squamous cells of undetermined significance). 5–17% will be diagnosed with CIN 2 or greater.
  - Option 1 – Reflex HPV typing (*preferred*)
    - (a) If HPV+, refer for colposcopy.
    - (b) If HPV−, repeat Pap in 1 year.
  - Option 2 – Repeat Pap at 6 and 12 months
    - (a) If either Pap abnormal, refer for colposcopy.
    - (b) If both Paps normal, return to routine screening.
    - (c) Consider using intravaginal estrogen cream in postmenopausal women with signs of atrophy.
  - Option 3 – Immediate colposcopy
    - (a) If no CIN identified, repeat Pap 1 year.
    - (b) Preferred option for immunosuppressed women
- For women under age 21, if screening has been done:
  Follow-up with annual Pap is recommended.
  - If repeat Pap is HSIL, refer for colposcopy.
  - At the 24-month follow-up if Pap is ASC-US or greater, refer for colposcopy.
- HPV testing is unacceptable in adolescents and if done should not influence decision making.
- For pregnant women:
  - Acceptable to defer colposcopy until 6 weeks postpartum.
- ASC-H (atypical squamous cells, cannot rule out high-grade disease). 24–94% will be diagnosed with CIN 2 or greater.
  - Refer for colposcopy, if no lesion identified ECC preferred.
    - (a) If no CIN identified, either repeat Pap at 6 and 12 months or do HPV test in 1 year.
    - (b) Repeat colposcopy for any positive result.
- AGC-NOS (atypical glandular cells, not otherwise specified). 9–38% will be diagnosed with CIN 2, AIS, or greater. 3–17% will have invasive cancer.
  - Refer for colposcopy with endocervical sampling and HPV sampling.
  - If atypical endometrial cells on Pap, perform endometrial biopsy first.
  - Do colposcopy and endometrial biopsy in women greater than 35 and in women with unexplained vaginal bleeding.
  - If all tests negative for neoplasia, repeat Pap and HPV test every 6 months until four consecutive, negative Paps; if initial HPV test is positive, repeat Pap and HPV test at 12 months if initial HPV test is negative. Close follow-up for 24 months is recommended.

- AGC-favor neoplasia or AIS (adenocarcinoma-in-situ). 27–96% will be diagnosed with CIN 2 or greater.
  - Refer all patients for colposcopy with endocervical sampling.
  - Endometrial biopsy if indicated. (See previous discussion in this section.)
  - If testing negative for neoplasia, refer for diagnostic excisional procedure.
  - Following with repeat Pap smears is unacceptable.
- LSIL (low-grade intraepithelial lesion). 12–16% will be diagnosed with CIN 2 or greater.
  - Option 1 – Colposcopy with endocervical sampling
    - (a) If colposcopy negative, either repeat Paps at 6 and 12 months or do HPV test at 12 months (preferred).
    - (b) If colposcopy positive, treat as appropriate.
  - Option 2
    - (a) Adolescent women, if screening performed: Repeat Pap in 12 months recommended.
      - * If Pap is HSIL, refer for colposcopy; if LSIL or less, repeat Pap in 12 months.
      - * At 24 months, if Pap remains LSIL or greater, refer for colposcopy.
    - (a) Postmenopausal women:
      - * Option 1 – Reflex HPV type the Pap sample; if positive, refer for colposcopy.
      - * Option 2 – Repeat Paps at 6 and 12 months.
      - * Option 3 – Colposcopy
    - (a) Pregnant women:
      - * Option 1 – Colposcopy is *preferred* in non-adolescent women.
      - * Option 2 – Defer colposcopy until 6 weeks postpartum acceptable.
- HSIL (high-grade intraepithelial lesion). 70–75% will be diagnosed with CIN 2 or greater.
  - Refer all patients for colposcopy and endocervical sampling.
    - (a) If colposcopy negative for CIN 2 or 3, diagnostic excisional procedure is preferred.
    - (b) In adolescent women, colposcopy and cytology every 6 months for 24 months is *preferred*.
- Combination screening: HPV+, cytology normal. 4% will have CIN 2 or greater.
  - Repeat Pap and HPV test at 12 months.
  - Refer for colposcopy if any repeat test is positive.
- Endometrial cells
  - If premenopausal, no further action is required.
  - If postmenopausal, do endometrial biopsy.

Procedure Note

(Provider to fill-in blanks/circle applicable choice when given multiple choices and customize as needed.)

> *The patient was placed in the dorsal lithotomy position and a speculum was inserted. The cervix was well visualized. Pap smear was obtained using _____ (insert collection device) and _____*
> *(insert either conventional Pap processing or liquid based cytology). No cervical, vaginal, or vulvar lesions were seen.*

Coding

Pap and Physical

CPT® Codes (Current Procedural Terminology, AMA, Chicago, IL)
99395 (age 18–39), 99396 (age 40–64), 99397 (age 65 or greater)
Medicare Pap and Pelvic Codes
G0101 and Q0091

ICD 9-CM-Diagnostic Codes (International Classification of Diseases, 9th Revision, Clinical Modification, Center for Disease Control and Prevention)
V76.47 for any Pap done

Postprocedure Patient Instructions

Instruct the patient that her Pap results will be mailed to or called into her. Reassure her that spotting can be normal after a Pap smear.

Case Study Outcome

The patient is at low risk for cervical cancer and has a history of consistent Pap smears. She may decrease her Pap frequency to every 2–3 years. Either conventional Pap or liquid-based cytology is appropriate. She may consider the combination of HPV testing and cervical cytology, with Pap no more often than every 3 years.

Patient Handout

(Provider to customize as needed.)

What is a Pap smear?
- It is a test in which cells are taken from the cervix and examined under a microscope to look for signs of cancer or precancer.

How is the Pap smear done?
- An instrument called a speculum is inserted into the vagina in order to see the cervix. A brush is then rotated over the cervix to collect a sample.

How often do I need to have a Pap smear?
- If you are less than 30, you should have a Pap smear every other year.
- If you are over 30 and have had regular Pap smears, you may be able to get Paps every 3 years, depending on your risk factors for cancer.

When should I start getting Pap smears?
- Women should begin getting Pap smears at age 21.

When can I stop getting Pap smears?
- If you have had regular Pap smears and are not at high risk for cervical cancer, you can stop Pap smears after age 65.

What are the risk factors for cervical cancer?
- Almost all cervical cancer is caused by the HPV virus, which is sexually transmitted.
- Risk factors include multiple sexual partners, early age of first sexual intercourse, personal history of HPV infection, partner with HPV infection, previous abnormal Pap smear, illnesses that suppress the immune system, and smoking.

If I have had a hysterectomy, do I still need to get Pap smears?
- You do not need to get Pap smears unless you have a history of cervical cancer.

What is HPV?
- HPV stands for Human Papilloma Virus. It is the virus that causes genital warts. Certain types can also cause precancer and cancer of the cervix. HPV is transferred from person to person through sex.

What can I do to keep from getting HPV?
- Practice safe sex.
- There is now a vaccine for HPV approved for girls and young women between ages 9–26 that protects against the most common types of the virus that cause cancer.

Should I be tested for HPV?
- Your doctor may recommend HPV testing as part of a screening program.
- A test for HPV is also often done to monitor abnormal Pap smears.

Is there a treatment for HPV?
- There is no medicine that will get rid of the virus. Most of the time your body's immune system will fight off the virus over time. If there are severe changes in the cells on your Pap smear, the abnormal cells can be surgically removed or frozen.

What can I expect after a Pap smear?
- Some women have a small amount of spotting after a Pap smear; consider wearing a sanitary pad for the next 24 h.
- Expect either a phone call or a letter from your provider describing the results of your Pap smear, and when you should return to the office for your next Pap.

References

1. United States Preventive Services Task Force. Screening for cervical cancer.
2. Amer College of Obstetricians and Gynecologists. *Cervical cytology screening. Practice Bulletin 45.* Washington, DC:ACOG, 2003.
3. Bernstein SJ, Sanchez-Ramos L, Ndubisi B. Liquid-based cervical cytologic smear study and conventional Papsnicolaou smears: a metaanalysis of prospective studies comparing cytologic diagnosis and sample adequacy. *Am J Obstet Gynecol* 2001;185:308–317.
4. Nance KV. Evolution of pap testing at a community hospital – a ten year experience. *Diagn Cytopathol* 2007;35:148–153.
5. Sweeny BJ, Haq Z, Happel JF, Weinstein B, Schneider D. Comparison of the effectiveness of two liquid based papanicoleau systems in the handling of adverse limiting factors, such as excessive blood. *Cancer* 2006;108(1):27–31.
6. Twu NF, Chen YJ, Want PH, Yu BKJ, Lai CR, Chao KC, Yuan CC, Yen MS. Improved cervical cancer screening in premenopausal women by combination of Pap smear and speculoscopy. *Eur J Obstet Gynecol Reprod Biol* 2007;133(1):114–118.
7. Loiudice I, Abbiati R, Boselli F, Cecchini G, Costa S, Grossi E, Piccoli R, Villani C. Improvement of Pap smear sensitivity using a visual adjunctive procedure: a cooperative Italian study on speculoscopy (GISPE). *Eur J Cancer Prev* 1998;7(4):295–304.
8. Wright TC, Massad L, Dunton C, Spitzer M, Wilkinson E, Solomon D. 2006 Consensus guidelines for the management of women with abnormal cerical cancer screening tests. *Am J Obstet Gynecol* 2007;197(4):346–355.
9. Amer College of Obstetricians and Gynecologists. Cervical Cytology Screening. Practice Bulletin 109. Washington, DC: ACOG, December 2009.
10. Wright TC, Cox JT, Massad LS. 2001 Consensus guidelines for the management of women with cervical cytological abnormalities. *JAMA* 2002;287:2120–2129.

Additional Resources

Articles

Solomon D, Davey D, Kurman R. The 2001 Bethesda System terminology for reporting results of cervical cytology. *JAMA* 2002;287:2114–2119.

Web Sites

www.ahrq.gov.
www.asccp.org.

Chapter 8
Vaginal Discharge

Barbara Jo McGarry

Introduction

The complaint of vaginal discharge is very common in primary care settings. Symptoms include discharge with or without odor, which may be accompanied by dysuria, vulvar, and/or vaginal itching or burning. A careful history that includes inquiry about new or multiple sexual partners, type of birth control, sexually transmitted infection prevention measures, current health status, medications used, and vaginal preparations used will help with the diagnosis. The practitioner must evaluate the vaginal mucosa with a speculum exam and obtain a sample of the vaginal discharge. In addition, it is important to determine whether the woman may have an upper tract infection by performing a bimanual examination. The discharge should be evaluated by doing a pH test, a whiff test, and saline and potassium hydroxide (KOH) wet mount slides viewed under the microscope. There are several commercial kits available that help to identify the most common causes of vaginal discharge; examples of these include Affirm® (Becton, Dickinson, & Co, Franklin Lakes, NJ) and FemExam® (Cooper Surgical, Trumbull, CT).

The most common pathological causes of vaginal discharge are Vulvovaginal Candidiasis (VVC), Bacterial Vaginosis (BV), and Trichomoniasis. VVC and BV are not sexually transmitted. Trichomonas vaginitis is a sexually transmitted protozoan organism. The vaginal discharge associated with VVC is classically thick, white, and of a cottage cheese consistency. The vaginal mucosa is generally erythematous [1]. In bacterial vaginosis, the hallmark complaint is discharge with a fishy odor. The discharge is generally thin and white-gray, and the vaginal mucosa is either normal or may be mildly inflamed. The discharge associated with trichomonas is frothy and cream-colored to greenish. A foul odor is also

B.J. McGarry
Department of Family Medicine, Robert Wood Johnson Medical School,
University of Medicine and Dentistry of New Jersey, 1 Robert Wood Johnson Place, MEB 278,
New Brunswick, NJ 08903, USA
e-mail: mcgarrbj@umdnj.edu

S.M. Sulik and C.B. Heath (eds.), *Primary Care Procedures in Women's Health*,
DOI 10.1007/978-0-387-76604-1_8, © Springer Science+Business Media, LLC 2010

associated with the discharge of trichomoniasis. Generally, patients complain of inflammatory symptoms of itching and burning. The vaginal mucosa and cervix can be quite erythematous. Minute punctuate hemorrhages on the cervix ("strawberry cervix") (Fig. 8-1) may be present in 10% of women diagnosed with trichomoniasis [2].

Diagnosis of BV is done using Amsel's Criteria. Three of the following four criteria are required to make a diagnosis: a thin nonclumping, homogeneous gray-white discharge, a vaginal pH greater than 4.5, more than 20% of cells are clue cells (Fig. 8-2) that are present on a saline wet mount (most reliable single indicator of BV), and a positive whiff test (presence of amine odor with addition of KOH to the discharge) [3].

Microscopic examination of the discharge associated with VVC (Fig. 8-3) will show hyphae and buds when discharge is combined with 10% KOH solution. In trichomoniasis (Fig. 8-4), saline wet mount will show the motile pear-shaped organisms. See Fig. 8-5 for microscopic examination of normal discharge.

There are several commercial kits available to assist in the diagnosis of vaginitis. The BD Affirm™ VPIII Microbial Identification Test (Becton, Dickinson, & Co, Franklin Lakes, NJ) is a DNA probe test intended for use in the detection and identification of *Candida* species, *Gardnerella vaginalis*, and *Trichomonas vaginalis* nucleic acid in vaginal fluid specimens from patients with symptoms of vaginitis/vaginosis. A speculum exam without water or lubricant should be performed to obtain the sample of vaginal fluid from the posterior vagina and the lateral walls of the vagina. The sample is then processed in the office if the equipment is purchased or alternatively sent to the lab for testing. This test has a sensitivity of >83% and a specificity of >97% [4]. The FemExam® pH and Amines TestCard™

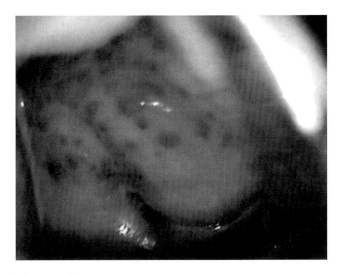

Fig. 8-1 Strawberry cervix

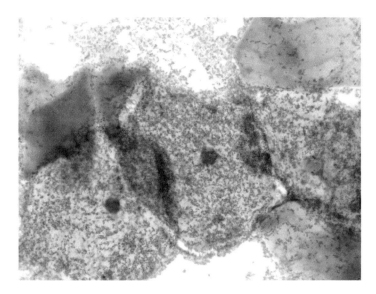

Fig. 8-2 Clue cells on vaginal smear on a gram stain specimen. These cells appear clear on a non-stained specimen

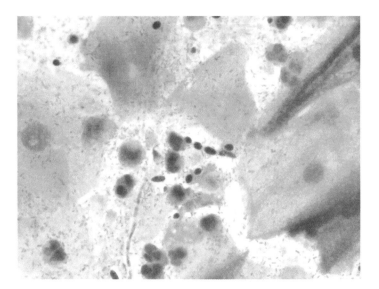

Fig. 8-3 Budding yeast and hyphae on a gram stained specimen

(Cooper Surgical, Trumbull, CT) is also an in-office test that shows the presence of elevated vaginal fluid pH (pH > 4.7) and detects the presence of amines. A swab containing unprocessed vaginal fluid is rubbed across the test area and the test results are ready in 2 min. The test has a sensitivity of 90% and a specificity of 97% [5]. This test is particularly useful for making the diagnosis of bacterial vaginosis.

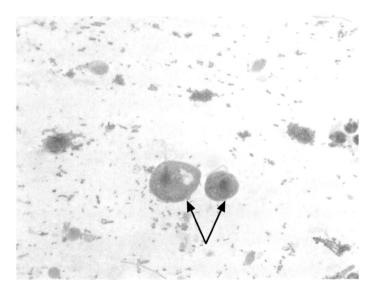

Fig. 8-4 Trichomonads on vaginal smear on a gram stained specimen

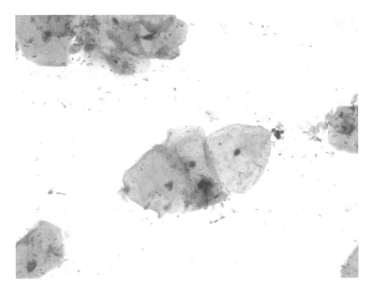

Fig. 8-5 Gram stain of normal vaginal discharge

Treatment regimens vary for the different causes of vaginitis. In general, preferred treatment for BV is with a 7-day regimen of metronidazole either orally or
intravaginally. The 2 g single-dose therapy has the lowest treatment success and
is no longer considered appropriate [6]. Conversely, trichomoniasis responds well

to single dose therapy. It is recommended that both sexual partners be treated simultaneously when trichomonas has been diagnosed [7]. Clindamycin, used as an alternative treatment for BV, has an efficacy of 94% cure rate in a single randomized trial (compared to metronidazole 500 mg orally twice daily for 7 days, which had 96% cure rate) [8]. Oral and intravaginal antifungals have similar cure rates; short-course therapy for VVC will cure 80–90% of women who complete the regimen. Non-albicans strains are more challenging, with no known preferred treatment. Both boric acid suppositories and flucytosine vaginal cream have been studied and show varied efficacy, with better response to flucytosine vaginal cream for *Candida glabrata* [9].

Case Studies

Case A

A 32-year-old G3P3 who comes in complaining of a 2-week history of foul-smelling vaginal discharge. She describes the discharge as whitish and profuse. She feels the need to wear a panty liner at times. She denies having any vaginal sores or bumps. She does not find her vagina to be particularly itchy or sore. She emphatically insists that her only sexual partner is her husband of 12 years. She is otherwise well and has no chronic medical problems and does not take any medications. Her LMP was 2 weeks ago and was normal. She denies any other associated symptoms.

Case B

A 29-year-old woman complaining of multiple episodes of vaginal discharge and itching. She has used multiple over-the-counter preparations to try and help her symptoms. She has found these products moderately helpful in the past, but this time she feels that the usual creams are not helping. She describes the discharge as thick and white. She finds her vaginal area to be very itchy. She has had two sexual partners in the past year, but insists that she always uses condoms for protection. She denies any other associated symptoms.

Case C

This is an 18-year-old woman who comes in for an emergency visit to your office for an itchy vaginal discharge that began 4 days ago. She works as a swimsuit model and is very concerned about "this smelly, constant discharge." She also complains of itching and burning in her vaginal area. She is healthy and is on no medications. She has had several sexual partners in the past year. She denies any other associated symptoms.

Diagnosis (Algorithm 8-1)

Vaginal Discharge

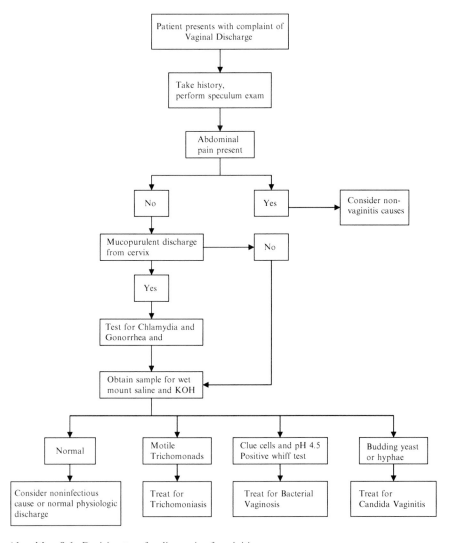

Algorithm 8-1 Decision tree for diagnosis of vaginitis

Differential Diagnosis (Algorithm 8-1)

- Vulvovaginal Candidiasis
- Bacterial Vaginosis
- Trichomoniasis
- Gonorrheal Cervicitis
- Chlamydial Cervicitis
- Noninfectious Causes of Vaginitis:
  - Atrophic vaginitis
  - Irritant/chemical vaginitis
  - Normal Physiologic Discharge

Indications (Algorithm 8-1)

- Vaginal Discharge
- Vaginal Irritation
- Vaginal Odor

Contraindications

None

May need to use very sensitive exam techniques in virginal females and post-menopausal females. Consider avoiding the speculum exam if it is not tolerated, and do vaginal swab.

Equipment (Fig. 8-6)

- Vaginal speculum
- Nonsterile gloves
- Cotton swab applicators
- Test Tube with saline
- Microscope with 10× and 40× magnification
- 10% KOH solution
- Microscope Glass Slides and cover slips
- Nitrazine paper – narrow range PH paper
- Gonorrhea and chlamydia antigen culture tubes
- Commercial Kits (optional):
  - BD Affirm™ VPIII Microbial Identification Test
  - The FemExam® pH and Amines TestCard™.

Fig. 8-6 Nonsterile equipment set-up for vaginal discharge: (a) ph paper (pHydrion™ Papers, Micro Essential Labs, Brooklyn, NY); (b) FemExam® (Cooper Surgical, Trumbull, CT) specimen card with swab; (c) Affirm® (Becton, Dickinson, & Co, Franklin Lakes, NJ) specimen collection container, KOH, swab; (d) Gonorrhea/Chlamydia collection container with swabs; (e) saline and KOH for microscopic evaluations with glass slides; (f) gloves

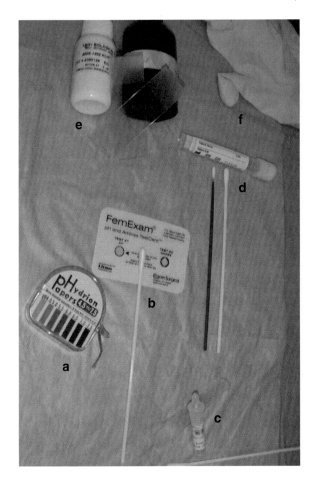

Procedure (Algorithm 8-1)

1. Place the patient in the dorsal lithotomy position after noting any abdominal or pelvic tenderness on abdominal examination.
2. Carefully note any irritation of the labia. Note any discharge, smell, open sores, or masses.
3. Insert speculum into vagina.
4. Note quality, color, character of discharge. Also note erythema or open sores in vagina or on cervix. Note whether the discharge is primarily coming from the cervical os or whether it is diffusely in the vagina.
5. Use cotton swab to take sample of discharge from lateral vaginal walls. Consider whether it is useful to do a chlamydia and gonorrhea culture. If the discharge is

primarily coming from the os, and if the patient has had unprotected intercourse, consider doing a culture.

6. Place cotton swab into test tube that contains a few drops of saline solution. Cap the test tube.
7. Use cotton swab to take another sample of discharge from lateral vaginal walls, and then use nitrazine paper to determine pH of discharge sample. Normal vaginal pH is 3.8–4.5. Bacterial Vaginosis (BV), trichomoniasis, and atrophic vaginitis often increase the vaginal pH above 4.5. Remove speculum and perform a bimanual pelvic exam. If there are symptoms of pain, reinsert speculum and obtain a gonorrhea and chlamydia culture if not already obtained.
8. Take test tube to your office laboratory while your patient is changing.
9. Perform the whiff test. Add several drops of potassium hydroxide (KOH) to a sample of the vaginal discharge. A strong fishy odor from the mixture suggests Bacterial Vaginosis or Trichomonas vaginalis.
10. Make the KOH slide by placing a sample of the vaginal discharge on the slide and mix with a few drops of the 10% KOH solution. The KOH destroys bacteria and cells from the vagina, leaving yeast hyphae and spores (if present) that indicate a yeast infection.
11. Make the wet mount slide by placing a sample of the vaginal discharge on a slide and mix with saline solution. The prepared slide is then examined under a microscope for bacteria, yeast cells, trichomonads, white blood cells that indicate an infection, or clue cells that indicate Bacterial Vaginosis (BV). These are best seen by 40× magnification.

Complications and Risks

- Pain and tenderness during exam
- Extreme anxiety (consider whether patient has been victimized)

Tricks and Helpful Hints

- Women with some forms of vaginal discharge, especially candida vaginitis, may actually have very little lubrication. Consider using extra time when inserting the speculum.
- Many women have more than one Sexually Transmitted Infection (STI) at the same time. Consider doing cultures on those who are at risk for STIs.
- Women with trichomoniasis should be instructed to avoid intercourse with sex partner until partner is treated.
- Women should be counseled to avoid alcohol when taking metronidazole.

- Clindamycin vaginal cream is oil-based and can weaken latex condoms or diaphragms during use of the cream and for 5 days after use.
- VVC is usually not sexually transmitted; therefore, male partners do not need treatment.
- All vaginal creams/suppositories used for VVC can weaken latex condoms and diaphragms.

Interpretation of Results

See Algorithm 8-1 for decision tree for diagnosis of vaginitis.

Procedure Note

(Provider to fill in blanks/circle applicable choice when given multiple choices and customize as needed.)

> *On speculum examination of the vagina and cervix, samples of vaginal discharge were obtained with cotton tipped applicators. The whiff test was performed. The sample was examined with KOH slide and with a saline wet mount preparation. Microscopy revealed clue cells, trichomonads, or yeast and hyphae. Nitrazine paper revealed the pH to be ___.*

Coding

CPT® Codes (Current Procedural Terminology, AMA, Chicago, IL)

87210	Smear, primary source with interpretation; wet mount for infectious agents
58999	KOH and Wet Smear

Medicare Codes

Q0111	(HCPCS code) Wet mounts, including preparations of vaginal, cervical or skin specimens for saline slide
Q0112	For the slide with KOH

ICD 9-CM-Diagnostic Codes (International Classification of Diseases, 9th Revision, Clinical Modification, Center for Disease Control and Prevention)

616.10	Vaginitis NOS
112.1	Candidal vaginitis
616.10	Bacterial vaginosis
131.01	Trichomonas vaginitis
627.3	Atrophic vaginitis
623.5	Vaginal discharge
625.9	Vulvar pain
625.9	Vaginal pain

Postprocedure Patient Instructions

Patient should be instructed to call if symptoms persist after treatment. The following treatments may be prescribed:

- Trichomoniasis:
    - 2 g metronidazole orally (po) at once or tindazole (Tindamax) 2 g po ×1 dose.
    - For persistent trichomonas disease: Metronidazole 500 mg po twice daily (BID) ×7 days.

- Bacterial Vaginosis:
  - Metronidazole 500 mg PO BID for 7 days; Efficacy 86% at 5–7 days; 78% at 4 weeks.
  - Metronidazole 0.75% gel 5 g vaginally BID for 5 days; Efficacy 81% at 5–7 days; 71% at 4 weeks.
  - Clindamycin 2% cream 5 g vaginally nightly for 7 days; Efficacy 85% at 5–7 days; 82% at 4 weeks.
  - Alternative regimens:
    (a) Clindamycin 300 mg PO BID for 7 days.
    (b) Clindamycin 100 mg ovules inserted into the vagina nightly ×3 days.
- Candida: Fluconazole (Diflucan) 150 mg po ×1 dose
  - Alternative oral regimens:
    (a) Itraconazole 200 mg PO BID for 1 day
    (b) Ketoconazole 200 mg PO BID for 5 days [6]
  - Intravaginal regimens:
    (a) Butoconazole 2% cream – 5 g as a single dose
    (b) Clotrimazole 1% cream – 5 g intravaginally nightly ×7–14 days
    (c) Clotrimazole 100 mg vaginal tablet – 1 tablet nightly ×7 days or 2 tablets nightly ×3 days
    (d) Miconazole 2% vaginal cream – 5 g nightly ×7 days or 100 mg vaginal suppository nightly ×7 days or 200 mg suppository nightly ×3 days or 1,200 mg suppository ×1 night
    (e) Nystatin 100,000 unit vaginal tablet nightly ×14 days
    (f) Tioconazole 6.5% ointment – 5 g intravaginally in a single dose
    (g) Terconazole 0.4% cream – 5 g intravaginally nightly ×7 days or 0.8% cream 5 g intravaginally nightly ×3 days or 80 mg vaginal suppository for 3 days
- Non-albicans Candida species:
  - Optimal treatment regimen is unknown.
  - Topical or oral treatment with a nonfluconazole azole drug for 7–14 days.
  - May respond to boric acid 600 mg intravaginally daily for 14 days
  - Alternative treatment: topical flucytosine cream 5 g intravaginally nightly ×14 days

Case Study Outcome

Case A

The nitrazine paper showed a pH of 5.0. The KOH slide did not show any buds or hyphae. The whiff test released a strong fishy odor. The saline wet mount showed many clue cells. The diagnosis of Bacterial Vaginosis was made, and the patient was treated with metronidazole 500 mg PO twice daily for 7 days. She was advised to abstain from alcohol during the time of treatment to avoid nausea, vomiting, and abdominal pain.

Case B

The nitrazine paper showed a pH of 3.5. The KOH slide showed many buds and hyphae. The whiff test did not produce any strong odors. The saline wet mount showed some white blood cells, but no clue cells. The diagnosis of Candida Vaginitis was made, and the patient was treated with Diflucan 150 mg orally one time.

Case C

The nitrazine paper showed a pH of 5.4. The KOH slide did not show any buds or hyphae. The whiff test did not produce any strong odors. The saline wet mount showed many motile pear-shaped organisms. The diagnosis was trichomoniasis, and the patient was treated with 2 g of metronidazole orally at once. She was advised that trichomoniasis is a sexually transmitted infection, and so her sexual partner should be treated at the same time. She was advised to abstain from alcohol during the time of treatment to avoid nausea, vomiting, and abdominal pain.

Postprocedure Patient Handout

(Provider to customize as needed.)

Candida

You have an infection of *Candida albicans*, commonly known as yeast. Yeast is *not* a sexually transmitted infection (STI); you did *not* catch it from anyone, and your partner does not need to be treated. It is caused by a change in the pH of the vagina, which is usually acidic and keeps yeast from growing. A variety of antibiotics, diabetes, pregnancy, and your menstrual period may change the pH and make it more likely for yeast to grow. In addition, there are some preventable measures that may help in avoiding another infection. Wearing cotton underwear, wiping front to back after urination, and avoiding douching may help. The medications are safe to use while pregnant and nursing.

Occasionally, women have chronic yeast infections. If you have not improved after the course of medication given to you, please return to your clinician.

Bacterial Vaginosis

You have Bacterial Vaginosis, also known as Gardnerella Vaginitis. It is the most common vaginal infection. It is caused by an overgrowth of the anaerobic bacteria that are commonly present in the vagina. BV is *not* a STI; you did *not* catch it from anyone, and your partner does not need to be treated. The infection can cause a thin vaginal discharge and sometimes a distinct fishy odor. It can be treated with oral pills or vaginal creams or gels. While it is safe to take the medication in pregnancy, there is less information about using the medication while nursing. If you are nursing, please discuss with your clinician.

If you are taking metronidazole by mouth, be sure not to drink alcohol while on the medication and for 24 h after you take the last dose of medication. If you are using the clindamycin vaginal cream or ovules, be aware that the cream may cause condoms to break. Use another form of birth control while on the cream and for 3 days afterward.

Some women may experience a yeast infection at the same time or after the treatment of bacterial vaginosis. If so, you may need treatment with an antifungal medication after the treatment of the BV. If you have any questions, please call your clinician.

Trichomonas vaginalis

You have an infection of *T. vaginalis* ("trich" or "tric"). Trich is a protozoal organism that is sexually transmitted. Trich causes a thin, watery yellow-greenish discharge that can have fishy odor. It can cause itching of the vagina and vulva ("lips") and burning during urination. It can also be present with very few symptoms for a very long time.

You and your partner should be treated for Trich at the same time to avoid passing the infection back to each other. It is important to avoid drinking alcohol while you are on the medication and for 24 hours afterward. Trich infections can be avoided by having your partner use condoms. Treatment is safe in pregnancy. Please let your clinician know if you are nursing.

Trich can be present with other vaginal infections and other STIs. Please make an appointment with your clinician to discuss screening for other STIs if you have not done so during your visit today or if other symptoms occur after treatment.

References

1. Anderson MR, Klink K, Cohrssen A. Evaluation of vaginal complaints. *JAMA* 2004;291(11):1368–1379.
2. Wölner-Hanssen P, Krieger J. Clinical manifestations of vaginal trichomoniasis. *JAMA* 1989;261:571–576
3. Amsel R. Totten PA, Spiegel CA, Chen KC, Eschenbach D, Holmes KK. Nonspecific vaginitis: diagnostic criteria and microbial and epidemiologic associations. *Am J Med* 1983;74:14.
4. Brown HL, Fuller DD, Jasper LT, Davis TE, Wright JD. Evaluation of the affirm VPIII test in the detection and identification of trichomonas vaginalis, Gardnerella vaginalis, and Candida species in vaginitis/vaginosis. *Infect Dis Obstet Gynecol* 2004;12(1):17–21.
5. West B, Morison L, Schim van der Loeff M, Gooding E, Awasana AA, Demba E, Mayaud P. Evaluation of a new rapid diagnostic kit (FemExam) for bacterial vaginosis in patients with vaginal discharge syndrome in The Gambia. *Sex Transm Dis* 2003;30(6):483–489.
6. Bacterial vaginosis. In Handbook of antimicrobial therapy. New Rochelle: The Medical Letter, 2005 edn, pp 201–203.
7. Trichomonas vaginalis infections. In Guidelines for the management of sexually transmitted infections. Geneva: WHO publication, 2003.
8. Kane KY, Pierce R. Clinical inquires: what is the most effective way to treat bacterial vaginosis in nonpregnant women? *J Fam Pract* 2001;50(5):399–400.
9. Sobel JD, Chaim W, Chaim W, Nagappan V, Leaman D. Treatment of vaginitis caused by candida glabrata: use of topical boric acid and flucytosine. *Am J Obstet Gynecol* 2003;189(5):1297–1300.

Chapter 9
Cervical Polyp Removal

Sandra M. Sulik

Introduction

Cervical polyps are pedunculated masses that vary in size from several millimeters to centimeters, are usually found in the endocervical canal, and protrude from the cervical os (Fig. 9-1). Occasionally, polyps protruding from the cervical os are endometrial in origin. Cervical polyps are often single, but they can be multiple. They are usually bright red, spongy in nature, and friable.

Most often asymptomatic, polyps are commonly found on the routine women's health exam. They can also be detected on colposcopy, seen as filling defects on hysterosalpingogram, and seen on abdominal and transvaginal ultrasound. Women with polyps can also present with intermenstrual spotting, postcoital bleeding, persistent leukorrhea, postmenopausal bleeding, or heavy menses. The cause of polyps is unknown, although they may be a secondary reaction to cervical inflammation or hormonal stimulation and are thus seen more often with increasing age, inflammation, trauma, and pregnancy. Cervical polyps are most frequently seen in peri- and postmenopausal women in the third through fifth decades of life. Symptomatic polyps tend to be more common in premenopausal women. More pathological conditions are also associated with symptomatic polyps and tend to occur more commonly in the postmenopausal age group. While malignant potential is rare, if symptomatic in the postmenopausal woman, Dilatation and Curettage (D&C) should be considered as part of the evaluation [1].

Several studies [2–4] have noted an association of endocervical polyps with endometrial polyps. One study showed that approximately 25% of women with endometrial polyps had cervical polyps. Combination oral contraceptives reduced the incidence of cervical polyps in this population from 2.5 to 8.3%. Postmenopausal women with polyps had a 56.8% incidence of cervix-related

S.M. Sulik (✉)
Department of Family Medicine, SUNY Upstate Medical Center, St. Joseph's Family Medicine Residency, Syracuse, NY 13203, USA
e-mail: smsulik@aol.com

S.M. Sulik and C.B. Heath (eds.), *Primary Care Procedures in Women's Health*,
DOI 10.1007/978-0-387-76604-1_9, © Springer Science+Business Media, LLC 2010

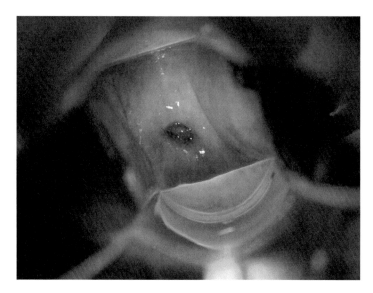

Fig. 9-1 Endocervical polyp

endometrial polyps [2]. Because of this association between endometrial and cervical polyps, some advocate that the removal of cervical polyps should be done with hysteroscopy, which would allow for the evaluation of the endometrial cavity. This would help clarify the initial diagnosis as well as allow for precise visualization of the polyp peduncle and treat concurrent asymptomatic intrauterine pathology [2].

Histologically, cervical polyps are composed of endocervical epithelium with a fibrovascular stalk. Most are benign, some will show squamous metaplasia or squamous dysplasia, and malignancy is very rare. All polyps should be sent to pathology for evaluation.

Case Study

A 45-year-old female presents to your office for her annual exam and Pap smear. Review of systems reveals regular menses, with occasional spotting after intercourse. No other spotting noted. On pelvic exam, a cervical polyp is found.

Diagnosis (Algorithm 9-1)

Cervical Polyp

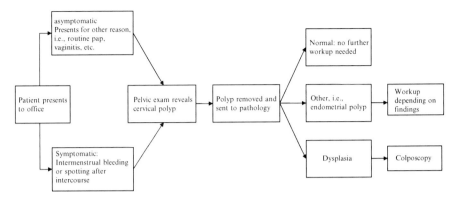

Algorithm 9-1 Decision tree for endometrial polyp removal

Differential Diagnosis (Algorithm 9-1)

- Cervical polyp
- Condyloma
- Nabothian cyst
- Prolapsed myoma
- Cervical malignancy
- Squamous papilloma
- Sarcoma
- Retained products of conception

Indications (Algorithm 9-1)

- Intermenstrual spotting or bleeding
- Spotting after intercourse
- Usually removed to prevent irritation, bleeding or discharge

Contraindications

- Pregnancy: delay removal until postpartum, unless significant bleeding exists
- Inability to see the base of the polyp
- Bleeding or coagulation disorder
- Uncooperative patient

Optional Additional Equipment (Fig. 9-2)

- Vaginal speculum
- Nonsterile gloves
- Long Kelly or ring forceps
- Topical anesthetic
- Formalin container

Optional Additional Equipment (Fig. 9-3)

- Endocervical curette (ECC) and/or endocervical brush
- Tischler biopsy forceps
- Colposcope
- Monsel's solution or Silver Nitrate sticks

Procedure

1. Insert speculum into the vagina and identify polyp.
2. Place long Kelly or ring forceps as close to the base of the polyp as possible and clamp. Some practitioners clean the cervix with betadine prior to removal of polyp. Can use topical anesthetic prior to removal as well.
3. Twist the polyp in one direction until it easily breaks off.

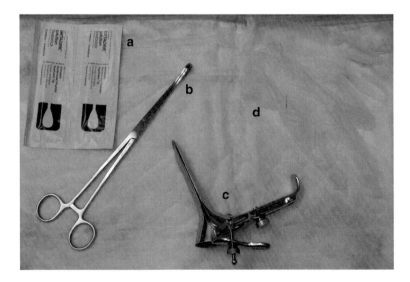

Fig. 9-2 Nonsterile equipment for endocervical polyp removal: (a) Betadine® Solution Swabsticks (Purdue Pharma, Stamford, CT); (b) Ring forceps; (c) Pederson speculum; (d) Gloves

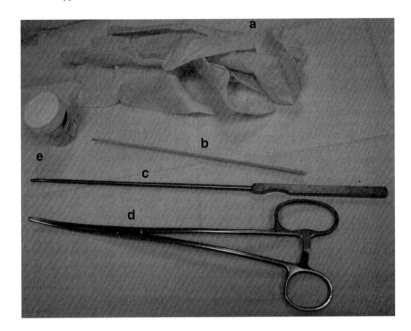

Fig. 9-3 Optional Equipment for endocervical polyp removal: (a) Nonlatex, nonsterile gloves; (b) Endocervical brush; (c) Endocervical curette; (d) Long Kelly forceps; (e) Cytology fixative jar

4. An ECC curette can be used to curette the base of the endocervical canal in order to remove any polyp remnants. An endocervical brush can also be used.
5. Send specimen to pathology for review.
6. Silver nitrate or Monsel's solution can be used to treat any bleeding.

Complications and Risks

- Bleeding/spotting
- Recurrence
- Infection (rare)

Tricks and Helpful Hints

Use the colposcope to identify the base of the polyp and then remove the polyp using a Tischler biopsy forceps.

Interpretation of Results (Algorithm 9-1)

- Report usually indicates benign tissue.
- If dysplasia noted on polyp, consider colposcopy.
- Any abnormal finding (i.e., sarcoma) requires additional therapy.

Procedure Note

(Provider to customize as needed.)

> *The patient was placed in the lithotomy position, a speculum was inserted into the vagina, and the cervix was identified. The polyp was identified. A long Kelly was placed at the base of the polyp, and the polyp was removed in its entirety by gentle twisting. An ECC curette was used to remove any polyp fragments in the endocervical canal. The specimen was sent to pathology. The patient tolerated the procedure without difficulty.*

Coding

CPT® Codes (Current Procedural Terminology, AMA, Chicago, IL)

There is no separate CPT code for cervical polyp removal

57500	Cervix uteri biopsy
57505	Endocervical curettage
58100	Endometrial sampling with or without Endocervical sampling, without cervical dilation, any method

ICD 9-CM-Diagnostic Codes (International Classification of Diseases, 9th Revision, Clinical Modification, Center for Disease Control and Prevention)

622.7	Polyp of cervix
621.0	Endometrial polyp
219.0	Benign neoplasm of the cervix
78.11	Condyloma acuminatum

Postprocedure Patient Instruction

The patient should be told to avoid douching or intercourse until all bleeding/spotting has resolved. Any excessive bleeding should be reported immediately, and the patient should be re-evaluated. Pathology is usually benign, and no further treatment is usually necessary. Routine follow up with annual exam is recommended.

Case Study Outcome

The polyp was easily removed with minimal bleeding. Pathology revealed normal benign epithelium.

Postprocedure Patient Handout

(Provider to customize as needed.)

- Cervical polyps are small pieces of tissue that are found within the canal of your cervix. While these are usually benign tissue pieces, the sample is always sent to the pathologist for review to ensure that no cancer or other abnormality is present.
- Today, your clinician removed a cervical polyp from your cervix. You should expect to have some minimal spotting/bleeding. This should not be heavier than a normal period.
- If you experience heavier bleeding, please call your physician/clinician right away.
- Cramping is usually transient, but if it persists, please take three Ibuprofen 200 mg tablets every 6 hours as needed, or Acetaminophen 650 mg every 4–6 hours as needed.
- You should avoid intercourse, douching, or tampon use for several days.
- Your clinician/physician will inform you of the results of the polyp when he/she receives the information from the pathologist.
- Please call the office if you have any problems or questions.

References

1. Neri A, Kaplan B, Rabinerson D, Ovadia J, Braslavsky D. Cervical polyp in the menopause and the need for fractional dilatationand curettage. *Eur J Obstet Gynecol Reprod Biol* 1995;62:53–55.
2. Coeman D, Van Belle Y, Vanderick G, DeMuylder X, Campo R. Hysteroscopic findings in patients with a cervical polyp. *Am J Obstet Gynecol* 1993;169(6):15163–15165.
3. Spiewankiewicz B, Stelmachow J, Sawicki W, Cendrowski K, Kuzlik R. Hysterocsopy in cases of cervical polyps. *Eur J Gynaecol Oncol* 2003;24(1):67–69.
4. Vilodre LC, Bertat R, Petters R, Reis FM. Cervical polyp as risk factor for hysterocopically diagnosed endometrial polyps. *Gynecol Obstet Invest* 1997;44(3):191–195.

Additional Resources

Articles

5. Abramovici H, Bornstein J, Pascal B. Ambulatory removal of cervical polyps under colposcopy. *Int J Gynaecol Obstet* 1984;22(1):47.
6. Golan VT, Ber A, Wolman I, David MP. Cervical polyp: evaluation of current treatment. *Gynecol Obstet Invest* 1994;37(1):56.

Chapter 10
Diaphragm and Cervical Cap

Jennifer W. McCaul

Introduction

Contraceptive diaphragms and cervical caps are two of the nonhormonal barrier contraceptive devices available for use today. Use of these devices has declined over several decades due to the increasing variety of other methods available, but they still have a place in providing contraception for certain carefully selected women. Caps and diaphragms are good contraceptives for women who are unable to tolerate hormones; they are both inexpensive and are durable. They are also intermittently used contraceptives which may be an advantage for those who require contraceptives on an infrequent basis.

The diaphragm is a silicone or latex flexible dome that fits over the cervix and into the vaginal fornix during intercourse, providing a barrier to sperm. The diaphragm must be properly fitted to each patient. Effectiveness of the diaphragm is user-dependent, and failure rates have been estimated at approximately 18% for this method (varying from 1 to 30%), assuming spermicide use with the diaphragm [1].

There are several types of diaphragms available today (Table 10-1, Fig. 10-1): arching spring, flat spring, coil spring, and wide seal. The arching spring diaphragm, such as the latex Ortho All Flex® (Ortho Pharmaceuticals, Raritan, NJ), folds into a half moon shape for insertion and does not require an introducer for insertion. Two types of arching spring diaphragms allow folding everywhere along the rim (dual spring) or only at a designated area of hinge (single axis hinge). The arching spring diaphragm's firm rim makes it the best choice for women with decreased pelvic support and it is the most popular type in the United States [2]. It is available in nine sizes from 55 to 95 mm.

The flat spring diaphragm has a thin rim, forms an oval when compressed, and requires an introducer to insert it. It is most appropriate for smaller women with narrow pelves and good pelvic musculature [2]. This type is popular in the United Kingdom.

J.W. McCaul (✉)

Assistant Professor, St. Joseph's Family Medicine Residency, St. Joseph's Hospital, 301 Prospect Avenue, Syracuse, NY, 13203, USA
e-mail: jennifer.mccaul@sjhsyr.org

S.M. Sulik and C.B. Heath (eds.), *Primary Care Procedures in Women's Health*, DOI 10.1007/978-0-387-76604-1_10, © Springer Science+Business Media, LLC 2010

Table 10-1 Types of diaphragms and indications for their use

Type of diaphragms	Characteristics	Indications	Brand name and supplier
Arcing spring	Fold in half moon shape	Average woman	Koro-Flex® : London
	Rim tends to be the most firm	Good for mild pelvic relaxation	International
Dual spring	Folds everywhere around the rim	Can be used with retroverted uterus	Ortho All-Flex® : Ortho Pharmaceuticals (55–105 mm)
	Folds only at a single axis	Can be obtained at pharmacy with prescription	
Single axis spring		Can be difficult to remove if axis rotates (single axis spring only)	
Flat spring	Thin delicate rim folds into flat oval	Harder to insert	Ortho-White®: Ortho Pharmaceuticals (55–105 mm)
	Requires plastic introducer	Less pressure on the urethra	
		Shallow arch behind pubic symphysis	
Coil spring	Soft, flexible rim	Deep pelvic arch	Ortho Coil Spring®: Ortho Pharmaceuticals (50–105 mm)
	Folds everywhere around rim	Avoid in patient with pelvic relaxation	Koromex®: London International
Wide seal	Silicone-based	Latex allergy	Milex® Wide-Seal Omniflex Coil Spring
	Wide flange of thin silicone at rim	Must be ordered from Milex	Wide-Seal Arching Spring
	Available with arching spring or coil spring		(60–95 mm): CooperSurgical

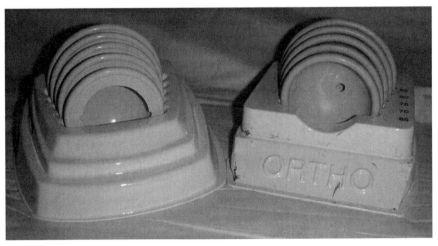

Fig. 10-1 Types of diaphragm kits: Milex® (CooperSurgical, Trumbull, CT) and ortho (Ortho Pharmaceuticals, Raritan, NJ) fitting kits

The coil spring diaphragm, such as the latex Ortho Coil Spring® (Ortho Pharmaceuticals, Raritan, NJ), has a rim that is more flexible than the arching spring but firmer than the flat spring. It can be used with or without an introducer. It is better suited to women without pelvic muscle relaxation [2].

The Milex® Wide-Seal Omniflex (CooperSurgical, Trumbull, CT) wide-seal diaphragm is silicone-based and has a thin skirt of silicone around the base of the rim to improve the seal and help hold spermicide. It also has an arching spring.

Some evidence exists that there is moderate protection provided against transmission of Sexually Transmitted Infections (STIs), mainly due to physical protection of the cervix, which is thought to be more susceptible to infections. This may not be the case for HIV infection, as there is some evidence favoring increased risk of transmission with use of spermicidal jelly, due to change in vaginal bacterial flora. Studies have been largely observational or case-controlled, and there are multiple confounding factors. In addition, diaphragm users may initially tend to be in a lower-risk group [1].

The cervical cap (available since 1988 although not widely used) is smaller than a diaphragm and more thimble-shaped with a deeper well. Many types of caps are in production worldwide, but only the silicone FemCap™ (FemCap Inc., Del Mar, CA) (Fig. 10-2) is FDA-approved for use in the US. Cervical caps are similarly sized by a provider, but can require more expertise to be properly fit. They are available in three sizes: small (22 mm), medium (26 mm), and large (30 mm). In general, the 22 mm size is indicated for nulligravid women, the 26 mm for women who have been pregnant but have not had vaginal birth, and the 30 mm for women who have given birth vaginally. Requiring less spermicide than a diaphragm, the cap is placed more tightly around the cervix. The FemCap™ dome covers the cervix, and the brim fits into the vaginal fornix to collect semen [3]. There is a strap to facilitate removal. It must be left in place for a minimum of 8 h after intercourse. However, it is approved for continuous use up to 48 h in the United States (72 h in the UK). Due to an increased risk of abnormal cervical cytology with cervical cap use, they are relatively contraindicated in the patient with a known abnormal Pap smear.

Annual contraceptive failure rates have been estimated at 17.4–30% with typical use, and may be as high as 40% if the patient has previously given birth vaginally [1, 4].

Cervical caps are more appropriately chosen for nulliparous patients due to the higher rate of failure in women with vaginal birth prior to fitting. Failure rates in parous women approach 17% at 6 months, approximately twice that of the nulliparous groups [3]. Cervical caps are less likely to be associated with an increased frequency of urinary tract infection, and unlike diaphragms, the fit is unaffected by weight changes [2]. Cervical caps may be a better barrier choice than diaphragms for patients with anterior wall relaxation. Lea's Shield® (Yama Inc, Union, NJ), approved by the FDA in 2002, is similar to the cervical cap but does not require sizing. It has an extrapolated 15% annual failure rate (based on 6-month preliminary study data) [5].

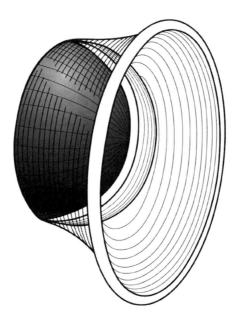

Fig. 10-2 FemCap™ (FemCap Inc., Del Mar, CA) diagram

The silicone device is held in place by the vaginal walls and acts by covering the cervix and sealing to it when air escapes from the integrated valve.

Careful patient selection is crucial when choosing either the diaphragm or cervical cap, and the ideal patient is comfortable with insertion and removal of the device and is willing to use the device with every act of coitus. Adolescents are rarely a good choice for diaphragms or cervical caps because of the level of maturity required for their use and the decreased level of protection from sexually transmitted with infections [6].

Case Study

A 26-year-old nulliparous patient in a monogamous longstanding relationship. She presents to your office today for her Pap smear and physical exam and asks you about changing her birth control method. She and her partner have been using condoms but would like a method that allows a little more spontaneity. She intends on having children in the next 1–2 years. In the past, she gained a great deal of weight on depo-provera, and she does not want to use this method again. She is a smoker and wants to avoid oral contraceptives because she has heard about the risks. Her aunt told her about her diaphragm, and she wants to know if this method is still available.

Diagnosis (Algorithm 10-1)

Barrier contraception screening/fitting.

Indications (Algorithm 10-1)

- Desire for nonhormonal, immediately reversible, female-controlled method of birth control.
- Women who feel at ease with touching themselves vaginally.
- Nulliparous women are especially suited for cervical caps or diaphragms.
- Cervical caps may be a better choice for women concerned about urinary tract infections or who have anterior wall relaxation.
- Women in whom hormonal methods are contraindicated.

Contraindications

Unreliable patient

Diaphragm Contraindications

- Significant pelvic organ prolapse (However, arching spring diaphragms may be helpful for mild pelvic relaxation), cystocele, rectocele, or uterine prolapse.
- Frequent urinary tract infections.
- Allergy to spermicide, latex, or silicone.
- Vaginal or cervical lacerations or significant friability.
- History of toxic shock syndrome.
- Inability to insert or use properly.
- History of HIV or high risk of HIV transmission.
- Inability to clean device, store device, or transport device to location of use.
- Requires fitting by provider and must be refit after pregnancy, abortion, or weight change of >20 pounds.

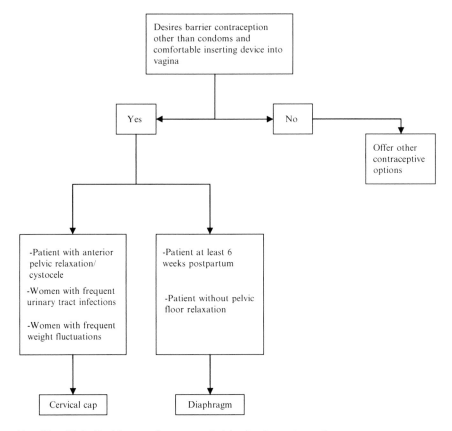

Algorithm 10-1   Decision tree for women desiring barrier contraception

Cervical Cap Contraindications

- Immediate postpartum or postabortal period (Patient should be at least 6 weeks postpartum or 2 weeks post abortion.)
- History of toxic shock syndrome
- Cervical polyps or other anatomic barrier to fitting properly
- Inability to insert or use properly
- Inability to clean device, store device, or transport device to location of use

Relative Contraindications

- Abnormal cervical cytology
- Should not be used during menses due to theoretical risk of endometriosis and toxic shock

- Presence of sexually transmitted disease
- Multiparous women due to decrease in effectiveness
- Up to 20% of women cannot be fitted with the four available sizes [2]

Equipment

Diaphragm (Fig. 10-3)

- Diaphragm fitting kit or fitting ring kit
- Nonsterile gloves
- Vaginal speculum
- Water-based lubricant (Surgilube®)
- Diaphragm introducer if using flat spring or coil spring

Cervical Cap

- Cervical caps in three sizes to be provided to the patients
- Vaginal speculum

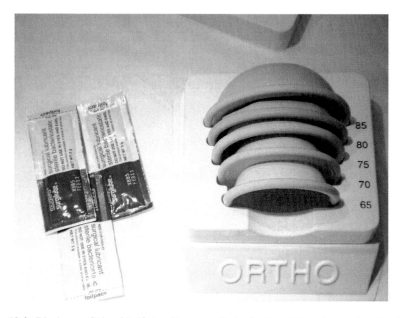

Fig. 10-3 Diaphragm fitting kit (Ortho Pharmaceuticals, Raritan, NJ) and water-based gel for fitting (Surgilube® water-based lubricant, E. Fougera & Co, Melville, NY)

- Nonsterile gloves
- Water-based lubricant
- Informational materials and video for patient review

Procedure

Diaphragm Fitting

1. Patient should be known to have normal cervical cytology prior to proceeding.
2. Have patient empty bladder and place her in the dorsal lithotomy position. Insert vaginal speculum and examine cervix and vaginal vault for any lacerations, abrasions, polyps, or signs of infection, which would contraindicate placement, and then remove speculum.
3. To estimate size of diaphragm needed, insert the index and middle finger into the vaginal vault so that the middle finger is placed at the posterior fornix. Place the thumb of the same hand against the symphysis pubis (Fig. 10-4).

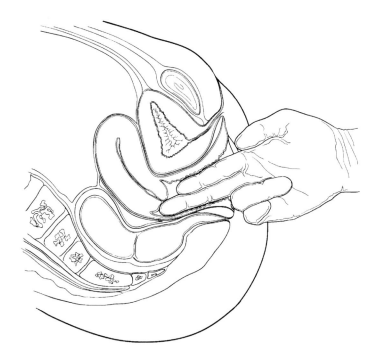

Fig. 10-4 Measure from the posterior fornix to the symphysis pubis to determine size of diaphragm

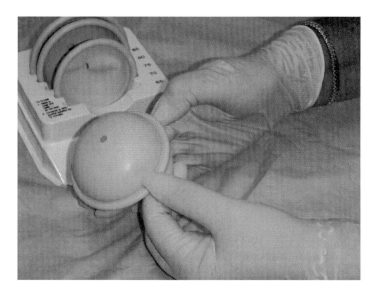

Fig. 10-5 Estimate the diaphragm size

4. Keeping the thumb against the index finger, remove the entire measuring hand, and measure the distance from the tip of the thumb to the tip of the middle finger. This distance represents the estimated necessary diaphragm size. Most women fit a 70 or 75 mm size.
5. Choose the estimated size diaphragm from the fitting kit (Fig. 10-5) and insert it into the vaginal vault by folding it in half (an introducer may be used for flat or coil spring diaphragms) and directing it posteriorly while separating the vulva with the other hand (Fig. 10-6a).
6. Palpate edges of diaphragm to ensure that it fits snugly behind the pubic symphysis, covers cervix entirely, and reaches the posterior fornix (Fig. 10-6b).
   • If necessary, choose a larger or smaller size to meet these criteria and try again.
7. Instruct the patient to feel for proper placement of the diaphragm in the vagina and to remove it by hooking the index finger behind the anterior rim and pulling straight down. Remind her to place one tablespoon of spermicidal jelly on the rim and inside the diaphragm.
8. Instruct patient to practice insertion and removal in exam room.
   Once she is able to insert it, have her leave the diaphragm in and then check her placement.
9. Prescribe diaphragm for patients with type and size noted on prescription.
10. Clean fitting set between fittings by disinfecting in a bleach solution; silicone-based devices can be autoclaved.

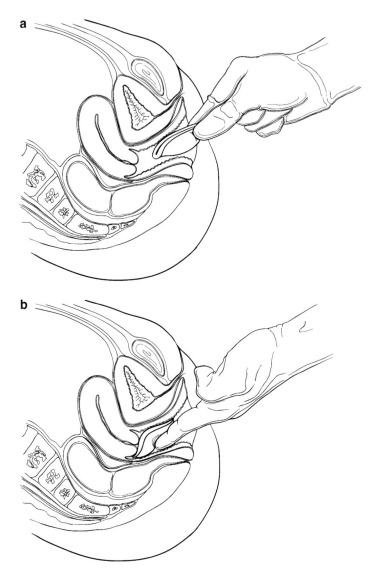

Fig. 10-6 (**a**) Fold diaphragm in half and insert in a downward fashion. (**b**) Check for fit of the diaphragm by sweeping finger to the back of the posterior fornix and fitting one finger tip between the symphsis pubis and the diaphragm

Cervical Cap Fitting

1. Have patient empty their bladder and place the patient in the dorsal lithotomy position.
2. Insert the vaginal speculum and examine the cervix for lacerations, polyps, or other structural abnormalities.

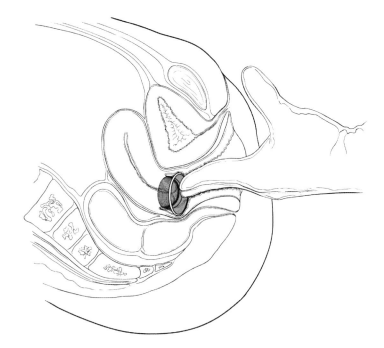

Fig. 10-7 Check fitting of FemCap™ (FemCap Inc., Del Mar, CA) once the patient has inserted it

3. Remove speculum, then perform pelvic exam to check cervical size.
   • Choose cervical cap size on the basis of exam and obstetrical history.
4. Have patient view the instructional materials provided by the manufacturer.
5. Allow patient to insert her own FemCap™ based on the instructional materials.
   • Insertion positions include squatting, one leg up, or dorsal lithotomy.
6. Check placement by digital exam to ensure cervix is completely covered (Fig. 10-7) and that the cap is not dislodged easily by movement or with a Valsalva maneuver.
7. Ensure that patient can remove the FemCap™ on her own.
8. Instruct patient on how to use ½ to ¾ teaspoon spermicide in the groove facing the vaginal vault prior to use.

Complications and Risks

• Unintended pregnancy (not as effective as other types of contraception).
• Frequent urinary tract infection (diaphragm only).
• Toxic shock syndrome (risk is 2.4 cases per 100,000 women, particularly when left in place more than 24 h) [7].
• Improper fitting resulting in failure of method.
• Cervical or vaginal lacerations, ulcerations, or abrasions.

- Dislodgement during intercourse (more common with cervical cap).
- Vaginal discharge or odor can develop if left in place too long.
- Partner discomfort with or awareness of the device.
- Penile abrasions.

Tricks and Helpful Hints

Diaphragm

- Have the patient perform a Valsalva maneuver and walk around the exam room after fitting to make sure there is no discomfort and the diaphragm does not dislodge.
- Ensure that the patient is comfortable with insertion and removal of the device on her own while she is in your office, and have her demonstrate proper application of one tablespoon of spermicide into the dome and around the rim of the device. Too much lubricant can make the diaphragm slippery and frustrating to insert for both provider and patient.
- Patient should be instructed to urinate before insertion and again after intercourse to avoid urinary tract infection.
- Consider a prescription if needed for emergency contraception given higher failure rate of barrier devices.
- Diaphragms can be obtained with a prescription at the pharmacy.
- If ordering a silicone diaphragm, this must be ordered from the company (CooperSurgical).

Cervical Cap

- Consider a prescription for emergency contraception given higher failure rate of barrier devices.
- Women with a long, short, or anterior cervix may not be amenable to fitting with a cervical cap and will need to use another method.
- The FemCap™ should always be inserted prior to any sexual arousal.
- Removal can be facilitated by squatting and bearing down.
- Cervical caps are generally supplied by a clinician's office. The clinician charges for the cervical cap as well as the fitting.

Procedure Note

(Provider to fill in blanks/circle applicable choice when given multiple choices and customize as needed.)

Diaphragm

> *The patient was placed in the dorsal lithotomy position. Vaginal speculum was inserted and the cervix and vagina were visually inspected and found to be normal. Diaphragm size was estimated by manual exam measurement. Fitting diaphragm was inserted to ensure proper size selection and # _____ (size) was prescribed. Patient was instructed in insertion, care, use, and removal, and demonstrated the ability to independently insert and remove the diaphragm. The patient tolerated the procedure well.*

Cervical Cap

> *The patient was placed in the dorsal lithotomy position. Vaginal speculum was inserted and the cervix and vagina were visually inspected and found to be normal. Manual vaginal examination was performed to estimate the size of the cervix. The patient's FemCap™ size was selected on the basis of obstetrical history and examination. The patient viewed the instructional materials and was able to adequately insert her own FemCap™ with the provided instructions. FemCap™ placement was checked by manual exam and size found to be appropriate. Patient demonstrated ability to independently remove the device. Patient tolerated the procedure well.*

Coding

Diaphragm

CPT® Codes (Current Procedural Terminology, AMA, Chicago, IL)

Diaphragm or cervical cap fitting with instructions	57170
Supply of Diaphragm	99070

ICD 9-CM-Diagnostic Codes (International Classification of Diseases, 9th Revision, Clinical Modification, Center for Disease Control and Prevention)

Insertion of diaphragm	96.17

Cervical Cap

CPT® Codes (Current Procedural Terminology, AMA, Chicago, IL)
Initial office visit, annual examination   99243
Follow-up visit   99214

ICD 9-CM-Diagnostic Codes (International Classification of Diseases, 9th Revision, Clinical Modification, Center for Disease Control and Prevention)
Diagnostic ICD-9 for cervical cap fitting   V25.49

Post-procedure Patient Instructions

Diaphragm

- Ensure that patient receives proper training regarding the insertion and removal of the device while in the office.
- Teaching points to review before the patient leaves the office:
  - Patient should insert the device 2 h prior to intercourse.
  - Patient can insert up to 6 h prior, but if that is done, an applicator of spermicide should be added at time of intercourse [6].
  - Device should be left in place for 6 h after intercourse but can stay in place up to 24 h.
  - Only water-based lubricants and spermicides should be used with the diaphragm.
  - Patient should check for dislodgement after intercourse and reposition if it occurs with insertion of an additional applicator of spermicide.
  - If additional episodes of intercourse take place, the device should be left in place and an additional applicator of spermicide should be inserted into the vagina.
  - Instruct patient to inspect diaphragm for holes or tears prior to each use by holding it up to the light.
  - Diaphragm should be cleaned after each use with mild soap and water, wiped dry, and kept in its case, avoiding extremes of temperature during storage.

Cervical Cap

- Patient should return in 2 weeks for a follow-up visit with the cap in place to ensure correct usage.
- Pap smear must be performed within 3 months of initiation of use and treated as indicated. If cytology is normal, the patient can resume yearly exams.
- Instruct patient not to use during menstruation.
- Instruct patient to check position after intercourse to ensure it has not dislodged.

Case Study Outcome

After discussing the specifics of the diaphragm barrier method. The patient was willing to try it. She felt that the risk of pregnancy was acceptable and was willing to use emergency contraception in the event of device failure. The patient was examined and found to be appropriate for a 65 mm arching diaphragm. Review of her gynecological and obstetrical history revealed no contraindications to diaphragm usage. The patient was instructed in its proper use and care and provided with a prescription and a follow-up appointment to ensure proper use.

Postprocedure Patient Handout

(Provider to customize as needed.)

Contraceptive Diaphragm Fitting

You have been fitted for a contraceptive diaphragm today. In order to obtain your diaphragm, please bring your prescription to the pharmacy to be filled. In order to be effective, your diaphragm must be used properly with spermicide during EVERY act of intercourse. Approximately one tablespoon of spermicide should be applied into the bowl and around the rim of the diaphragm. Use only water-based spermicides and lubricants with the diaphragm in place.

Your diaphragm may be inserted up to 6 h prior to intercourse, but new spermicide should be added into the vagina just prior to intercourse if insertion is more than 2 h before. It can be left in place up to 24 h but MUST be left in place for 6 h afterward. If repeated acts of intercourse take place within the 24 h, leave the diaphragm in place and insert additional spermicide prior to each episode. Check diaphragm placement for dislodgement after each episode. In the case of the diaphragm becoming dislodged, do not remove it. Reposition it and add an additional applicator of spermicide. Diaphragms should not be used while menstruating for more than fifteen hours due to the increased risk of toxic shock syndrome.

Clean your diaphragm with gentle soap and water after use, dry it, and keep it in its box. It must not be stored in extreme heat or cold. Examine the diaphragm for holes or tears by holding it up to the light prior to each use.

Cervical Cap Fitting

You have been fitted for a cervical cap today. Your cervical cap will be supplied by your physician. In order to be effective, your cervical cap must be used properly with spermicide during EVERY act of intercourse. Use approximately ¾ teaspoon of spermicide in the bowl and around the rim of the cervical cap.

Insert your cervical cap as directed by your provider 1–2 h prior to intercourse. It may be left in place up to 8 h after intercourse but can be left in for up to 48 h if necessary. If additional acts of intercourse take place within the 48 h time period, then insert another applicator of spermicide. Always check your cervical cap's placement after intercourse to ensure it has not dislodged. If it does, reposition it and add an applicator of spermicide. Make sure to break suction prior to device removal by dimpling the dome and twisting to avoid injury to the cervix.

Clean your cervical cap with gentle soap and water, pat it dry, and store it in its pouch. The cap should not be used during menstruation, and alternate methods should be used at that time.

References

1. Minnis A, Padian N. Effectiveness of female controlled barrier methods in preventing sexually transmitted diseases and HIV: current evidence and future research directions. *Sex Transm Infect* 2005;81:193–200.
2. Mayeaux E, Apgar B. Barrier contraceptives: cervical caps, condoms and diaphragms. In Pfenninger J, Fowler G (eds): *Procedures for primary care*. St. Louis, MO: Mosby, 1994:993–999.
3. FDA Summary of safety and effectiveness data. FemCap™. March 28, 2003.
4. Weiss B, Bassford T, Davis T. The cervical cap. *Am Fam Physician* 1991;43(2):517.
5. FDA Summary of safey and effectiveness data. Lea's Shield™. March 14, 2002.
6. Barbieri R. How to fit and use a diaphragm for contraception. Up to Date: 2009; www.uptodate.com/gynecology/gyncologic procedures
7. Allen R. Diaphragm fitting. *Am Fam Physician* 2004;69:97–100, 103, 105–106.

Additional Resources

Articles

Cook L, Nanda K, Grimes D. Diaphragm versus diaphragm with spermicides for contraception (review). *Cochrane Library* 2007, Issue 1.
Gallo MF, Grimes DA, Shulz KF. Cervical cap versus diaphragm for contraception (review). *The Cochrane Library* 2007.
Trussell J, Leveque J, et al. The economic value of contraception: a comparison of 15 methods. *Am J Public Health* 1995;85(4):494–503.

Web Sites

Ortho-McNeil Pharmaceutical Company: www.ortho-mcneil.com.
Lea's Shield: www.leasshield.com.
FemCap: www.femcap.com.
Milex: www.milexproducts.com.

Chapter 11
Copper Intrauterine Device

Elizabeth H. McNany

Introduction

The Intrauterine Device (IUD) is the most commonly used form of reversible contraception throughout the world [1], and in some countries it accounts for 40% of the contraception used by women [2]. In the United States (US), current use is 0.8% of the contraceptive population [3]. Prior to issues with infection and infertility with the Dalkon Shield in the 1970s, use in the US approached 10%. The newer IUDs are safe and effective forms of birth control when used in appropriate patients. Not only effective in preventing pregnancy with a failure rate of 0.42%, but if used for at least 5 years, it is one of the least expensive forms of birth control [4]. There are two IUDs currently in use in the US, the copper T 380A (in place for up to 10 years) and the levonorgestrel intrauterine system (in place for up to 5 years).

Appropriate patient selection is crucial when offering a copper IUD. A detailed history should be obtained, and the patient must have a thorough understanding of the use of the copper IUD. Knowledge of the patient's risk of sexually transmitted infections, the pattern of her menstrual cycle, her risk and history of pelvic inflammatory disease, her use of contraception in the past, and her future wishes regarding childbearing is essential [5].

It is important that a woman have a clear understanding of possible adverse events with the insertion and use of an IUD. She needs to understand what signs and symptoms to look for and when to seek medical attention. This should be emphasized by the clinician, and a patient handout should be given to the patient for reference.

E.H. McNany
Assistant Professor, Department of Medical Education, St. Joseph's Family Medicine Residency, Syracuse, NY 13202, USA
e-mail: Elizabeth.McNany@sjhsyr.org

S.M. Sulik and C.B. Heath (eds.), *Primary Care Procedures in Women's Health*,
DOI 10.1007/978-0-387-76604-1_11, © Springer Science+Business Media, LLC 2010

Historically, there has been great concern about ectopic pregnancy and IUD use. A recent meta-analysis showed that the use of an IUD does not increase the risk of ectopic pregnancy in a woman because the IUD generally prevents pregnancy effectively. If a woman gets pregnant with an IUD in place, however, she is more likely to have an ectopic pregnancy than a woman without an IUD [6].

Case Study

A 27-year-old patient, presents to the office requesting an IUD. She has been on oral contraceptives for the past 10 years. She is not good about taking them regularly and would like something more permanent. She has had a stable partner for the past 10 years, and they do not wish to have a child within the next few years. Her periods are regular, she has never had a sexually transmitted infection, and her Paps are normal. She is interested in a copper IUD, as she prefers a nonhormonal method.

Indications (Algorithm 11-1)

- Multiparous and nulliparous women at low risk for sexually transmitted infections
- Women who desire long-term reversible contraception
- Failure of a previous birth control method due to noncompliance
- Previous uncomplicated use of IUD
- Contraindications to hormonal contraception
- Emergency contraception within 5 days of intercourse for a woman who meets other criteria
- Women with the following medical conditions:
  - Diabetes
  - Breastfeeding
  - Breast cancer
  - Clotting disorders

Contraindications [7–9] (Algorithm 11-1)

Absolute Contraindications

- Pregnancy
- Puerperal sepsis
- Immediate placement postseptic abortion

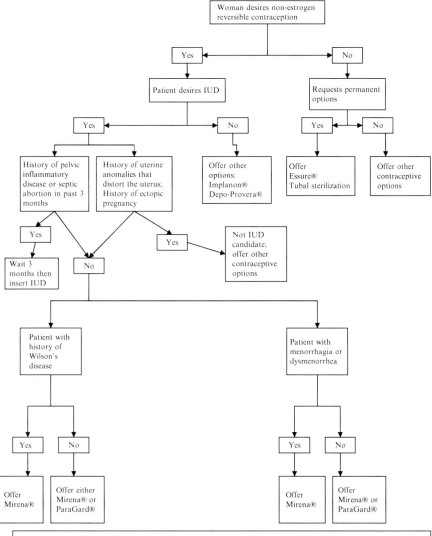

Algorithm 11-1   Decision tree for determining a nonhormonal contraception method

- Unexplained vaginal bleeding
- Malignant gestational trophoblastic disease
- Endometrial cancer
- Uterine anomalies that distort the anatomy
- Uterine fibroids that distort the shape of the uterus

- Current PID or history of PID in past 3 months
- Current purulent cervicitis or infection with gonorrhea or chlamydia
- Known pelvic tuberculosis
- Cervical cancer awaiting treatment
- Wilson's disease

Relative Contraindications (Algorithm 11-1)

- Excessively heavy periods or marked dysmenorrhea
- Small uterine cavity (higher risk of expulsion if uterus <6 cm)

Equipment (Fig. 11-1)

- ParaGard® T 380A (Duramed Pharmaceuticals, Cincinnati, OH)
- Speculum
- Basin with cotton balls moistened with antiseptic solution
- Cervical tenaculum
- Uterine sound

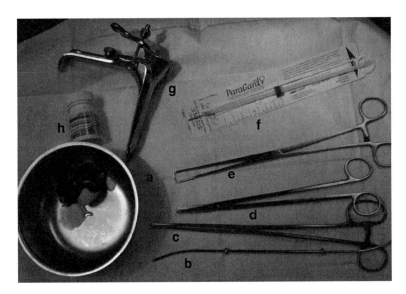

Fig. 11-1 Equipment set-up for Copper IUD. (a) Metal basin with cotton balls soaked in iodine; (b) Sterile uterine sound; (c) Sterile long Kelly forceps; (d) Long scissors; (e) Sterile cervical tenaculum; (f) Sterile ParaGard® (Duramed Pharmaceuticals, Cincinnati, OH) IUD Contraceptive; (g) Sterile Graves speculum; (h) Topical cervical anesthetic (Hurricane®, Beutlich LP Pharmaceuticals, Waukegan, IL)

- Sterile gloves
- Nonsterile gloves
- Sterile towel for tray top
- Long suture scissors
- Topical anesthetic (Hurricane®, Beutlich LP Pharmaceuticals, Waukegan, IL)
- Ring forceps

Procedure

1. Prior to placement:
   - Discuss thoroughly with the patient the risks, benefits, and expectations for follow-up after placement, and obtain signed consent.
   - Document negative pregnancy test.
   - Screen high-risk patient for gonorrhea and chlamydia. American College of Obstetrics and Gynecology (ACOG) does not recommend screening the low-risk patient [7].
   - Recommend NSAID use 1 hour prior to placement.
2. Perform a bimanual exam to check for position of the uterus.
3. Insert a warm vaginal speculum (large enough to easily visualize the cervix).
4. Clean the cervix with antiseptic solution:
   - Apply topical anesthetic to cervix (if tenaculum is going to be used).
5. Remove nonsterile gloves and put on sterile gloves. *The next four steps should be done using sterile technique.* Use sterile uterine sound to determine the depth of the uterus. Uterus should be between 6 and 9 cm to continue with the placement of IUD. Stabilize cervix, if needed, by the application of single-tooth tenaculum to anterior lip of cervix.
6. Have your assistant place contents of IUD package on sterile towel. Alternatively, do this step prior to changing into sterile gloves, making sure the contents of the package drop onto the sterile towel in a manner that maintains the sterile field.
   - Insert the solid white inserter rod so that it just touches the tip of the vertical arm of the IUD (Fig. 11-2). Fold the horizontal arms down and place inside the tube. (Do not do this step more than 5 min prior to placement.) Insert the arms no further than necessary to ensure retention.
   - Adjust the blue flange on the inserter rod to the depth of the uterus as determined by sounding, measuring from the top of the folded IUD to the blue flange. Be sure that the horizontal arms of the T of the IUD are parallel to the horizontal orientation of the long axis of the blue flange (Fig. 11-3). If needed, use the tenaculum to stabilize the cervix and insert the IUD through the cervical canal into the uterus up to the blue flange (Fig. 11-4). Ask an assistant to hold tenaculum in place (if using) and hold the solid white rod steady in the non-dominant hand. Using the dominant hand, pull back on the clear insertion tube 1–2 cm. The solid colored rod should *not* move (Fig. 11-5).

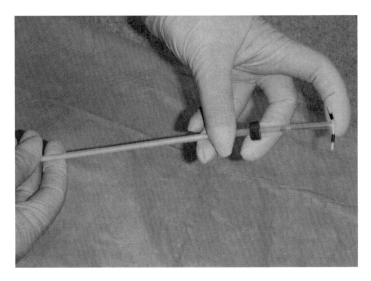

Fig. 11-2 Insert the white rod into the insertion tube and move up to the tip of the IUD. Keep a finger on the IUD to prevent it from falling out of the insertion tube

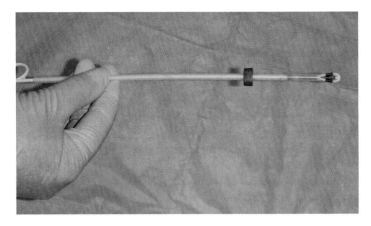

Fig. 11-3 Fold down the arms into the insertion tube just enough to hold in place. Adjust the blue flange to the measured uterine length

7. Once the IUD is released, gently push the tube inserter toward the fundus until slight resistance is felt to assure high placement of the IUD.
   - Hold the insertion tube steady and withdraw the solid white rod.
   - Slowly and gently withdraw the insertion device, leaving only threads protruding from the cervix.
8. Cut the threads protruding from the cervical os to 3–5 cm in length (Fig. 11-6) and document length in records.
   - It is best to leave threads longer because they can be shortened at the follow-up visit if necessary.

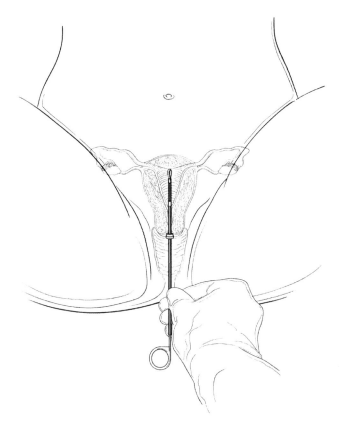

Fig. 11-4 Insert the IUD into the uterus until it meets the fundus (measured by the blue flange)

9. Show the patient on how to check for strings after each menstrual period and prior to intercourse.
10. Be sure to give the patient the handout provided by the company that gives information about when to contact healthcare provider.
11. Schedule a follow-up appointment with patient after first menstrual period to assess placement.
12. If there is any concern about whether IUD is properly placed, an ultrasound can be done to assess placement (this is rarely needed).

Complications and Risks

- Cramping and bleeding:
  - This leads to 12% of the removal requests in the first year [9]. The cramping can be treated with nonsteroidal anti-inflammatory medications (NSAIDs),

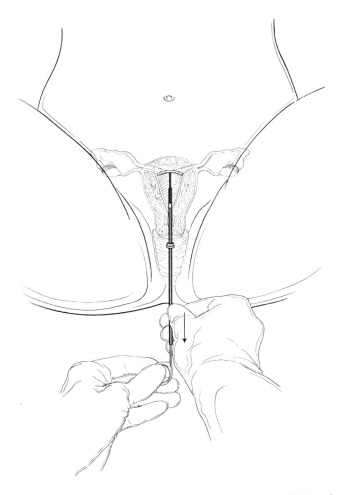

Fig. 11-5 Holding the white rod steady, pull the insertion tube toward the clinician. Once the IUD is released, push the insertion tube back up to the blue flange to anchor the IUD in the fundus of the uterus. Then, remove the rod and insertion tube

but if symptoms persist for more than 3–4 cycles, consider prescribing a short course of estrogen or oral contraceptive pills. If bleeding persists, removal can be considered [5].

- Expulsion:
  - Most common in the first year at a rate of 5.7% [9]
  - Typically occurs during menses. Emphasize importance of checking for the strings on a regular basis [5].
  - If the location of the device is uncertain, an ultrasound can determine the location of the IUD.

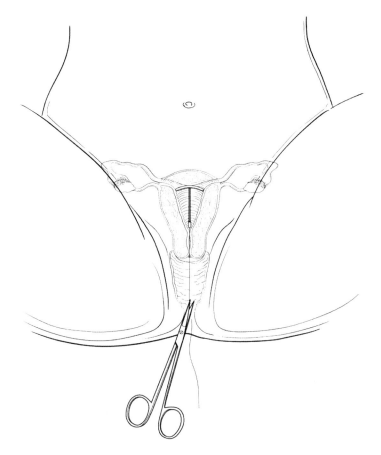

Fig. 11-6 Cut the strings 3–5 cm from the os and give the strings to the patient so she knows what they feel like on self-examination

- – Expulsion rates are lower the later in the menstrual cycle the device is inserted [10].
- – Uterine cavity less than 6 cm can increase the risk of expulsion, perforation, and bleeding, while greater than 9 cm increases the risk of expulsion.
- • Pelvic inflammatory disease (PID):
  - – Can potentially lead to infertility. Farley and colleagues showed that a woman is at greatest risk of PID in the first 20 days after the IUD is placed [11]. They also showed that the insertion process itself and the woman's background risk of Sexually Transmitted Infection (STIs) are most strongly linked to the development of PID. Women who are at low risk for STIs have little risk of PID with IUD use after the initial 20 days post insertion [11]. There is no indication of prophylactic antibiotics at the time of insertion to reduce PID. A recent meta-analysis confirmed that prior antibiotic use conferred little benefit [12].

- Uterine Perforation
  - Uterine perforation is rare (occurring in 0.1–0.3%). Must be corrected surgically with the removal of the IUD and repair of the uterus [5]. Proper technique and uterine sounding are important to help prevent this from occurring.
- Pregnancy
  - If pregnancy is confirmed and the IUD is in place, the IUD should be removed as soon as possible. Risks include: ectopic pregnancy, spontaneous abortion, premature delivery, sepsis, septic shock, and rarely death [9]. With the IUD in the uterus, the risk of spontaneous abortion is 50–60%, with half of these occurring in the second trimester, decreasing to 20% when the IUD is removed. Septic abortion is 26 times more common in women with an IUD in place [5].
- Other adverse events:
  - Anemia
  - Backache
  - Dysmenorrhea
  - Dyspareunia
  - Leukorrhea
  - Prolonged menstrual flow
  - Menstrual spotting
  - Urticarial allergic skin reaction
  - Vaginitis [9]

Tricks and Helpful Hints

- Advance a large cotton-tipped applicator (Scopette®, Birchwood Labs, Eden Prairie, MN) in with the uterine sound. The applicator's cotton swab will stop at the cervix; continue to advance the sound to the fundus of the uterus. Then remove the applicator and the sound simultaneously with the same hand. The distance from the top of the cotton applicator to the top of the sound is a clear indication of the uterine depth.
- Show the device through the packaging to the patient prior to insertion in order to reassure her of the small size and configuration of the device.
- If the IUD is contaminated or dropped, call the manufacturer, who will replace it free of charge.

Procedure Note

(Provider to customize as needed.)

> *Complications, risks, and benefits of IUD discussed. Pregnancy test performed and patient is not pregnant. Bimanual examination performed; speculum applied, and cervix visualized without difficulty. Cervix washed with antiseptic three times. Tenaculum placed under local anesthetic. Uterus sounded to 6–9 cm size. IUD inserted without difficulty. Strings cut to appropriate length. Strings given to patient to feel, and instructions given on how to check for the strings. Patient tolerated procedure well.*

Coding

CPT® Codes (Current Procedural Terminology, AMA, Chicago, IL)

58300	Insertion of IUD
J7300	Charge for cost of copper IUD

ICD 9-CM-Diagnostic Codes (International Classification of Diseases, 9th Revision, Clinical Modification, Center for Disease Control and Prevention)

V 25.1	Encounter of contraceptive management, insertion of intrauterine contraceptive device
V 25.42	Intrauterine contraceptive device, checking, reinsertion, or removal of intrauterine device

PostProcedure Patient Instructions [9, 13]

- Educate the patient on how to check for strings after each menstrual period and prior to intercourse.
- Be sure to give the patient the handout provided by the company that gives information about when to contact healthcare provider. Emphasize the major concerns:
  - Patient must check for the threads of the IUD after each menstrual period. If not palpable, she should contact her healthcare provider.
  - Remind the patient to report any of the following: Excessive pain, malodorous discharge, excessive bleeding, fever, prolonged pelvic discomfort or pain during intercourse, genital lesions, suspicion of STIs, missed period, or any other concerns she may have.
- Schedule a follow-up appointment with patient after first menstrual period to assess placement.

Case Study Outcome

Patient had an IUD inserted without difficulty in her provider's office. She was delighted to discontinue her oral contraceptive pills, and reported no difficulty with her IUD.

Postprocedure Patient Handout

(Provider to customize as needed.)

- Check for the threads from the IUD after each menstrual period, and if you cannot feel them, contact your provider immediately.
- You may have increased bleeding during your periods and spotting between periods the first 2–3 months after placement. Typically, these symptoms improve with time, but if they persist contact your provider.
- You may have cramping associated with the placement of the IUD, but if the pain is severe, let your provider know.
- When to contact your provider:
  - If you think you are pregnant
  - If you cannot feel the threads from the device or the length has changed
  - If you have severe menstrual bleeding
  - If you have pelvic pain during sex
  - If you have unusual vaginal discharge or genital sores
  - If you have unexplained fever
  - If you may have been exposed to STIs
  - If you or your partner becomes HIV positive

References

1. Anonymous. IUDs: an update. *Popul Rep B* 1995;6:1–35.
2. Mauldin WP, Segal SJ. IUD use throughout the world: past, present and future. In Bardin CW, Mishell DR Jr (eds) *Proceedings from the Fourth International Conference on IUDs.* Boston, MA: Butterworth-Heinemann, 1994, pp 1–10.
3. Piccinino LJ, Mosher WD. Trends in contraceptive use in the United States: 1982–1995. *Fam Plann Perspect* 1998;30:4–10, 46.
4. Trussell J, Leveque JA, Koenig JD, London R, Borden S, Henneberry J, LaGuardia KD, Stewart F, Wilson TG, Wysocki S. The economic value of contraception: a comparison of 15 methods. *Am J Public Health* 1995;85(4):494–503.
5. Canavan TP. Appropriate use of the intrauterine device. *Am Fam Physician* 1998;58(9):2077–2084, 2087–2088.
6. Xiong X, Buekens P, Wollast E. IUD use and the risk of ectopic pregnancy: a meta-analysis of case-control studies. *Contraception* 1995;52:23–34.
7. World Health Organization. *Medical eligibility criteria for contraceptive use*, 3rd edn. Geneva: WHO, 2004.
8. ACOG Practice Bulletin, Intrauterine Device, Number 59, January 2005.
9. Paragard package insert, FEI Products LLC, last revision September 2005.
10. White MK, Ory HW, Rooks JB, Rochat RW. Intrauterine device termination rates and the menstrual cycle day of insertion. *Obstet Gynecol* 1980;55:220–224.
11. Farley TM, Rosenberg MJ, Rowe PJ, Chen JH, Meirik O. Intrauterine devices and pelvic inflammatory disease: an international perspective. *Lancet* 1992;339:785–788.
12. Grimes DA, Schulz FK. Antibiotic prophylaxis for intrauterine contraceptive device insertion. *Cochrane Database Syst Rev* 1999, Issue 3. Art. No.: CD001327. DOI: 10.1002/14651858. CD001327.
13. Johnson BA. Insertion and removal of intrauterine devices. *Am Fam Physician* 2005;71(1): 95–102.

Additional Resources

Website

Supplier: Duramed Pharmaceuticals: www.paragard.com

Chapter 12
Levonorgestrel Intrauterine System Insertion

John L. Bucek

Introduction

The Levonorgestrel-Releasing Intrauterine System (LNG IUS) is a safe, effective form of contraception. The number of women choosing an Intrauterine Device (IUD) as their form of contraception is increasing in the United States due to the fact that the LNG IUS is one of the least expensive, safest, and most effective methods of reversible contraception.

The LNG IUS prevents pregnancy through several mechanisms, including thickening of the endocervical mucus and suppressing the endometrial lining of the uterus [1]. It also causes a type of foreign body reaction in the uterine cavity and may have effects on tubal motility. Taken together, these changes impair sperm survival and effectiveness. Tubal washing studies demonstrate that LNG IUS is not an abortifacent; rather, its contraceptive action is prevention of conception [2].

The cost of LNG IUS use is concentrated at the time of initiation of the method. The provider fee and the device cost vary, but can be a barrier for obtaining an IUS. In some practices, patient charges can be high as $900–$1,000 on the day of device insertion. However, when amortized over the average time of use, the LNG IUS is one of the least expensive contraceptive methods.

Its side effect profile is very favorable compared to other methods. For the vast majority of users, the levonorgestrel effects are limited to the local uterine environment. As a result, LNG IUS users experience ovulation 85% of the time and do not experience the side effects typical of methods that block ovulation. Discontinuation rates are used to compare overall acceptance of contraceptive methods [2]. LNG IUS has a rate comparable to that of the Copper IUD systems and is superior to most other methods other than tubal ligation [1].

J.L. Bucek
Somerset Medical Center, Somerset Family Medicine Residency Program,
110 Rehill Avenue, Somerville, NJ, 08807, USA
e-mail: jbucek@somerset-healthcare.com

S.M. Sulik and C.B. Heath (eds.), *Primary Care Procedures in Women's Health*,
DOI 10.1007/978-0-387-76604-1_12, © Springer Science+Business Media, LLC 2010

Its effectiveness in usual use is nearly identical to its effectiveness in ideal use. The Pearl Index for LNG IUS is 0.14; the first-year pregnancy rate for LNG IUS is 0.1 per 100 users [1]. The LNG IUS also significantly reduces the ectopic pregnancy rate for users of the method.

The LNG IUS is associated with changes in the pattern of menses for most users. During the first 6 months of use, many women experience more days of bleeding than before insertion. This tapers off after 6 months, until about 20% of women experience amenorrhea. During the 5-year life of the LNG IUS, all users experience a reduction in the number of days per month with bleeding. Properly counseling patients about what to expect in regard to bleeding is key to achieving patient acceptance and continuation of the method. FDA-approved in 2009 for the treatment of menorrhagia, many clinicians find that the LNG IUS may significantly decrease the bleeding in menorrhagia, especially in women who are peri-menopausal [3].

Case Study

A 26-year-old woman, who is now G 2 P 1011, returns to your office 6 months after her delivery. She is breastfeeding twice a day and wants to discuss a contraceptive method that she can use for 2–3 years. She thinks she will wait that long before trying to become pregnant again. She took oral contraceptives for a short time in the past and discontinued them due to headaches and stomach symptoms. She has used condoms at times on and off and is not satisfied with that method. She has been together with the father of the baby for 3 years, and they do not have any partners outside this relationship. Her Pap smears at the first prenatal visit and at the postpartum visit were both normal. She has no history of CIN or HPV, and her other infection screening in pregnancy was normal.

Diagnosis

Our patient with apparently normal fertility wants reversible contraception. Her risk factors and history suggest that she is not at high risk for exposure to sexually transmitted infections. She would like to avoid pregnancy for 2 or more years. The side effect profile, cost, and efficacy of LNG IUS make it an excellent option for this patient.

Indications (Algorithm 12-1)

- Reversible contraception
- Monogamous
- Prefers continual contraception
- Prefers not to take oral contraceptives on a daily basis

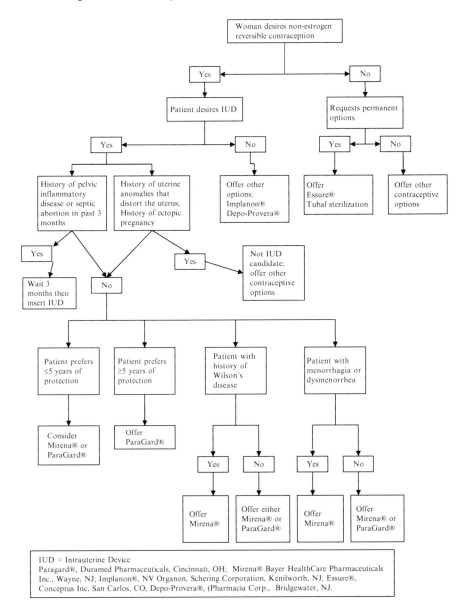

Algorithm 12-1 Candidates for IUD placement

Contraindications (Algorithm 12-1)

- Pregnancy
- Current Sexually Transmitted Infection (STI) or cervicitis
- Multiple partners
- Abnormal uterine anatomy (some patients with fibroids may be candidates)

- History of Pelvic Inflammatory Disease (PID) within 3 months
- Endometritis within 3 months
- Cervical Dysplasia or Cancer (if abnormal Pap is found after IUD is in place, diagnostic work up may continue before IUD is removed)
- Uterine cavity less than 6 cm or greater than 9 cm depth (associated with higher expulsion rates)

Relative Contraindications

Sensitivity to prior exposure to systemic levonorgestrel

Equipment (Fig. 12-1)

- Levonorgestrel Intrauterine System
- Nonsterile exam gloves
- Sterile gloves
- Urine pregnancy test
- Speculum
- Light source

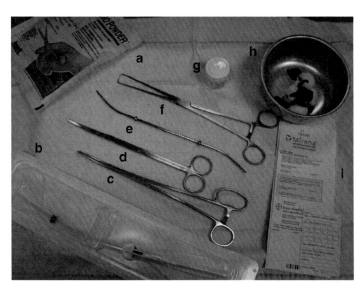

Fig. 12-1 Sterile tray for Levonorgestrel IntraUterine System insertion: (a) Sterile nonlatex gloves; (b) Mirena® (Bayer HealthCare Pharmaceuticals Inc., Wayne, NJ); IUD in sterile package; (c) Long Kelly forceps; (d) Long scissors; (e) Sterile uterine sound; (f) Sterile cervical tenaculum; (g) Specimen jar (if needed for Pap); (h) Metal basin with sterile cotton balls soaked in iodine; (i) Mirena® permit and patient card

- Iodine/povodine solution
- Tenaculum
- Uterine sound
- Ring forceps
- Gauze
- Large Cotton swabs (with long shaft for use in speculum). Scopettes® (Birchwood Labs, Eden Prairie, MN)
- Long-handled scissors

Procedure

1. Patients should receive the LNG IUS manufacturer's patient education to review before the procedure. Pamphlets and a video are available. Review the patient's cervical cancer screening with her. Review the patients STI risk and any screening for STIs done preprocedure. Review risks, benefits, and side effects with the patient. Ask if she has any questions about LNG IUS use.
2. Confirm that the patient is not pregnant with the urine pregnancy test. Sign the consent form and ask the patient to sign the consent form with a witness present.
3. Perform a bimanual exam to estimate the uterine size and to confirm the position and direction of the uterine cavity.
4. Place a speculum and visualize the cervix.
5. Replace your exam gloves with a new pair of sterile gloves.
6. Swab the cervix with antiseptic. Use large swabs or gauze folded in the ring forceps and paint the cervix with the iodine solution three times to sterilize the outer cervix.
7. Grasp the anterior lip of the cervix with the tenaculum about 1.5 cm from the os. Close the tenaculum slowly until one tooth is engaged.
8. Gently pull on the tenaculum to straighten the endometrial cavity before sounding the uterus. Maintain this traction when inserting the sound. Determine the endometrial cavity size with the uterine sound
9. Open the IUD package and maintain the IUD in a sterile state (Fig. 12-2). Figure 12-3 reviews terminology for IUD insertions system.
10. Free the string as directed in the package insert.
11. Push the slider on the inserter to the limit away from you. Confirm that the arms of the IUD are horizontal (Fig. 12-4).
12. Pull the strings at the base of the inserter until the LNG IUS system is drawn into the inserter. Lock the strings into the handle of the inserter (Figs. 12-4–12-6).
13. Set the marker/flange on the inserter to the uterine depth you found with the sound (Fig. 12-7).
14. Insert the IUD into the uterine cavity. Stop when the flange is 1.5 cm away from the cervix (Fig. 12-8).
15. Pull the slider 1 cm to allow the arms of the IUD to open. There is a mark on the inserter indicating that it has been pulled 1 cm back (Figs. 12-9 and 12-10).

Fig. 12-2 Remove IUS from
sterile packaging using
sterile technique (reprinted
with the permission of Bayer
HealthCare Pharmaceuticals
Inc., Wayne, NJ)

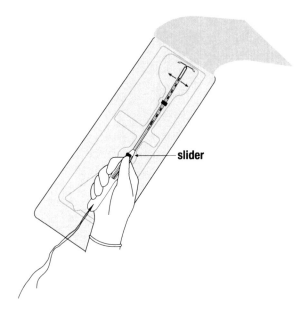

Fig. 12-3 Terminology for IUD
insertion system (reprinted with
the permission of Bayer
HealthCare Pharmaceuticals Inc.,
Wayne, NJ)

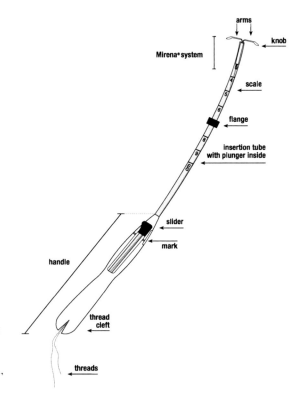

Fig. 12-4 Advance slider to furthest
away position, pulling strings to place
IUS into insertion system (reprinted with
the permission of Bayer HealthCare
Pharmaceuticals Inc., Wayne, NJ)

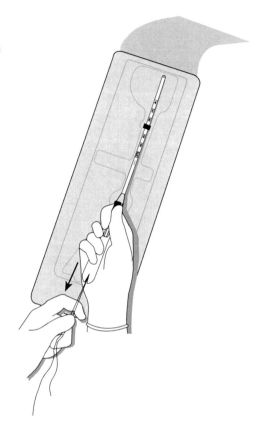

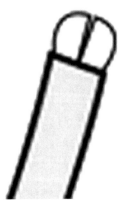

Fig. 12-5 Horizontal arm tips fold superiorly into insertion tube
(reprinted with the permission of Bayer HealthCare
Pharmaceuticals Inc., Wayne, NJ)

Fig. 12-6 Lock strings into place (reprinted with the permission of Bayer HealthCare Pharmaceuticals Inc., Wayne, NJ)

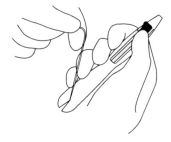

Fig. 12-7 Adjust flange to depth of uterine sound (reprinted with the permission of Bayer HealthCare Pharmaceuticals Inc., Wayne, NJ)

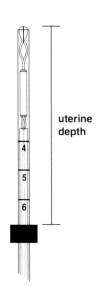

uterine depth

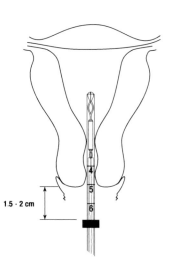

1.5 · 2 cm

Fig. 12-8 Insert system to within 1–2 cm of flange marker (reprinted with the permission of Bayer HealthCare Pharmaceuticals Inc., Wayne, NJ)

Fig. 12-9 Extend arms horizontally by pressing slider to mark on handle (reprinted with the permission of Bayer HealthCare Pharmaceuticals Inc., Wayne, NJ)

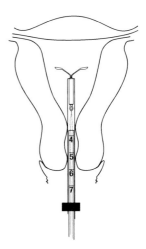

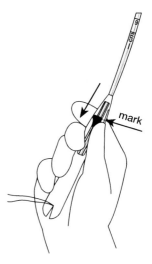

Fig. 12-10 Close-up of mark on handle (reprinted with the permission of Bayer HealthCare Pharmaceuticals Inc., Wayne, NJ)

16. Advance the whole inserter until the flange is at the os. This will place the open arms at the top of the uterine fundus (Fig. 12-11).
17. Pull the slider all the way to the limit toward you. Confirm that this has released the strings (Fig. 12-12).
18. Remove the IUD inserter.
19. Trim the strings with the scissor so that 2–3 cm will remain (Fig. 12-13).
20. Remove the tenaculum and inspect for bleeding. Apply gentle pressure with a swab to achieve hemostasis.
21. Remove the speculum and do a bimanual exam to feel for uterine position and tenderness.

Fig. 12-11 Advance handle so that flange touches endo-cervical os (reprinted with the permission of Bayer HealthCare Pharmaceuticals Inc., Wayne, NJ)

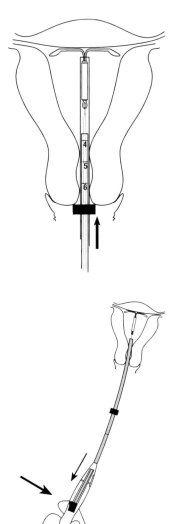

Fig. 12-12 Push slider toward inserter, allowing strings to release (reprinted with the permission of Bayer HealthCare Pharmaceuticals Inc., Wayne, NJ)

Complications and Risks

- Uterine perforation (rare)
- Infection (risk of salpingitis is 1/1,000.)
- Pain during placement

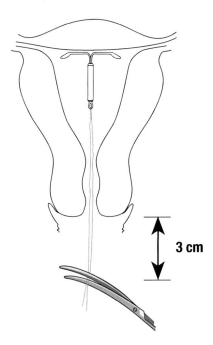

Fig. 12-13 Cut string 2–3 cm beyond os (reprinted with the permission of Bayer HealthCare Pharmaceuticals Inc., Wayne, NJ)

- Bleeding and cramping (common up to a week postprocedure)
- Spotting and irregular bleeding during first 6 months
- Eventual amenorrhea

Tricks and Helpful Hints

- Show patients a nonsterile IUS and let them hold it when counseling them. Seeing how small and flexible an IUD is may reduce patient fear.
- Have the patient take 400–800 mg ibuprofen an hour before IUS insertion. This may reduce postprocedure cramping.
- Some providers prefer to do IUS insertions when patients are menstruating. This is not necessary and may be very inconvenient for patient and provider. The levonorgestrel-releasing intrauterine system can be inserted during any day of the menstrual cycle; however, it is imperative to document negative pregnancy test.
- Before gripping the cervix with the tenaculum, you may want to pause the procedure and use lidocaine or Hurricane to anesthetize the anterior cervix or to perform a paracervical block. This will reduce the pain and discomfort.
- When maintaining traction on the tenaculum you may need to monitor the speculum to ensure that it is not displaced.

- When advancing the sound, use torque to advance the tip. Put a very gentle bend in the sound and twist the tip from side to side to advance it. This is safer than pushing the tip in. If you meet resistance at the level of 3–4 cm, consider that you may be at the endocervix or at the fold near where the cervix joins the uterine body. Check to see if more traction is needed to straighten the uterus.
- Marking the maximum advance of the sound visually is difficult. Insert the long end of a swab adjacent to the sound and align the tip of this with the exocervix. Then, pull the sound and the swab out together. The tip should line up with the sound mark that corresponds to the uterine depth
- Rinse the cut end of the IUD string and allow the patient to hold it so she can see what it feels like on her fingertip. This may facilitate finding the strings when the IUD is in place.

Procedure Note

(Provider to fill in blanks/circle applicable choice when given multiple choices and customize as needed.)

- *Recent Pap shows no dysplasia and cultures show no signs of sexually transmitted infections.*
- *Patient has no history of recent STIs and is monogamous.*
- *Patient understands the risk of bleeding, infection, pain/cramping, and the patient knows alternatives. She consented to IUD placement in writing after having opportunity to ask questions.*

  Bimanual exam performed:

- *Speculum placed; cervix normal looking and midline.*
- *Cervix visualized and swabbed three times with betadine.*
- *Tenaculum clamped onto anterior lip of cervix; uterus sounded to _____ cm.*
- *Levonorgestrel IUS placed without complications.*
- *Arms deployed in a high fundal position.*
- *String trimmed and string palpation described to patient. Bimanual exam after placement demonstrates no/minimal uterine tenderness.*

Coding

CPT® Codes (Current Procedural Terminology, AMA, Chicago, IL)
58300   IUD insertion
58301   IUD removal

ICD 9-CM-Diagnostic Codes (International Classification of Diseases, 9th Revision, Clinical Modification, Center for Disease Control and Prevention)
V25.1   IUD insertion
V45.51   Presence of IUD

PostProcedure Patient Instructions

Instruct patient to: Return in 1 month for IUS check if string not palpated; no unprotected sex until IUS placement confirmed by string palpation. Tell patient to check IUS string after each period. Instruct patient to use Ibuprofen today as needed for cramping and to call office if she develops purulent discharge, fever, chills, nausea, vomiting, or excessive bleeding.

Case Study Outcome

The patient selected the Levonorgestrel Intrauterine system, which was inserted without difficulty in the office. She tolerated the procedure well and remarked at her follow-up visit 1 year later that she was very satisfied with her selection.

PostProcedure Patient Handout

(Provider to fill in blanks/circle applicable choice when given multiple choices.)

You have just had a Levonorgestrel Intrauterine System (LNG IUS) inserted on _____(insert date). This contraceptive system is effective for 5 years. Your Levonorgestrel Intrauterine System should be removed prior to_____ (insert date 5 years from date of insertion).

Please remember to check for the LNG IUS string after every period.

Most women have no side effects from the LNG IUS, but common side effects include:

- Uterine cramping, which usually goes away within the first 3 months. Consider taking two 200 mg ibuprofen for pain up to every 6 h as needed.
- Change in bleeding pattern, including spotting and between period bleeding. Most women eventually have little or no period.
- Acne, breast tenderness, weight gain, and back pain occur rarely (less than 3.5% of the time).

Please call your clinician's office if:

- You develop a smelly discharge or have a fever.
- Develop severe abdominal pain not relieved by ibuprofen.
- If the bleeding becomes excessive (more than one pad per hour or more than ten pads per day).
- You are interested in getting pregnant and wish for your provider to remove the LNG IUS. Please be aware that fertility returns immediately upon removal.

Please make a follow-up appointment in the office in 1 month.

_____

References

1. Grimes DA. Intrauterine devices. In Hatcher R (ed) *Contraceptive technology*, 18th edn. New York: Ardent Media, 2004.
2. Mirena® (levonorgestrel-releasing intrauterine system) product Monograph. Montville, NJ: Berlex, 2005.
3. Pfenninger JL, Fowler GC. IUD insertion. In *Procedures for primary care physicians*. St. Louis, MO: Mosby, 1994.

Additional Resources

Books

World Health Organization. *Medical eligibility criteria for contraceptive use,* 3rd edn. Geneva, Switzerland: World Health Organization, 2004.

Websites

http://www.who.int/reproductive-health/publications/mec/mec.pdf
www.mirena-us.com. Telephone: 866-647-3646

Chapter 13
Intrauterine Device Removal

Joel A. Kase

Introduction

One of the many benefits of utilizing intrauterine contraception is the typical ease with which the device can be inserted and removed. Following patient counseling, once the patient and provider have together formulated a decision to remove the device, retrieval of the apparatus can often be accomplished in a short office visit.

The two options for intrauterine contraception currently available for use in the United States, the levonogestrel-releasing system (Mirena®, Bayer HealthCare Pharmaceuticals Inc., Wayne, NJ) and the T 380A intrauterine copper contraceptive (ParaGard®, Duramed Pharmaceuticals, Cincinnati, OH), are licensed for use for up to 5 years [1] and 10 years [2], respectively.

Patients seek to have their Intrauterine Device (IUD) removed when they desire pregnancy or they have reached the maximum recommended time for utilization of the apparatus. Adverse reactions that most often prompt women to present for removal of their IUD include pelvic cramping and abnormal vaginal bleeding [3]. Other less common reasons for removal include concerns such as partner discomfort with intercourse, and the inability of the patient to self-palpate IUD strings.

Case Study

A 27-year-old female, gravida 2 para 1011, presents to the office concerned that she has not been able to feel her IUD strings over the past few weeks since her last period ended. Prior to her last menstrual cycle she had been able to palpate her

J.A. Kase (✉)
Division Chief for Public Health, Department of Family Medicine University of New England College of Osteopathic Medicine, Biddeford, ME 04005, USA
e-mail: jkase@une.edu

S.M. Sulik and C.B. Heath (eds.), *Primary Care Procedures in Women's Health*,
DOI 10.1007/978-0-387-76604-1_13, © Springer Science+Business Media, LLC 2010

strings since placement of the device 15 months earlier, and she had always been able to do so without difficulty. The patient had experienced minimally increased bleeding and cramping with menses in the first few months following placement of the IUD; however, these symptoms resolved, and she has had no other concerns with her contraception until now. The patient and her husband have unprotected sex regularly, and they remain mutually monogamous.

Review of systems reveals continued regular menses, with no spotting in between periods and no symptoms suggestive of pregnancy. On pelvic exam, a normal appearing cervix is identified, without evidence of IUD strings passing through the external os, with no abnormalities identified on bimanual exam. A urine pregnancy test is negative.

If in fact her IUD is still in place, the patient does not want to have the device removed. She and her husband have been in the process of discussing when they would plan to have their next child.

Arrangements were made to have a pelvic ultrasound performed for confirmation of IUD presence (Figs. 13-1, 13-2). The IUD was noted to be in a satisfactory intrauterine position. The patient felt comfortable not being able to check her strings monthly since her periods continued to be very regular.

Diagnosis and Indications

- Patient adverse reaction:
  - Pelvic pain

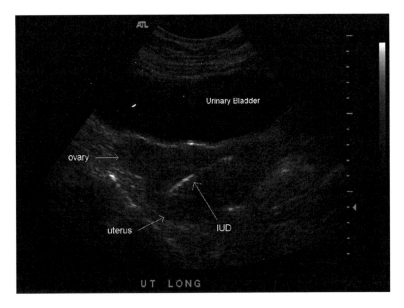

Fig. 13-1 Longitudal view of intrauterine device in uterus

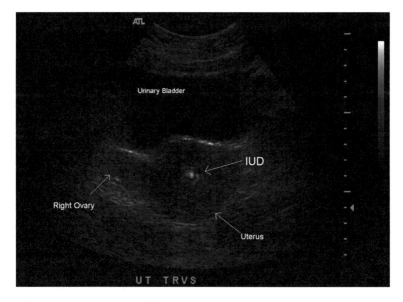

Fig. 13-2   Cross-sectional view of IUD in uterus

- – Back pain
- – Dysmenorrhea
- – Meno- or menometrorrhagia
- – Partial IUD expulsion
- Documented or suspected genital tract/pelvic infection
- Pregnancy
- Patient desires pregnancy
- Patient has reached the maximum recommended time for use
- Patient has reached menopause
- Patient dissatisfaction
- Partner discomfort with intercourse
- Inability to palpate IUD strings

Contraindications

IUD removal in the presence of pregnancy should be performed by an experienced clinician following appropriate patient counseling and review of informed consent.

Equipment (Fig. 13-3)

Equipment for Straightforward IUD Removal

- Vaginal speculum
- Non-sterile gloves
- Ring forceps

Equipment for Potentially Complicated IUD Removal, Including Evaluation of Absent Strings

- Vaginal Speculum
- Non-sterile gloves
- Cytobrush, cytobroom, or two sterile cotton swabs
- Antiseptic solution
- Single-toothed tenaculum
- Alligator clamp or IUD hook
- Endocervical speculum
- Ring forceps
- Uterine sound

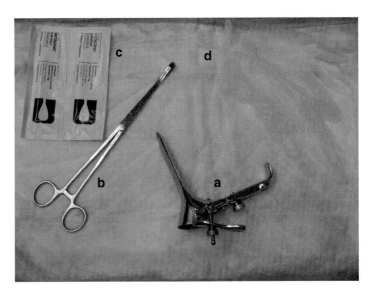

Fig. 13-3 Set-up for IUD removal: (a) Pederson speculum; (b) Ring forceps; (c) Betadine® Solution Swabsticks (Purdue Pharma, Stamford, CT); (d) gloves

Optional Equipment

- Colposcope
- Monsel's solution
- Silver nitrate sticks
- Topical anesthetic

Procedure

When IUD Strings Are Visualized

1. Perform pregnancy test.
2. Perform a bimanual examination to determine the size and position of the uterus.
3. Insert a speculum into the vagina to bring the cervix into view.
4. Grasp the IUD strings with ring forceps and gently apply steady traction (Fig. 13-4).
5. Encourage the patient to take a deep breath and exhale slowly, allowing for enhanced relaxation of the pelvic floor musculature as the IUD is withdrawn through the cervix (Fig. 13-5).

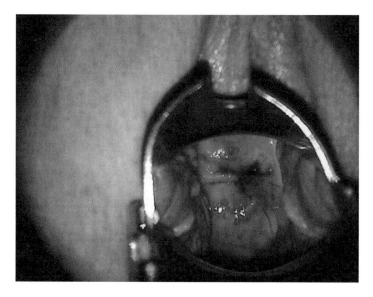

Fig. 13-4   Vaginal view of IUD string prior to removal

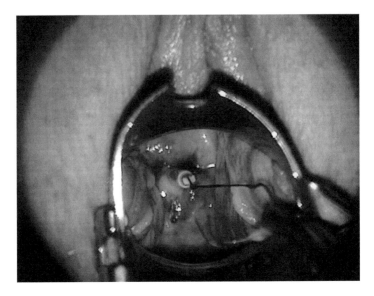

Fig. 13-5 Vaginal view of IUD during removal

When IUD Strings Are Absent (Algorithm 13-1)

1. Perform a pregnancy test.
2. Perform a bimanual examination to determine the size and position of the uterus.
3. Insert a speculum into the vagina to bring the cervix into view. Cleanse the cervix with antiseptic solution prior to instrumentation.
4. Grasp the anterior lip of the cervix with a single-toothed tenaculum in order to maintain gentle traction to facilitate instrumentation.
5. Insert a cytobrush into the os, twirling as it is withdrawn, in the hopes of snagging the strings to permit removal of the device.
   - Alternatively, two sterile cotton swabs may be inserted, and then twirled as they are withdrawn, in an attempt to snag the strings.
   - The cervix may be dilated with a uterine sound, and an endocervical speculum inserted to facilitate visualization of the strings; an alligator clamp may then be passed to attempt grasping the strings.
6. Visualization of the cervix with a colposcope may aid in more difficult removals.
7. When retrieval has been attempted unsuccessfully, the patient may then require having the IUD removal performed with hysteroscopy in the operating room under anesthesia.

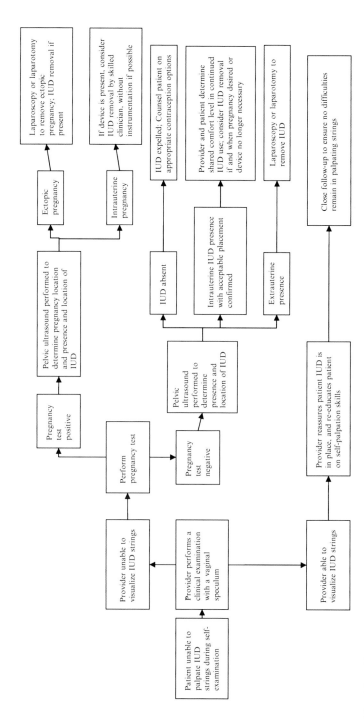

Algorithm 13-1 Decision tree for absent IUD strings. Note that some IUDs available outside the United States do not have strings

Tricks and Helpful Hints

- Advising a woman to take NSAIDs such as ibuprofen or naproxen prior to her appointment may help limit discomfort experienced during and following the procedure.
- Although less commonly utilized, specially designed instruments for IUD removal are commercially available, including the IUD hook and IUD extractor.
- It may be necessary to apply a single-toothed tenaculum to the anterior lip of the cervix in order to stabilize the cervix and uterus prior to instrumentation. Once the tenaculum has been removed, pressure can be applied to the puncture sites with a large swab to control any oozing of blood; silver nitrate or Monsel's solution can be used to treat any excessive bleeding.

Interpretation of Results

See the Algorithm 13-1, which illustrates possible options for proceeding when IUD strings are absent [4].

Procedure Note

(Provider to customize as needed.)

> *The patient was placed in the lithotomy position, a speculum was inserted into the vagina, and the cervix was identified. The IUD strings were noted to be passing through the external os. The strings were grasped with a ring forceps and gentle traction was applied. The IUD was retrieved without incident. The patient tolerated the procedure without difficulty.*

Coding

CPT® Codes (Current Procedural Terminology, AMA, Chicago, IL)
58301   Removal of intrauterine device

ICD 9-CM-Diagnostic Codes (International Classification of Diseases, 9th Revision, Clinical Modification, Center for Disease Control and Prevention)
V25.42   Surveillance of previously prescribed contraceptive methods; checking, reinsertion, or removal of intrauterine device
996.32   Mechanical complication of genitourinary device; due to intrauterine contraceptive device
996.76   Other complications of internal (biological) (synthetic) prosthetic device, implant and graft; due to genitourinary device, implant, and graft

Postprocedure Patient Instructions

The patient should be advised that she may experience mild cramping and minimal vaginal spotting and/or discharge in the first 12–24 h following removal. Although no further follow-up is usually necessary, any excessive bleeding should be reported immediately and the patient re-evaluated. Couples should be reminded of the subsequent rapid return to fertility once the apparatus has been removed [5]. In a randomized comparative study of the two currently available devices, the median time to pregnancy was 4 months for the levonorgestrel releasing intrauterine system and 3 months for the intrauterine copper contraceptive [6].

Case Study Outcome

The patient presented to the office 4 months later for removal of her IUD, as she and her husband had decided that they were now emotionally and financially prepared to conceive again. The patient's periods had remained regular, although she continued not to be able to feel her IUD strings following menstruation. Upon repeat examination, the IUD strings could still not be visualized. Attempts were made at retrieval utilizing a cytobrush and then sterile swabs, though these were both unsuccessful. Following administration of a paracervical block, the cervix was dilated with the passing of a uterine sound. Another attempt at retrieval was then made utilizing an alligator clamp, with successful identification of the strings and subsequent removal of the IUD.

Postprocedure Patient Handout

(Provider to customize as needed.)

- Today your clinician removed your intrauterine device. You may expect minimal vaginal spotting or discharge, and possibly mild abdominal cramping. You should not experience bleeding heavier than a normal period.
- If you experience heavier bleeding, foul smelling vaginal discharge, persistent abdominal pain, or fevers, please call your clinician right away.
- Abdominal cramping is usually temporary. You may wish to take three Ibuprofen 200 mg tablets every 6 h, or two acetaminophen 325 mg tablets every 4–6 h, as needed.
- As a reminder, immediately following removal of your Intrauterine Device (IUD), you are now able to get pregnant if you have vaginal sex without the use of a condom or other barrier method. In fact, the majority of women trying to conceive are able to successfully become pregnant in the first year after removal of their IUD.
- Please call the office if you have any problems or questions.

References

1. Berlex, Inc. Mirena® prescribing information. September, 2004.
2. FEI Products, LLC. ParaGard® prescribing information. September, 2005.
3. Canavan TP. Appropriate use of the intrauterine device. *Am Fam Physician* 1988;58(9):2077–2084.
4. Intrauterine device. ACOG Practice Bulletin No. 59. American College of Obstetricians and Gynecologists. *Obstet Gyenocol* 2005;105:223–232.
5. Shulman LP, Westhoff CL. Return to fertility after reversible contraception. *Dialogues Contracept* 2006;10(1):1–3.
6. Belhadj H, Silvin I, Diaz S, Pavez M, Tejada AS, Brache V, Alvarez F, Shoupe D, Breaux H, Mishell DR Jr, et al. Recovery of Fertility after use of the levonorgestrel 20 mcg/d or copper T 380 Ag intrauterine device. *Contraception* 1986;34:261–267.

Additional Resources

Web Sites

866-PARAGARD. www.paragard.com.
866-647-3646. www.mirena-us.com.

Chapter 14
Natural Family Planning

Dawn Brink-Cymerman

Introduction

Natural Family Planning (NFP) is one of the oldest practiced methods of birth control. Also known by the names Periodic Abstinence, Rhythm Method, and Fertility Awareness Method, it can be used either for pregnancy prevention or planning and is acceptable to all major religious groups. Although it is not a popular method of birth control, there are couples who still choose to practice natural family planning and may request the assistance and support of their health care provider. In motivated patients with appropriate instruction, NFP may be an effective method of preventing or spacing pregnancies. Eighty-five percent of women will get pregnant within a year of having intercourse without contraception. With perfect use, 2–5% of women who have been instructed and use the symptothermal or the ovulation method will become pregnant [1]. However, perfect use is uncommon and many women do not use NFP appropriately, or choose not to continue using this method [2].

There are several methods of NFP, including the Calendar Method, the Lactational Amenorrhea Method, the Basal Temperature Method, the Cervical Mucus Method, the Creighton Method, the Symptothermal Method, and the Standard Days Method/2 Days Method.

The Calendar Method is the original natural method and is based solely on calculation of the days of a woman's cycle. This method is based on the theory that a woman ovulates approximately 14 days prior to menses. Most women have variations of one to several days in their cycle, therefore predicting the day of menses is difficult. This is even more difficult in women with irregular cycles. Although the Calendar Method may be appropriate for women with regular cycles, additional means of assessing ovulation may be necessary for women with irregular cycles.

D. Brink-Cymerman (✉)
Assistant Professor, Department of Family Medicine, SUNY Upstate, St. Joseph's Family Medicine Residency, 4104 Medical Center Drive, Fayetteville, NY, 13066, USA
e-mail: dawn.brink-cymerman@sjhsyr.org

S.M. Sulik and C.B. Heath (eds.), *Primary Care Procedures in Women's Health*,
DOI 10.1007/978-0-387-76604-1_14, © Springer Science+Business Media, LLC 2010

The Lactational Amenorrhea Method (LAM) can be used by breastfeeding women in the postpartum period. This method should only be considered by women who are exclusively breastfeeding eight to ten times per day and at least one time during the night. This assures hormone levels remain high enough to suppress ovulation [3]. LAM should not be used after the initial 6 months postpartum as fertility can return prior to the onset of menses.

The Basal Temperature Method is based on the change in the early morning basal temperature at the time of ovulation when the cycle comes under the influence of progesterone. Intercourse is avoided from the onset of menses through the ovulation period. This lengthy period of abstinence is unacceptable to some couples. The basal body temperature rises under the influence of progesterone, with most ovulatory cycles having a lower temperature in the first half of the cycle and a higher temperature with the onset of ovulation. At the time of ovulation, the temperature usually rises by 0.4°F and remains elevated until menses. Patients should be instructed that their fertile period lasts until the temperature is elevated for at least 3 days.

The Cervical Mucus Method (also called Ovulation Method) is a method that instructs a woman to check her cervical mucus pattern on a daily basis to determine the time of ovulation. She learns to recognize patterns of mucus by sensations on the vulva and visual inspection and avoids intercourse during the ovulation period. Probabilities of pregnancy are 3.1% in the first year with perfect use and 86.4% during imperfect use. It is crucial that couples who choose this method follow some very important rules, which include no intercourse during mucus days, no intercourse during times of stress, and no intercourse within 3 days after the peak of fecundity [1].

The different types of mucus are based on glucose composition. Changes in cervical mucus occur at the beginning and end of the fertile period even in irregular cycles. Secretions should be observed by how they look, by touch, and by feel. Women chart their mucus changes in order to be aware of their fertile period. There is variation in mucus composition woman to woman, but each individual has a pattern that remains fairly stable. Ultrasound studies have confirmed that these symptoms accurately identify the timing of ovulation [4]. The World Health Organization (WHO) is interested in finding birth control methods that are inexpensive but effective for use in third-world countries. A study supported by WHO found that 93% of women were able to determine the state of the cervical mucus regardless of educational level and cultural influences [5].

The Creighton Model of birth control is a modification of the Cervical Mucus Method and was developed at the Pope Paul VI Institute by Dr. Thomas Hilgers in 1980. It was intended as a natural procreativity education method that allowed a couple to know when their fertile periods occurred. When a couple uses this method, they meet with an instructor over a period of approximately 1 year in order to accurately learn to recognize the changes in cervical mucus and body changes that indicate fertility. The vulvar mucus is observed, and intercourse is avoided during the 3 days prior to until 2 days after the peak vulvar mucus [6]. Proponents of the method quote studies that state the failure rate is less than 1% per year; however, some couples who became pregnant during the study were deliberately not counted as failures as investigators believed the couples intended pregnancy [7].

The Symptothermal Method is a combination of monitoring symptoms that indicate fertility, using the basal body temperature to assess for ovulation and using calendar calculations to assess peak fertility. In this method, women assess cervical mucus and observe symptoms of fertility, such as midcycle cramping and breast tenderness, to help determine the period prior to ovulation that they may engage in intercourse. Women also use calendar calculations to monitor fertile periods and also monitor basal body temperatures to indicate when ovulation has occurred and that they have passed through the fertile period of the menstrual cycle. By combining these methods, couples may avoid the prolonged periods of abstinence required by other NFP; however, a higher level of instruction is necessary for its appropriate use. Monitoring cervical mucus and observing symptoms of fertility such as midcycle cramping and breast tenderness aid a woman in determining the time prior to ovulation during which she may engage in intercourse without risking pregnancy. By combining symptom observation and basal body temperature monitoring, couples can avoid the prolonged period of abstinence recommended with the use of the basal body temperature method alone.

The Standard Days Method [8] is based on the probability of pregnancy and the timing of ovulation. Studies have shown that a woman's fertile period is approximately 6 days: 5 days before ovulation and for 24 hours after ovulation. After 24 hours, there is decreased probability of pregnancy. Thus, the fertile window in a woman's cycle is 6 days. Data have also shown that ovulation occurs in the middle of the cycle when the cycles last between 26 and 32 days [9]. Couples avoid intercourse on days 8–19 of every cycle to avoid pregnancy. With correct use, the failure rate is approximately 4% with actual rates that approach 9% [9]. CycleBeads® (Cycle Technologies, Inc., Washington, DC) are a color coded string of beads to help women keep track of their cycles. To use the beads, a rubber ring is moved over the beads each day of the cycle to track where she is in the cycle. The colors of the beads indicate fertile and nonfertile days.

There are many trials that look at the efficacy or failure rate of the various methods of Natural Family Planning. Advocates of the particular method report high levels of success, but trials are generally poorly done and reporting of failures of a particular method are suspect.

Case Study

A 22-year-old woman and her partner present at the office to discuss birth control. They have not been sexually active prior to this time and are planning to be married in 3 months. They would like to put off pregnancy for 1–2 years yet and would like to have a method that is consistent with their religious beliefs. In their premarital counseling sessions, there was discussion of natural family planning methods.

Diagnosis (Algorithm 14-1)

Request for natural family planning methods

Indications (Algorithm 14-1)

- Women who prefer nonhormonal contraceptive method due to religious or financial reasons.
- Women who have contraindications due to concomitant diseases or side effects to hormonal birth control.
- Women requesting immediately reversible contraception.
- Women who wish an increased awareness of their own body's hormonal cycles, including fertility and infertility.

Contraindications, Complications, and Risks (Algorithm 14-1)

- High failure rate in couples who are not highly motivated.
- Requires periods of abstinence from intercourse.
- Less effective for women with irregular menstrual cycles.
- No protection against sexually transmitted infections.
- Interference in charting the correct temperature can be caused by illness, alcohol use, travel, or interrupted sleep (at least 3 h of sleep must occur). These events should be noted on the chart.
- Monitoring of cervical mucus may be inaccurate if a vaginal infection is present, with use of douches, vaginal creams or gels, or if there is an illness or use of medication.

Equipment

- Basal body temperature thermometer (Fig. 14-1).
- Chart for temperature and recording consistency of cervical.
- Mucus and menstrual bleeding (Fig. 14-2).

Procedure and Patient Instructions (Algorithm 14-1)

Calendar Method

1. Track several menstrual cycles to determine length. (Cycle determination is based on first day of menses as Day 1 of cycle.)

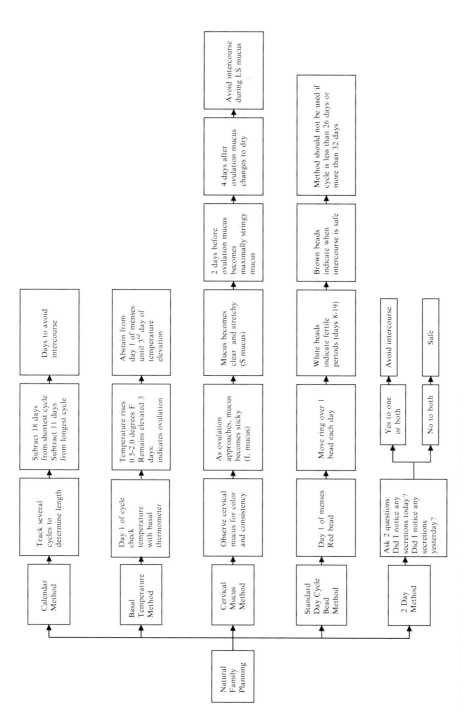

Algorithm 14-1 Decision tree for choosing a method of family planning

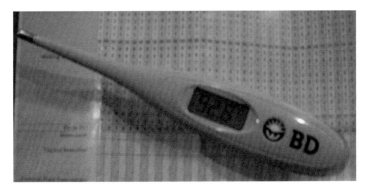

Fig. 14-1 Sample digital basal body temperature thermometer (Becton Dickinson & Co., Franklin Lakes, NJ)

2. Subtract 18 days from the shortest cycle.
3. Subtract 11 days from the longest cycle.
4. This determines the range of days to avoid intercourse.

Example:

- Month 1 cycle 30 days
- Month 2 cycle 28 days
- Month 3 cycle 32 days
- Month 4 cycle 28 days
- Woman subtracts 28 − 18 = 10
- Woman subtracts 32 − 11 = 21
- Patient would avoid intercourse between days 10 and 21.

Basal Temperature Method

1. Day 1 of cycle (menses) begins charting basal body temperature with a basal thermometer marked to detect small fluctuations in body temperature.
2. Temperature must be checked prior to getting out of bed at the same time each morning.
3. A rise in temperature of 0.5–2.0°F that remains elevated for 3 days indicates ovulation. Ovulation actually occurs just prior to the temperature elevation.
4. A true postovulatory rise lasts 10 days.
5. The period of abstinence should be from the first day of menses through the third day of temperature elevation to completely cover the fertile period.
6. Interference in charting the correct temperature can be caused by illness, alcohol use, travel, or interrupted sleep (at least 3 h of sleep must occur). These events should be noted on the chart.

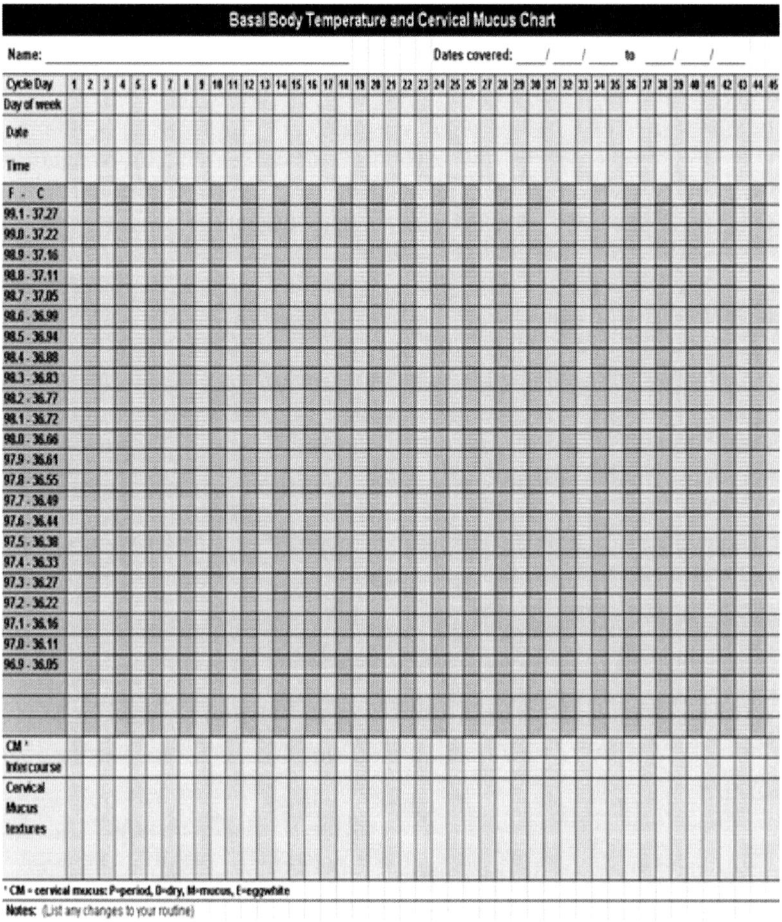

Basal Body Temperature and Cervical Mucus Chart

Name: _____   Dates covered: ___/___/___ to ___/___/___

Cycle Day	1	2	3	4	5	6	7	8	9	10	11	12	13	14	15	16	17	18	19	20	21	22	23	24	25	26	27	28	29	30	31	32	33	34	35	36	37	38	39	40	41	42	43	44	45
Day of week																																													
Date																																													
Time																																													

F - C
99.1 - 37.27
99.0 - 37.22
98.9 - 37.16
98.8 - 37.11
98.7 - 37.05
98.6 - 36.99
98.5 - 36.94
98.4 - 36.88
98.3 - 36.83
98.2 - 36.77
98.1 - 36.72
98.0 - 36.66
97.9 - 36.61
97.8 - 36.55
97.7 - 36.49
97.6 - 36.44
97.5 - 36.38
97.4 - 36.33
97.3 - 36.27
97.2 - 36.22
97.1 - 36.16
97.0 - 36.11
96.9 - 36.05

CM *
Intercourse
Cervical
Mucus
textures

* CM = cervical mucus: P=period, D=dry, M=mucus, E=eggwhite

Notes: (List any changes to your routine)

DAY 1 IS THE FIRST DAY OF MENSES.

Temperature Charting

Monitor temperature with a basal body temperature thermometer.

Take temperature at the same time each morning prior to getting out of bed or any other activity.

Plot temperature on the chart and connect with a line.

Temperature elevation of at least 0.2 degrees that remains for at least 3 days indicates ovulation.

Chart for a few months to see a pattern.

Interference in charting a correct temperature is caused by illness, alcohol use, travel, getting up during the night. Any of these variations should be noted on the chart.

Mucus Charting

Cervical mucus is charted by consistency.

Dry indicates a lack of cervical mucus (G).

Mucus is a sticky consistency that indicates ovulation is approaching (L).

Egg white consistency corresponds to a clear stretchy mucus that is present with ovulation (S and L).

Interference with cervical mucus evaluation occurs with vaginal infection, douches, vaginal creams

or gels, illness. or medications.

Fig. 14-2 Basal body temperature and cervical mucus chart

Cervical Mucus Method

1. Women should be instructed to observe their cervical mucus:
   Observe the mucus for color and consistency on undergarments or toilet paper. Highly fertile secretions are wet, slippery, clear, and stretchy. Ovulation can occur the day before, during, or after the day of the clear stretchy mucus.
2. At the end of menses: G mucus forms a plug in the cervix causing the woman to be dry or without cervical mucus discharge.
3. As ovulation approaches, G mucus decreases and L mucus increases. L mucus has a sticky, cloudy nature.
4. With increasing estrogen: S mucus increases and peaks on the day of peak estrogen during the cycle. The combination of S and L mucus causes clear, stretchy mucus that aids the survival of sperm and transport through the female genital tract.
5. Two days prior to ovulation, the stringy sensation is at a maximum.
6. Two hours prior to ovulation, the slippery sensation or wetness is at its most noticeable.
7. Four days after ovulation, the mucus pattern reverts back to dry or unchanging as the G mucus again develops under the influence of progesterone.

Monitoring of cervical mucus may be inaccurate if there is vaginal infection; use of douches, vaginal creams or gels; illness or use of medication.

The Standard Day (CycleBead® Method, Cycle Technologies, Inc., Washington, DC) (Fig. 14-3)

1. Women are considered fertile on days 8–19 of their cycle.
2. Women start on the first day of their menstrual cycle with the red bead.
3. Move the ring over one bead each day.
4. White beads indicate fertile periods.
5. Brown beads indicate non-fertile periods when intercourse is safe.
6. The dark brown bead indicates a cycle shorter than 26 days, and this method should not be used.
7. If the menses does not start by the end of the brown beads, the cycle is longer than 32 days, and this method should not be used.

2 Day Method

- Uses cervical secretions to determine fertility.
- Patient asks herself two questions:
  "Did I notice any secretions today?"
  "Did I notice any secretions yesterday?"

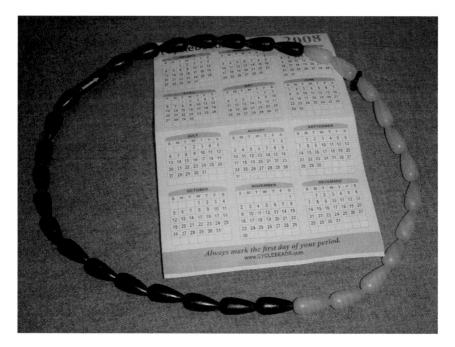

Fig. 14-3 CycleBeads® (Cycle Technologies, Inc., Washington, DC)

- If patient noticed secretions, either day she is potentially fertile and should avoid intercourse.
- If the answer is no to both questions, the probability of pregnancy is low and intercourse is safe.

Fertility rates are similar to the Standard Day Method.

Procedure Note

(Provider to customize as needed.)

> *The patient and her partner were counseled on the different methods of Natural Family Planning and made aware of the advantages and disadvantages of each, including the risk of pregnancy. The patient was instructed to chart her menstrual bleeding and symptoms throughout the month and to bring the chart with her to future visits so that the chart could be evaluated with the patient to aid in understanding of cyclic periods of fertility. The patient and partner will decide whether or not they want to include basal temperature monitoring as a part of their daily monitoring. They are encouraged to hire a natural family planning coach to give further instruction and training in the method they choose.*

Coding

CPT® Codes (Current Procedural Terminology, AMA, Chicago, IL)
Preventive Medicine Counseling:
99401-15 min
99402-30 min
99403-45 min
99404-60 min

ICD 9-CM-Diagnostic Codes (International Classification of Diseases, 9th Revision, Clinical Modification, Center for Disease Control and Prevention)
V25.09   Family Planning Advice

Case Study Outcome

After 1 year of use of Natural Family Planning, the couple continues to be satisfied with their choice of birth planning method. The patient has discontinued the use of basal temperature as her comfort level with the use of cervical mucus to determine that fertility has increased. She also considers it an added benefit that she has increased understanding of her fertility cycles and will be able to use that information to her advantage when she does desire pregnancy.

References

1. Jennings VH, Arevalo, M, Kowal D. Fertility awareness-based methods. In Hatcher RA (ed) *Contraceptive technology, 18th revised edition.* New York: Ardent Media, 2004;317–329.
2. Grimes DA, Gallo MF, Grigorieva V, Nanda K, Schulz K. Fertility awareness-based methods for contraception: systematic review of randomized controlled trials. *Contraception* 2005;72:85–90.
3. Tommaselli GA, Guida M, Palomba S, Barbato M, Nappi C. Using complete breastfeeding and lactational amenorrhoea as birth spacing methods. *Contraception* 2000;61(4):253–257.
4. Frank-Herrmann P, Gnoth C, Baur S, Strowitzki T, Freundl G. Determination of the fertile window: reproductive competence of women – European cycle databases. *Gynecol Endocrinol* 2005;20(6):305–312.
5. Ryder RE. Natural family planning: effective birth control supported by the Catholic Church. *BMJ* 1993;307:723–776.
6. Stanford JB, Smith KR, Dunson DB. Vulvar mucus observations and the probability of pregnancy. *Obstet Gynecol* 2003;101(6):1285–1293.
7. Hilgers TW, Stanford JB. Creighton Model NaProEducation Technology for avoiding pregnancy. Use effectiveness. *J Reprod Med* 1998;43:495–501.
8. Germano E, Jennings V. New approaches to fertility awareness based-methods: incorporating the standard days and 2Day methods into practice. *J Midwifery Womens Health* 2006;51:471–477.
9. Trussell J, Grummer-Strawn L. Contraceptive failure of the ovulation method of periodic abstinence. *Fam Plann Perspect* 1990;22(2):65–75.

Additional Resources

Articles

Bulletin of Ovulation Method Research and Reference Centre of Australia. Vol 29, No1, pp2–11.
Trussell J, Grummer-Strawn L. Further analysis of contraceptive failure of the ovulation method. *Am J Obstet Gynecol* 1991;165:2054–2059.
Wade ME, McCarthy P, Braunstein GD, Abernathy JR, Suchindran CM, Harris GS, Danzer HC, Uricchio WA. A randomized prospective study of the use-effectiveness of two methods of natural family planning. *Am J Obstet Gynecol* 1981;15:368–376.

Web Sites

Couple to Couple League: htpp://www.ccli.org/.
An in depth explanation of the method and assistance in finding an instructor can be found at the web site: www.CreightonModel.com.
www.irh.org/resources-SymptothermalMethod.htm.

Chapter 15
Implanon®*: Insertion and Removal

Jeffrey P. Levine

Introduction

The etonogestrel implant, Implanon® is a sterile 4-cm×2-mm single rod that is implanted subdermally and can provide up to 3 years of continuous effective contraception. Each rod contains 68 mg of the progestin etonogestrel encased in an ethylene vinylacetate copolymer skin [1]. It is supplied in a sterile, preloaded disposable applicator. The applicator greatly facilitates proper insertion in a superficial plane, reduces the risk of infection via contamination of the sterile rod, and allows insertion without the need for incision and concomitant risk of scarring. Implanon® was approved by the US Food and Drug Administration in July 2006, but has already been used by over 5 million women worldwide.

Implanon® is indicated for any woman of reproductive age seeking rapid, long-lasting (up to 3 years), safe, and highly effective contraception. Once inserted, the etonogestrel implant offers excellent patient convenience since its effectiveness is not user-dependent [2]. The implant can be removed at any time, with a rapid return to fertility. In particular, Implanon® is a consideration for patients who cannot use estrogen (e.g., smokers >35 years old [3]), and those willing to tolerate irregular menses, possibly for the full duration of use. Implanon® does not protect against sexually transmitted infections (STIs) and has not been evaluated in patients > 130% of their ideal body weight [1].

The etonogestrel implant is a highly effective contraceptive, with a Pearl Index of 0.38 per 100 women-years of use. However, efficacy depends on proper insertion. It has happened, rarely, that the implant has fallen from the needle or remained in the needle during insertion. Expulsion may also occur if the full length of the

---

*Implanon® is a registered trademark of Schering-Plough (Merck & Co., Inc., Whitehouse Station, NJ).

J.P. Levine (✉)
Department of Family Medicine, University of Medicine and Dentistry of New Jersey,
Robert Wood Johnson Medical School, 1 Robert Wood Johnson Place,
CN19, New Brunswick, NJ, 08903-0019, USA
e-mail: levinejp@umdnj.edu

needle is not inserted when placing the implant. Failure to insert the implant completely and correctly can lead to unintended pregnancy. Too deep an insertion can hinder removal, and failure to remove the implant within the recommended time period can result in an unintended pregnancy.

Complications at the implant site occurred among 3.6% of patients at any assessment during clinical trials, including during 1% of insertions and 1.7% of removals [1]. There has been one report of inability to remove the implant because it was inserted intravascularly. If infection at the implant site does not respond to appropriate treatment, the implant should be removed. In rare cases, injury to branches of the medial antebrachial cutaneous nerve has occurred during insertion or removal, the risk of which can be minimized by proper training and understanding of the position of these nerves [4].

Bleeding irregularities are the most common adverse events contributing to the discontinuation of use in clinical trials (11%) [1]. When compared with the six-capsule levonorgestrel implant Norplant® (Population Council, New York, NY) (currently no longer on the market), Implanon® had the same rate of bleeding, but the variability of the bleeding was higher with Implanon®. After 2 years of use, amenorrhea rate was higher with Implanon® than with Norplant® [5]. Less common reasons for discontinuation (<3%) include emotional lability, weight gain, headache, acne, and depression but none of these side effects were found to be significantly increased in clinical trials of Implanon®.

Patients who want to consider Implanon® should first undergo a thorough history and physical examination, including a gynecologic examination. They should be informed of both the risks and benefits of this form of contraception compared with other alternatives. The practitioner should document the counseling and patient consent process, and can provide a copy of the Patient Labeling to the patient for reference.

Appropriate timing of Implanon insertion is based on the patient's current contraceptive method and recent history of pregnancy, miscarriage, abortion, or postpartum breastfeeding status (Table 15-1). Ideally, the implant should be inserted within the first 5 days of menses. Patients who have the implant inserted at any other time during their menstrual cycle should first have a pregnancy test and use additional contraception for the first week. Implanon® can be inserted immediately after miscarriage, first-trimester abortion, or switching from another contraceptive method. It can also be inserted 3–4 weeks after second-trimester abortion or pregnancy (if not exclusively breastfeeding). Nursing mothers may safely use Implanon® any time after the fourth week postpartum; earlier use has not been studied.

Implanon® must be removed within 3 years of insertion. Before beginning the removal procedure, determine whether the patient wants to continue contraception with another implant, which can be inserted in the same location, immediately upon removal of the current implant. If the patient does not want to continue using the contraceptive implant and does not wish to become pregnant, alternative methods of contraception should be discussed and initiated. It should be emphasized to the

Table 15-1 Selecting the appropriate time for Implanon® insertion (If inserting according to times recommended here, no backup contraception is needed. However, insertion may be made at other times if pregnancy is first excluded and patient is advised to use backup contraception during the first week after insertion [1])

Patient's recent history	Date of insertion
No preceding hormonal contraceptive use in past month	Count 1st day of menstruation as Day 1. Insert between days 1 and 5, even if still menstruating.
Switching from a combination hormonal contraceptive	Insert: Anytime within 7 days after last active oral contraception tablet. Anytime during 7-day ring-free period of NuvaRing®. Anytime during 7-day Ortho-Evra® patch-free period of transdermal contraceptive system.
Switching from progestin-only method	Insert: On any day of the month when switching from progestin-only pill; do not skip any days between last pill and insertion. On same day as contraceptive implant removal. On same day as removal of progestin-containing IUD. On day when next contraceptive injection would be due.
Following first trimester abortion or miscarriage	Insert immediately following complete first trimester abortion. If insertion does not occur within 5 days following first trimester abortion, follow instructions under "No preceding hormonal contraceptive use in past month."
Following delivery or second trimester abortion	Insert 21–28 days postpartum, if not exclusively breastfeeding, or between 21 and 28 days following second trimester abortion. If more than 4 weeks have passed, pregnancy should be excluded and nonhormonal method of birth control should be used during first 7 days after insertion. If exclusively breastfeeding, insertion should take place after fourth postpartum week.

NuvaRing® (N.V. Organon, Merck & Co., Inc., Whitehouse Station, NJ)
Ortho Evra® (Ortho-McNeil-Janssen Pharmaceuticals, Titusville, NJ)
Adapted with acknowledgement to Merck & Co., Inc., and N.V. Organon. Implanon is a registered trademark of N.V. Organon

patient that her fertility will rapidly return following removal, and she should assume she can become pregnant immediately after removal.

A meta-analysis of six open studies and seven comparative trials found that insertion (average time: 1.1 min) and removal (average time: 2.6 min) procedures were four times faster with the single-rod etonogestrel implant versus the six-capsule levonorgestrel implant. The authors also concluded that "complications with insertion and removal are rare in the hands of medical professionals familiar with the techniques" [6]. Indeed, infection, expulsion, and local reactions are rare, especially when insertion is properly performed using the preloaded applicator.

This chapter describes the recommended Implanon® insertion and removal techniques. However, clinicians must actively participate in a formal live training program before performing insertion and removal in actual patients. In addition, they should review the insertion and removal instructions and package insert information prior to each related patient visit.

Case Study

A 35-year-old female, G3P3003, comes to your office for a routine gynecologic exam. She is in a monogamous relationship with her husband, with no history of STIs. They use condoms as their only method of contraception, but she admits that they are not consistent with using them. She has smoked cigarettes (~1 ppd) for the past 12 years and is not ready to quit. She has three daughters and is not planning to have more children in the next year. She has no complaints and denies any chronic medical problems. Her physical exam is completely normal.

Indications (Algorithm 15-1)

- Any women desiring reversible contraception.
- Smoking women over age 35 who desire reversible contraception.
- Women who desire contraception but cannot utilize estrogen.

Contraindications

Implanon® is contraindicated in patients with:

- Known or suspected pregnancy
- Current or past history of thrombotic disease
- Hepatic tumors, active liver disease
- Undiagnosed abnormal genital bleeding
- Known, suspected, or history of breast cancer
- Hypersensitivity to any of the components of Implanon®

Equipment (Fig. 15-1)

Before beginning, assemble everything needed for the insertion procedure. In addition to the blister pack containing the implant in its applicator, you will need:

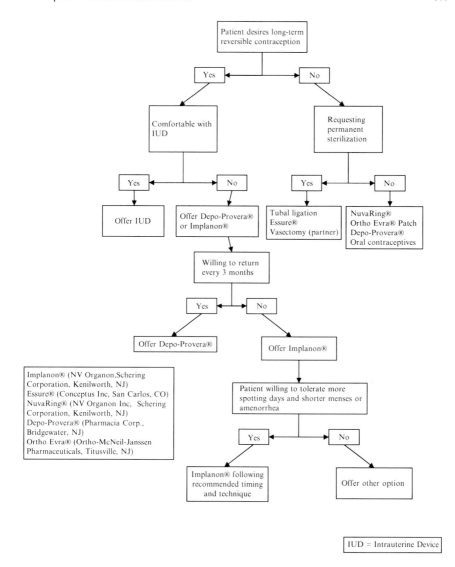

Algorithm 15-1 Decision Tree for Choosing Implantable Contraception

- Sterile gloves
- Antiseptic solution
- Local anesthetic (preferably 1% lidocaine)
- Needles (preferably 1.5 in. 25-gauge)
- Syringe (preferably 3 cc)
- Antiseptic solution

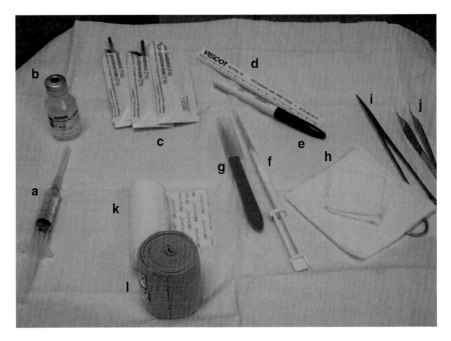

Fig. 15-1 Equipment list for insertion of Implanon®: (a) 5cc syringe; (b) Anesthetic lidocaine; (c) PDI® Povidone-iodine swabsticks (Orangeburg, NY); (d) ruler (Viscot Industries, East Hanover, NJ) enclosed with Implanon® kit; (e) Skin marker (Viscot Industries, East Hanover, NJ) enclosed with Implanon® kit; (f) Implanon® in applicator; (g) #11 blade surgical scalpel; (h) Cotton gauze 2×2 cm, 4×4 cm; (i) Hemostat; (j) Pick-ups; (k) Steri Strips™ (3M, St. Paul, MN); (l) Bandage for arm

- Surgical scalpel (preferably #11 or #15 blade)
- Sterile gauze (4×4 cm)
- Adhesive bandage or Steri Strips™
- Pressure bandage
- A sterile marker with tape measure (optional)
- Sterile gloves

At the time of insertion, it is important to confirm that the patient is not pregnant and does not have allergies to etonogestrel or the antiseptic or anesthetic [1].

Procedure

1. Schedule patient at the appropriate time for insertion (Table 15-1).
2. Obtain consent and perform urine pregnancy test.
3. Place patient in supine position on the exam table with her nondominant arm rotated externally so that her elbow is flexed and her wrist is parallel to her ear, alongside her head.

4. Identify the insertion site at the inner side of the upper, nondominant arm approximately 8–10 cm (3 to 4 inches) above the medial epicondyle of the humerus (Fig. 15-2a):
   • Use a sterile marker to make a dot where the implant will be inserted and then another about 2.5–3 in. proximal to the first, which serves as a direction guide (Fig. 15-2b).
5. Use antiseptic solution to clean the insertion site and then anesthetize the area, preferably with 1% lidocaine (epinephrine is not necessary), along the insertion track before beginning (≤1.0 cc should be sufficient) (Figs. 15-3 and 15-4).

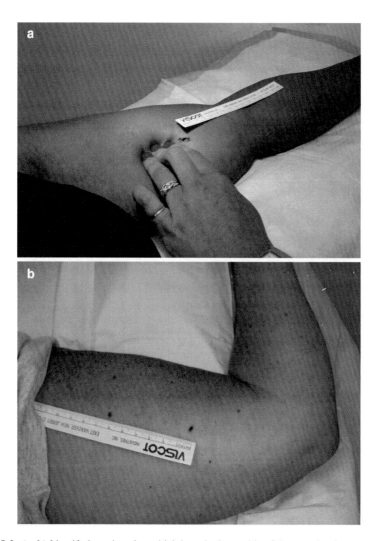

Fig. 15-2 (**a, b**) Identify insertion site, which is at the inner side of the non-dominant upper arm about 8–10 cm (3 to 4 inches) above the medial epicondyle of the humerus

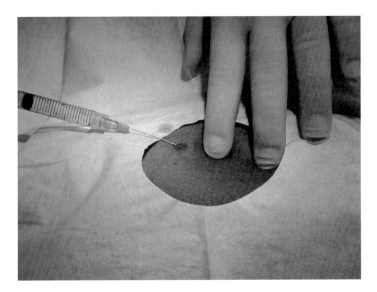

Fig. 15-3 Raise a wheal of anesthesia

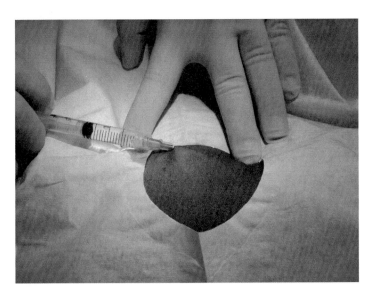

Fig. 15-4 Inject anesthesia along the insertion site

- It may be helpful to mark also the area where the anesthetic is injected so that the anesthetized area can easily be identified during the procedure.
6. Take the applicator from the blister pack and, without removing the shield, confirm that the implant rod (a white cylinder) is inside the tip of the needle (Fig. 15-5). If you do not see it, tap the needle shield against a firm sterile surface until the rod slides into the needle.

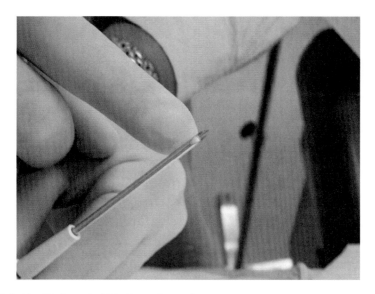

Fig. 15-5   Identify the rod within the applicator tip

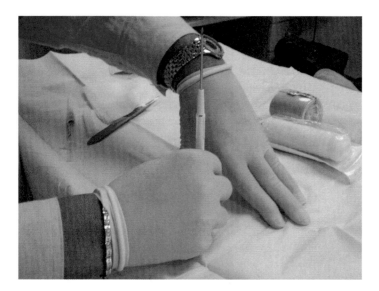

Fig. 15-6   Tap the rod back into the applicator

- Once you have confirmed the presence of the rod, lower it back into place by tapping the obturator against a firm surface until the rod returns down into the needle tip (Fig. 15-6).
  - Holding the applicator upright to avoid having the rod fall out of the needle, remove the needle shield. Make sure that the needle and rod remain sterile.

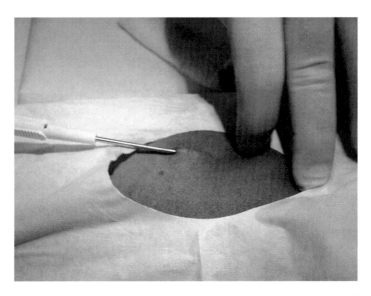

Fig. 15-7 Insert the applicator through the incision and tent up the skin to place intradermally.

7. Applying counter-traction to the skin around the site, insert only the tip of the needle with the beveled side up at a slight ($\leq 20°$) angle. Alternatively, a small nick in the skin can be made with the scalpel, then insert the tip of the needle thru the skin opening.
   - Next, lower the applicator until it is horizontal.
   - "Tent" the skin by lifting it with the tip of the needle, while still maintaining the needle in the subdermal connective tissue (Fig. 15-7).
   - In this position, gently and fully insert the entire needle, keeping it parallel to the skin surface in the superficial layer between the dermis and subdermal fat tissue [1].
8. Press the obturator support to break the applicator seal and turn the obturator 90° clockwise or counterclockwise (Fig. 15-8).
   - Keeping the obturator still, fully retract the cannula. The obturator keeps the implant in place within the needle while you retract the cannula and needle.
   - ***The obturator should <u>not</u> be pushed or retracted from the patient's arm at the same time as the cannula.*** Note that this insertion procedure is the reverse of that used for an injection but similar to that used in placing a copper intrauterine device.
9. When this procedure is performed as described, the rod will be left in the correct position.
10. After insertion, check that the white grooved tip of the obturator is visible inside the needle tip to confirm that the rod is no longer in the needle (Fig. 15-9).
11. Palpate the patient's arm immediately after insertion to verify the presence of both ends of the rod and, after covering the site with a small adhesive bandage, have the patient palpate the rod also (Fig. 15-10).

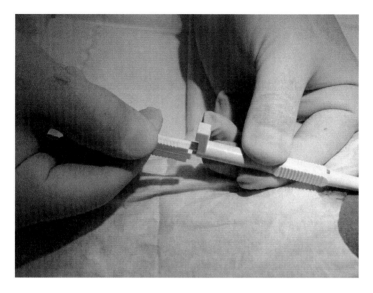

Fig. 15-8 Once completely inserted, break the obturator seal and rotate 90° in either direction

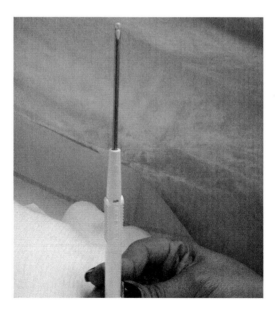

Fig. 15-9 Check the tip of the obturator to ensure that the rod has left the applicator and is present in the patient's arm and not still in the applicator

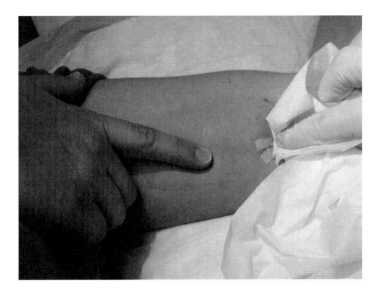

Fig. 15-10 Palpate the rod in place and have the patient palpate the rod as well

12. Once the presence of the rod has been confirmed, apply a pressure bandage with sterile gauze to reduce the risk of bruising. Instruct the patient to keep the top bandage on for 24 h, and the small bandage on for 3–5 days. Use acetaminophen if analgesics are needed [1].
13. Provide the patient with the completed User Card and affix the completed Patient Chart Label to the patient's records.
14. Dispose of the applicator in accordance with CDC guidelines for hazardous waste.

Removal Technique [6]

Use the same patient position and aseptic conditions for removal as for insertion.

Equipment for Removal

- A sterile scalpel (#11 blade preferred)
- Forceps (Kelly curved or mosquito clamps)
- Skin closure (Steri Strips™ (3M, St. Paul, MN)/butterfly closures)
- Antiseptic solution
- 3 cc syringe
- 25 gauge needle
- 1% Lidocaine
- Sterile gauze (4×4 cm)
- Sterile gloves
- Pressure bandage

Procedure for Removal

1. Check the patient's User Card or the Patient Chart Label to confirm which arm contains the implant and then locate the rod by palpation.
2. Wash the arm and apply antiseptic.
3. Mark the end of the rod closest to the elbow (distal end) with a sterile marker.
   • The incision for implant removal is performed at the same site/end as the insertion.
4. Anesthetize the arm where the incision will be made, with a very small amount of anesthetic; ≤ 0.5 cc should be sufficient as injecting more lidocaine may interfere with localizing the distal rod tip. Be sure to inject the anesthetic beneath the contraceptive rod to keep it close to the surface of the skin [1].
5. At the end of the implant closest to the elbow, make a 2–3 mm longitudinal incision (Fig. 15-11), and then gently push the implant toward the incision until you can see the tip (Fig. 15-12). Any fibrous sheath can be removed by blunt dissection. If the rod is encapsulated, make an incision into the tissue sheath before removing the rod.
6. Use forceps at the distal tip to pull the implant out gently (Fig. 15-13). After pushing the implant toward the initial incision, if the tip is still not visible, but is able to be grasped, it may be necessary to dissect the tissue around it (e.g., with a #15 blade or a curved forceps).
7. Gently insert the forceps into the incision to grasp the implant and then turn the forceps around, gently bending the rod. Use a second forceps to dissect the tissue around it and grasp the other end to complete the removal (Fig. 15-14).

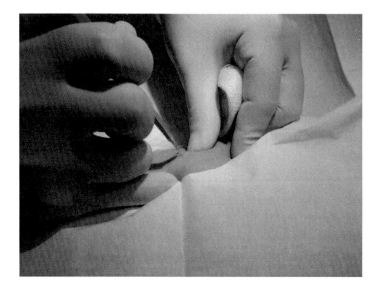

Fig. 15-11 Make a small incision at the base of the inserted rod

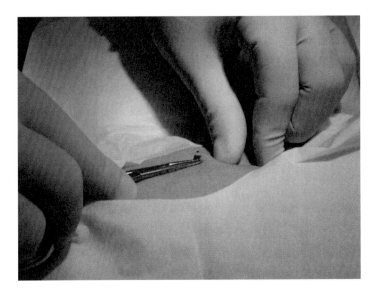

Fig. 15-12 Locate the rod and push the rod towards the incision site

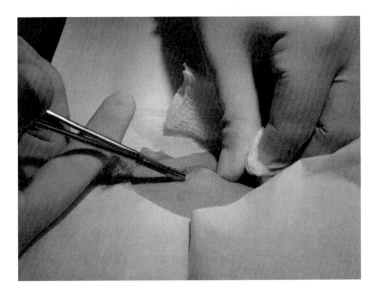

Fig. 15-13 Grasp the rod with curved forceps and pull toward the incision

8. Measure the rod to be sure that all of it (4 cm) has been removed.
9. Bandage with Steri Strips™ (3M, St. Paul, MN) (Fig. 15-15).
10. If the patient has chosen to continue Implanon®, the preferred method is to insert a new rod in the same location, using the same incision. Another option is to perform a new insertion into the other arm.

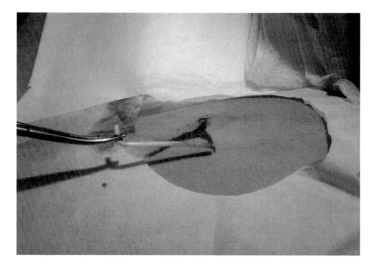

Fig. 15-14 Grasp the rod and pull out

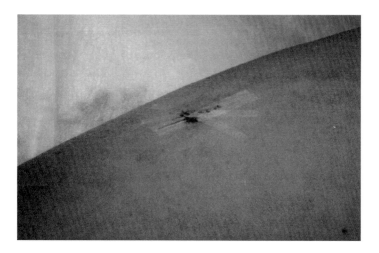

Fig. 15-15 Apply Steri Strips™ (3M, St. Paul, MN) to the insertion or removal site after completion of the procedure

11. Use a skin closure (butterfly/Steri Strips™) to close the incision and cover it with a pressure dressing using sterile gauze. Instruct the patient to keep the site clean, dry, and covered with the bandage for 3–5 days to reduce the risk of infection [1] (Fig. 15-15).

Complications and Risks

Implantation Site

- Failure to insert the implant: Undetected failure to insert rod, 1% occurrence, may lead to unintended pregnancy.
- Pain
- Redness
- Paresthesias
- Bleeding
- Hematoma
- Scarring
- Infection

Removal

- Difficult removal: Deep insertion may lead to difficult or impossible removals, which require a surgical procedure in the operating room. Deep insertion may cause nerve or vascular damage or migration of the rod.
- Breakage of implant during removal: May necessitate surgical removal.

Causes for Discontinuation

- Bleeding (most common: accounts for 11% discontinuation rate)
- Emotional liability (<3%)
- Depression (<3%)
- Weight gain (<3%)
- Headache (<3%)
- Acne (<3%)

Tricks and Helpful Hints

1. Patients should be reassured that the single-rod etonogestrel implant (Implanon®) is easier and requires less time to insert and remove than the six-capsule levonorgestrel implants (Norplant®), which are no longer marketed in the United States [7, 8].
2. If the 4-cm rod is not palpable after insertion or before removal, its presence should be verified using ultrasound with a ≥10 MHz linear array transducer [9].

Note that most gynecologic ultrasound transducers are <10 MHz and will not visualize the rod. In rare cases, when the implant cannot be visualized on ultrasound, Magnetic Resonance Imaging (MRI) may be utilized [9]. The rod is not radio opaque; therefore, it is not visible on x-ray or computed tomography (CT) scan. Ultrasound can also be used to conduct difficult removals. If no rod is visible on ultrasound or MRI, contact the manufacturer at 877-467-5266 (877-IMPLANON) for specific instructions on obtaining an etonogestrel level (not available in the United States) [1].

Procedure Note

(Provider to fill in blanks/circle applicable choice when given multiple choices and customize as needed.)

Insertion

Age: _____ G: _____ P: _____ LMP: _____ ; Urine Pregnancy: +/-
BP_____ Pulse _____ Weight _____
Current Contraceptive Method: _____
Date of Last Delivery/Termination: _____; Breastfeeding: Y/N
    Informed Consent for Implanon® insertion (consent form provided with each device) has been signed and all questions answered. Patient has no contraindications to this method. She desires long-term protection against pregnancy. Patient has no pregnancy or risk of pregnancy at the time of insertion. She has a documented Pap smear/clinical breast exam within past 12 months. Patient counseled about potential benefits, risks, side effects, and complications. Patient has no allergy to lidocaine, betadine, or tape.
Plans for backup contraception if needed:_____
Implanon® Lot #: _____ Expiration date: _____
    The ventromedial surface of _____ arm was cleansed with antiseptic solution and a sterile field created. Lidocaine 1% _____ mL with/without epinephrine was injected intradermally into the planned insertion site, 8–10 cm above medial epicondyle of the humerus. The implant was inserted according to the Implanon® system protocol. Both provider and patient were able to palpate the implant at the end of the procedure. Steri-strips™ (3M, St. Paul, MN) and compression dressing applied to insertion site. Complications: None/_____

_____

_____

Postinsertion

Patient aware of the need for backup method for 1 week if not inserted cycle day less than day 5. Patient Labeling/Education booklet (provided with each device) given to client.
Follow-up appointment: _____
Patient advised to call ASAP if any symptoms/signs of infection.
Patient aware Implanon® must be removed on or before://
Signature/Title:_____Date:_____

Removal

Age:_____ BP_____ Pulse _____ Weight _____
Consent for Implanon® removal has been signed and all questions answered.
Reason for contraceptive implant removal: _____
Plans for contraception after removal: _____
Implanon® Lot #: _____ Expiration date: _____
The ventromedial surface of _____ arm was cleansed with antiseptic
solution and a sterile field created. Lidocaine 1% _____ mL with/without
epinephrine was injected intradermally into the planned removal site. The implant was
removed completely according to the Implanon® system protocol. Patient was shown
removed implant. Steri-strips™ and compression dressing applied to insertion site.
   Removal Time: _____
   Complications: None/_____

_____

Postremoval

Contraceptive method
prescribed:_____
Follow-up appointment: _____
Patient advised to call ASAP if any symptoms/signs of infection.
Signature/Title:_____Date:_____

Coding

CPT® Codes (Current Procedural Terminology, AMA, Chicago, IL)
11981	Insertion of non-biodegradable drug delivery implant
11982	Removal of non-biodegradable drug delivery implant
11983	Removal with reinsertion of non-biodegradable drug delivery implant
Or	
11975	Insertion, implantable contraceptive capsules
11976	Removal, implantable contraceptive capsules
11977	Removal with reinsertion of implantable contraceptive capsules

ICD 9-CM-Diagnostic Codes (International Classification of Diseases, 9th Revision, Clinical Modification, Center for Disease Control and Prevention)

V25.5   Encounter for contraception management, insertion of
        implantable subdermal contraceptive
V25.43 Encounter for contraceptive management, surveillance of previously
        prescribed contraceptive methods (checking, reinsertion or removal
        of contraceptive device), implantable subdermal contraceptive

Postprocedure Patient Instructions

Patient labeling/education booklet is provided with each device.

Insertion

- Inform the patient of the need for backup method for 1 week if not inserted cycle day less than day 5 of menses.
- Advise the patient to call ASAP if any symptoms/signs of infection.
- Ensure that the patient is aware that the Implanon® must be removed on or before 3 years from the insertion date.
- Counsel patient to expect changes in their bleeding patterns that may be unpredictable and include: changes in bleeding frequency, duration, and/or amenorrhea. Patients with persistent bleeding should be seen to rule out pregnancy or pathologic conditions.

Removal

- Advise patient to call if any symptoms/signs of infection.
- Discuss other contraception needs or preconception counseling.

Case Study Outcome

Given the patient's desire for long-term, reversible, non-daily contraception, and fact that she is a 35-year-old 1 ppd smoker, she was recommended Implanon®, Depo-Provera®, or an intrauterine device. Given her previous satisfaction with Norplant®, she opted for Implanon®. The Implanon® was inserted without difficulty. The patient returned the following year after Implanon® insertion for a recheck visit. She reports some occasional spotting but no other complaints. She is extremely satisfied with the method and has not smoked in over 3 months.

Patient Handout[1]

The contraceptive implant (Implanon®) is a very effective, convenient, and safe form of contraception. A small operation under local anesthetic is needed to insert the implant under the skin. Each implant lasts 3 years.

What Is Implanon®?

Implanon® is a contraceptive implant, a small flexible rod that is inserted under the skin. It contains a progestin hormone. Implanon® lasts for up to 3 years. It is 99% effective.

How Does the Implanon® Work?

The progestin hormone in the implant is released slowly into the bloodstream at a steady rate. The progestin works mainly by stopping ovulation (the release of the egg from the ovary). It also thickens the mucus made by the cervix which forms a "mucus plug" in the cervix. This stops sperm getting through to the uterus (womb) to fertilize an egg. It also makes the lining of the uterus thinner. This means that if an egg was to fertilize, it is not likely to be able to attach to the uterus.

How Effective Is Implanon®?

Implanon® is more than 99% effective. This means that less than 1 woman in 100 who uses this method of contraception will become pregnant each year. (Compare this to when no contraception is used. More than 80 in 100 sexually active women who do not use contraception become pregnant within 1 year.)

What Are the Potential Advantages of Using Implanon®?

- You do not have to remember to take a pill every day.
- You only have to think about contraception every 3 years.
- It does not interfere with sex.
- It can be used when breastfeeding.
- Period pain is usually less than usual.
- It stops ovulation and thickens cervical mucus.

---

[1] This section (Patient Handout) is adapted with acknowledgement to Merck & Co., Inc. Implanon is a registered trademark of N.V. Organon.

- It can be used by some women who cannot take pills that contain estrogen.
- It may help protect against Pelvic Inflammatory Disease (PID). (The mucus plug in the cervix may help to prevent bacteria from traveling into the uterus.)

What Are the Potential Disadvantages of Using Implanon®?

The release of progestin will usually cause changes to the pattern of periods. During the first year, it is common to have irregular bleeding. Sometimes periods are heavier and longer than before. They usually settle back into a regular pattern after the first year, but may remain irregular. In some women, the periods become infrequent and light, or even stop altogether.

Some women worry about irregular or changed periods, but it does not mean anything is wrong and is of no consequence. However, unpredictable or irregular periods can be a nuisance.

Who Cannot Use Implanon®?

Your health care provider will discuss any current and past illnesses. Some illnesses may mean that you cannot use progestin-based contraceptives such as Implanon®. However, the number of women this affects is small.

Are There Any Potential Side Effects with Implanon®?

Some women report side effects such as mood changes, breast discomfort, fluid retention, weight gain, headaches, and increase in acne. These are uncommon, and, if they do occur, they tend to develop in the first few months only, and often resolve after 3–6 months if the implant remains. The area around the implant may be bruised and sore for a few days. You can apply an ice pack to the area and/or take some ibuprofen or acetaminophen to help the discomfort.

How Is the Implant Put Under the Skin?

- It is put in the inner side of the upper arm.
- It is usually first inserted within 5 days of a period starting. (This ensures that you are not pregnant.) It is effective from then on.
- An injection of local anesthetic is used to numb the skin. A small cut is made and the implant is placed under the skin. The wound is dressed and will soon heal just like any other small cut.

- The area around the implant may be bruised and sore for a few days, but this soon goes away.

When Is the Implant Taken Out?

The implant is usually removed at the end of 3 years, but may be removed sooner by patient request.

A replacement rod can be reinserted at the time of removal if so desired.

Once removed, the rod loses its effect immediately and another form of contraception should be used if pregnancy is not desired.

Further Information

Your health care provider and pharmacist are good sources of information if you have any questions. You may also call: 1-877-IMPLANON (1-877-467-5266) or visit www.IMPLANON-USA.com

References

1. Implanon® package insert. Organon USA Inc; Roseland, NJ; July 2006.
2. Levine JP. Nondaily hormonal contraception: establishing a fit between product characteristics and patient preferences. *J Fam Pract* 2004;53(11):904–913.
3. Amer College of Obstetricians and Gynecologists. ACOG Practice Bulletin No 73. *Obstet Gynecol* 2006;107:1453–1472.
4. Wechselberger G, Wolfram D, Pulzl P, Soelder E, Schoeller T. Nerve injury caused by removal of an implantable hormonal contraceptive. *Am J Obstet Gynecol* 2006;195(1):323–326.
5. Power J, French R, Cowan F. Subdermal implantable contraceptives versus other forms of reversible contraceptives or other implants as effective methods of preventing pregnancy. *Cochrane Database Syst Rev* 2007;(3):CD001326.
6. Mascarenhas L. Insertion and removal of Implanon®. *Contraception* 1998;58(6 suppl):79S–83S.
7. Klavon SL, Grubb GS. Insertion site complications during the first year of Norplant® use. *Contraception* 1990;41(1):27–37.
8. Dunson TR, Amatya RN, Krueger SL. Complications and risk factors associated with the removal of Norplant® implants. *Obstet Gynecol* 1995;85(4):543–548.
9. Shulman LP, Gabriel H. Management and localization strategies for the nonpalpable implanon® rod. *Contraception* 2006;73(4):325–330.

Additional Resources

Articles

Levine JP. Insertion and removal of the single-rod progestin-only contraceptive implant. *Female Patient* 2006;suppl:26–30.

Web Sites

Information about insertion and removal of Implanon® is available from the manufacturer by contacting Organon USA Inc at 1-877-467-5266 or www.implanon-usa.com.

Chapter 16
Pessary

Catherine I. Keating

Introduction

A pessary is a device that allows for nonsurgical treatment of pelvic organ prolapse and/or stress urinary incontinence. One of the oldest known medical devices, the pessary dates back to Hippocrates' pessary design: a pomegranate soaked in vinegar. Other historical pessaries include other fruits, items of bronze, cotton wool, linen, wax-coated cork and wood, and rubber [1]. Today, the pessary is made of latex or silicone in many different styles. There are two main types of pessaries: space filling and support.

Indications for pessary use include uterine or vaginal prolapse, cystocele, rectocele, enterocele, and stress urinary incontinence. Less common indications include incompetent cervix and the correction of a retroverted or incarcerated uterus. For the surgeon, the pessary can also be used for preoperative selection of patients with stress incontinence – correction of incontinence with the pessary can predict good postoperative correction of incontinence – or to allow for healing of prolapsed pelvic mucosa before surgery. The pessary was originally indicated for pregnant women, those wishing to have more children, or those who had contraindications to surgery. Today, however, a pessary is an excellent option for anyone who prefers nonsurgical treatment of their condition [2]. A woman's lifetime risk of undergoing surgery for urinary incontinence and/or prolapse by age 80 is 11.1% [3]. Comparison of patient satisfaction between pessaries and pelvic reconstructive surgery in women with pelvic organ prolapse has not been reported [4].

One-third of premenopausal women and up to 45% of postmenopausal women experience pelvic organ prolapse and/or urinary incontinence [5]. Different pessary styles are appropriate for different degrees, or stages, of prolapse. The pelvic organ Prolapse Quantification (POP-Q) defines Stage 1 as descent of the uterine

C.I. Keating (✉)
Family Health Network of Central New York, 17 Main St. Cortland, NY 13045, USA
e-mail: ckeating@familyhealthnetwork.org

S.M. Sulik and C.B. Heath (eds.), *Primary Care Procedures in Women's Health*,
DOI 10.1007/978-0-387-76604-1_16, © Springer Science+Business Media, LLC 2010

cervix to above 2 cm from the hymen, Stage 2 as descent to within 1 cm of the hymen, either externally or internally, and Stage 3 as descent beyond 2 cm below the hymen (Fig. 16-1) [6]. Reported successful use of pessaries ranges from 33.9 to 89% [7–10].

Although pessaries can successfully be used to treat most stages of prolapse, complete organ prolapse most often needs surgical repair. Recent studies have not shown an association between prolapse stage and outcome of a pessary trial [4, 10]. One study found that improvement in prolapse symptoms was limited to women with anterior vaginal wall prolapse [8]. Another showed that severe posterior vaginal wall prolapse was associated with discontinued pessary use. Patient characteristics associated with continued pessary use for pelvic organ prolapse are age greater than 65 years and poor surgical risks [11]. Unsuccessful pessary fittings and use are related to previous reconstructive surgery for prolapse or hysterectomy, obesity, increased parity, severe posterior prolapse, short vaginal length, and wide introitus [9, 10, 12, 13]. One study demonstrated that weight was not a negative or positive predictor of successful fitting and use [9]. Also, nulliparity does not provide absolute protection against prolapse [14]. Currently, there are no randomized controlled trials of pessaries for women with pelvic organ prolapse [15].

One complication of treating prolapse with a pessary is the unmasking of underlying urinary incontinence. One study showed that during treatment with a pessary for prolapse, 21% of patients developed de novo stress incontinence, 6% urge incontinence, and 4% developed difficulty with voiding. Despite these findings, 67% of treated patients reported improvement in prolapse or incontinence symptoms with pessary use [4].

Pessary treatment for stress urinary incontinence occurs by compressing the urethra against the upper posterior portion of the symphysis pubis and elevating the bladder neck. This results in an increase in outflow resistance and corrects the angle between the bladder and the urethra [16]. Women who have undergone prior incontinence surgery have a higher failure rate of pessary use for their incontinence [7].

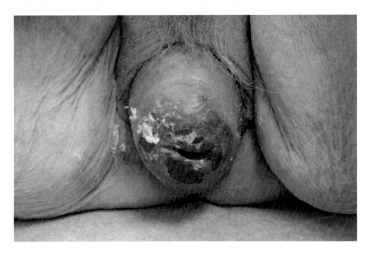

Fig. 16-1 Fourth-degree uterine prolapse

Pessary use should be individualized based on the patient's symptoms (Table 16-1) (Figs. 16-2–16-5). Women who are incontinent during daily activities can wear the pessary continually. For others who experience incontinence only during vigorous activities, the pessary can be worn as needed. One small study showed 5 of 14 subjects achieved complete continence during vigorous exercise [17].

Table 16-1 Pessary style choices based on symptom

1st and 2nd degree uterine prolapse	Ring, Donut, Milex® Inflatoball, Milex® Regula
Mild prolapse with cystocele	Ring with support, Shaatz
3rd degree uterine prolapse	Cube, Donut, Milex® Inflatoball, Gellhorn
3rd degree uterine prolapse with cystocele	Gehrung
Prolapse s/p hysterectomy	Ring with support
Mild cystocele	Ring with support, Dish with support, Hodge with support, Donut, Gehrung
Moderate cystocele	Gellhorn, Gehrung
Rectocele and enterocele	Gellhorn, Donut, Milex® Inflatoball, Cube, Gehrung
Stress incontinence	Incontinence Ring, Incontinence Dish
Incontinence during exercise	Cube, Hodge, Inflatoball, Ring, Ring with knob
Incontinence and cystocele	Hodge, Hodge with support

Milex®, CooperSurgical, Trumbull, CT
Data from Weber AM, Richter HE. Pelvic organ prolapse. *Obstet Gynecol* 2005;106(3):615–634; Viera AJ, Larkins-Pettigrew M. Practical use of the pessary. *Am Fam Physician* 2000;61:2719–2726, 2729; http://milexproducts.com

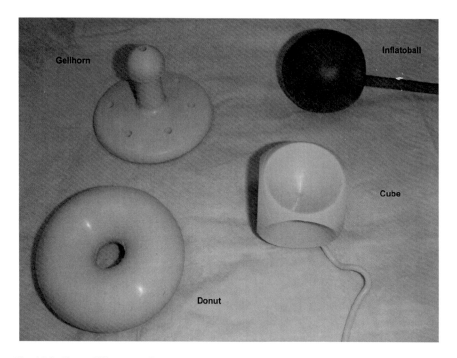

Fig. 16-2 Space-filling pessaries

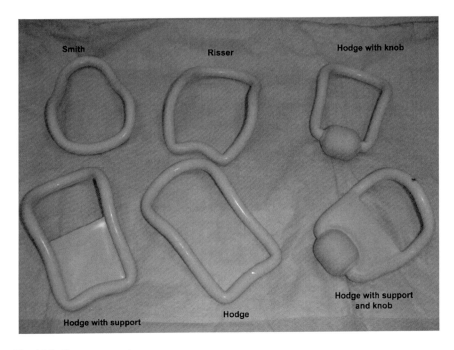

Fig. 16-3 Support pessaries

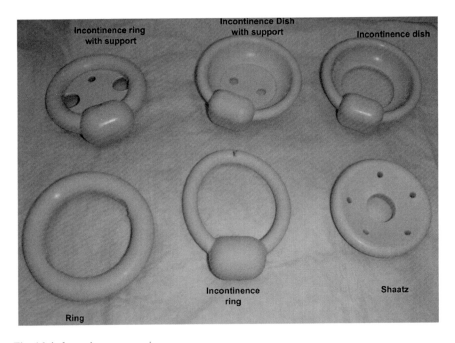

Fig. 16-4 Incontinence pessaries

Fig. 16-5 Saddle pessaries

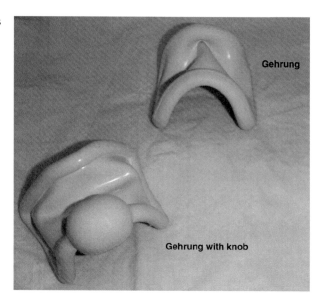

Case Study

Case A

A 36-year-old female with a past medical history significant for two vaginal deliveries following uncomplicated pregnancies presents to your office for a routine physical. After the last pregnancy, she noticed that she occasionally leaked urine when she laughed, coughed, or while she was running. She failed to mention her symptoms at a postpartum checkup because she thought they were normal, but a year later she is still troubled with the problem and would like to know about treatment options. She performs Kegel exercises only intermittently. Today, pelvic exam is completely within normal limits.

Case B

A 72-year-old female with a history of a cystocele presents for evaluation. Previously, she has been able to tolerate her symptoms of stress incontinence; however, today she is interested in available treatment options. On exam, patient has a grade I cystocele and slight atrophy of vaginal mucosa consistent with chronic estrogen deficiency.

Diagnosis (Algorithm 16-1)

- Stress incontinence
- Pelvic organ prolapse

Differential Diagnosis (Algorithm 16-1)

Urge incontinence

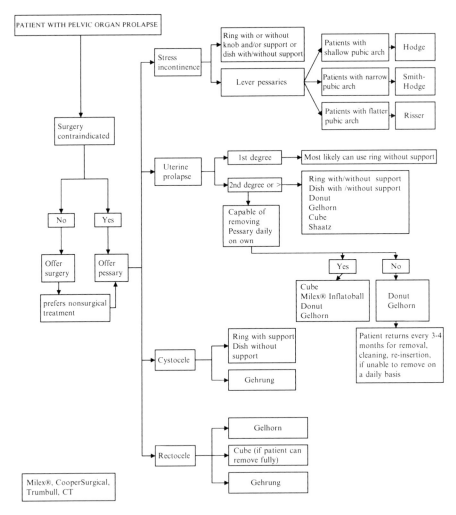

Algorithm 16-1 Decision tree for patient with pelvic organ prolapse

Indications (Algorithm 16-1)

- Pelvic organ prolapse
- Vaginal vault prolapse
- Cystocele
- Rectocele
- Enterocele
- Uterine prolapse
- Stress urinary incontinence
- Preoperative evaluation for stress incontinence
- Preoperative preparation for eroded prolapsed tissue

Contraindications

- Noncompliance
- Vaginal erosions
- Active vaginal or pelvic infections
- Silicon or latex allergy

Equipment (Figs. 16-6 and 16-7)

- Pessary fitting kit or actual pessaries for fitting (Table 16-1)
- Water-based lubricant

Procedure

1. Patient preparation
   (a) For pelvic organ prolapse, have patient empty her bladder.
   (b) For incontinence, fit patient with full bladder.
2. Place the patient in the lithotomy position.
3. Replace any prolapsed tissue.
4. Perform a bimanual exam to estimate pessary size (Fig. 16-8).
5. Lubricate tip of pessary and introitus with water-based lubricant.
6. Insert the pessary into the vagina in a downward fashion, avoiding the urethra.
7. Position the pessary properly (Figs. 16-9–16-16). The examiner's fingers should pass easily between the pessary and vaginal wall.

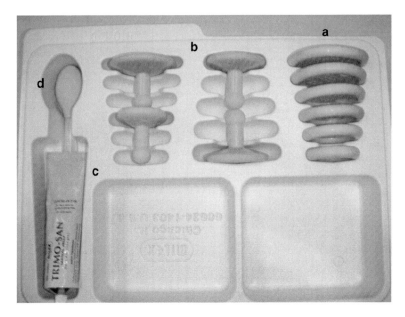

Fig. 16-6 Milex® pessary fitting kit (CooperSurgical, Trumbull, CT) with Ring (a) and Gellhorn (b) pessaries, Milex® Trimo-san Vaginal Jelly (CooperSurgical, Trumbull, CT) (c), and applicator (d)

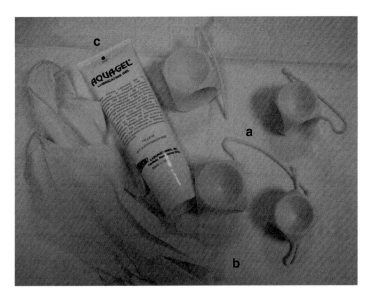

Fig. 16-7 Cube (a) pessary set up with gloves (b) and Aqua-Gel® Lubricating Gel (Parker Laboratories, Fairfield, NJ) (c)

   (a) Have the patient stand, walk, and valsalva.

   (b) If painful or uncomfortable, try next smallest size.

   (c) If it falls out or starts to slip out, try next largest size. The largest pessary that the patient can comfortably wear is generally the most effective.

8. Patient needs to void effectively before leaving the office to ensure there is no urethral obstruction.

9. Schedule follow-up visit within 1 week.

   (a) Remove pessary and inspect vagina for irritation, erosion, or allergic reaction.

10. For those unable to remove their own pessary, schedule routine removal and cleaning visits from 1 to 6 months depending on doctor and patient preference.

Complications and Risks

- Vaginal irritation/erosions/bleeding
- Vaginal discharge and odor
- Discomfort

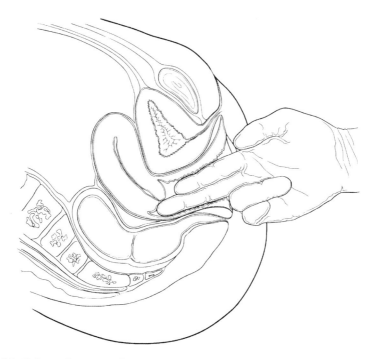

Fig. 16-8 Estimate the pessary size

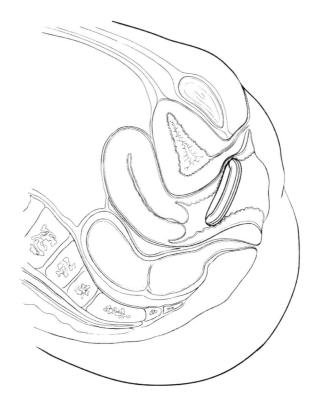

Fig. 16-9 Proper position of incontinence Ring pessary

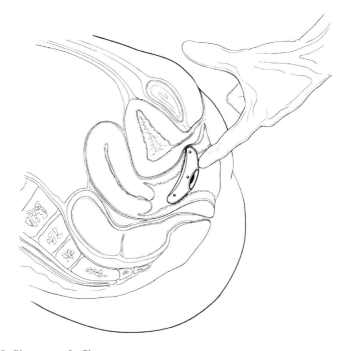

Fig. 16-10 Placement of a Shaatz pessary

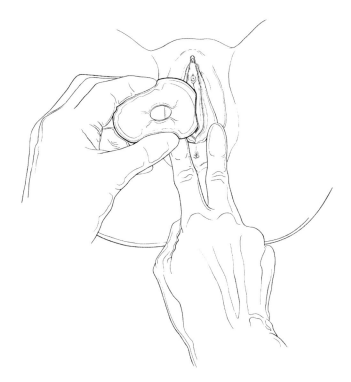

Fig. 16-11 Insertion of a Donut pessary

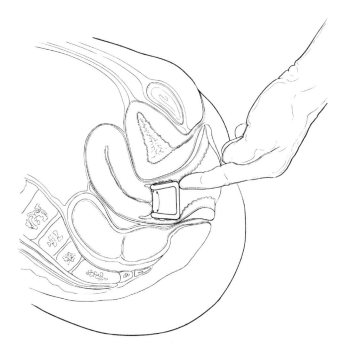

Fig. 16-12 Proper position of the Milex® Regula pessary (CooperSurgical, Trumbull, CT)

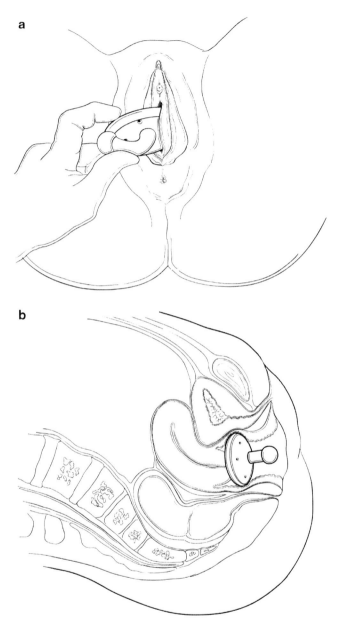

Fig. 16-13 (**a**) Gellhorn knob is folded on its side for easier insertion. (**b**) Proper position of inserted Gellhorn pessary

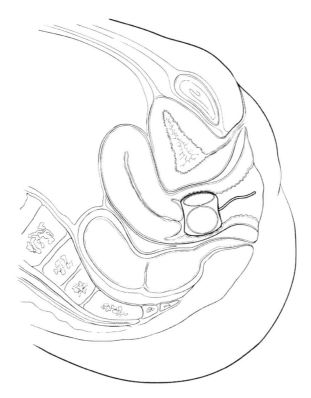

Fig. 16-14   Cube pessary in proper placement

- Infections:
  - Bacterial vaginosis
  - Actinomycosis
  - Urosepsis
- Rectovaginal fistula
- Incarceration
- Dislodgment
- Urinary tract or bowel obstruction
- Hydronephrosis
- Cervical/uterine herniation/entrapment
- Latex allergy

Tricks and Helpful Hints

- For patients with atrophic vaginal tissue, pretreat for 1–2 weeks with estrogen cream (1/2 applicator full at night prior to bedtime).
- Advise patients that usually many fittings are necessary to get the right size and shape pessary.

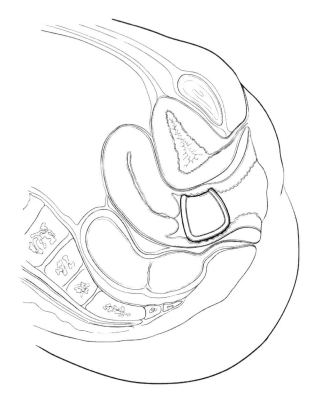

Fig. 16-15 Gehrung pessary placement

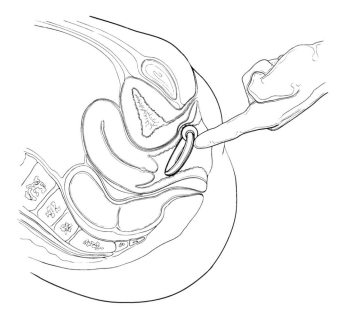

Fig. 16-16 Incontinence Ring with knob in proper position

- If the patient is not going to be removing the pessary daily, use an acidic vaginal gel, such as Milex® Trimo-san (CooperSurgical, Trumbull, CT), three times a week (may be ordered with the pessary) to prevent odor and discharge.
- For patients who use a diaphragm, their diaphragm size does not correlate with their correct pessary size. (Patients may use a diaphragm to help with incontinence or prolapse.)
- If one size is too large and the next smaller size is too small, try a different style pessary.
- In some patients with long-term pessary use, it may be necessary to switch to a smaller pessary over time.
- The Milex® Regula (CooperSurgical, Trumbull, CT) can be tried when expulsion of the pessary is a problem.
- The Milex® Inflatoball (CooperSurgical, Trumbull, CT) is a good choice for someone who needs a space-filling pessary but has a very narrow introitus and is capable of removing the pessary on a daily basis.
- The Cube can be difficult to remove and needs to be removed daily.

Procedure Note

(Provider to customize as needed.)

Risks and benefits of pessary use were reviewed with the patient. Patient was placed in the lithotomy position. (Prolapsed tissue was inspected and replaced.) Bimanual exam was performed to estimate pessary size. Chosen pessary was lubricated and gently inserted into the vagina. Fit was ensured as pessary filled vagina and one finger passed easily around it. (If too loose, larger size was tried. If uncomfortable or too tight, smaller size was tried.) Patient was asked to stand, ambulate, and valsalva with the pessary in place to ensure fit. Patient voided without difficulty with pessary in place. Follow-up appointment was given.

Coding

CPT® Codes (Current Procedural Terminology, AMA, Chicago, IL)

Pessary fitting	57160
Nonrubber pessary device	A4562
Rubber pessaries including latex	A4561

ICD 9-CM-Diagnostic Codes (International Classification of Diseases, 9th Revision, Clinical Modification, Center for Disease Control and Prevention)

Incontinence:	618.5
Stress urinary	625.6
Urge and stress	788.33
Incompetent cervix	654.5
Prolapse:	
Cystocele	618.0
Uterovaginal	618.4
Complete	618.3
Incomplete	618.2
Uterus (all degrees) without:	
Vaginal wall prolapse	618.1
Vaginal wall prolapse:	
Without uterine prolapse	618.0
With uterine prolapse:	
Complete	618.3
Incomplete	618.2
Posthysterectomy	618.5

Postprocedure Patient Instructions

Have the patient call if pessary becomes dislodged, falls out, or is uncomfortable or if the patient is having difficulty voiding or having a bowel movement with the pessary in place.

Follow up in 1–2 weeks for confirmation of fitting and vaginal exam to look for irritation, pressure sores, or allergic reaction.

Case Study Outcome

Case A

A size 3 Cube pessary was successfully inserted into the vagina and positioned. The patient tolerated the pessary well and was able to walk and valsalva without it falling out. She voided while at the office and was able to demonstrate removing the pessary. She understands the importance of taking the pessary out on a daily basis. She returns in 1 week for follow-up.

Case B

The patient is asked to use estrogen cream nightly for the next week. Upon returning the following week, the vaginal mucosa appears less atrophied. Attempts are made to fit a Dish with support, but these prove uncomfortable. Next, the Gehrung is fitted with the patient experiencing no loss of the pessary with walking or a valsalva maneuver. She also voids without difficulty. She is given a tube of Milex® Trimo-san and returns in 1 week for follow-up.

Postprocedure Patient Handout

(Provider to fill in blanks/circle applicable choice when given multiple choices and customize as needed.)

A pessary is a silicone or latex device placed inside your vagina. It can be used to help support your uterus (which can hang down from its original position), vagina (which can lose the firm support to its walls), bladder (which can push down into your vagina), or rectum (which can push up into your vagina). A pessary can also be used to help prevent the leakage of urine, which happens during coughing, sneezing, straining, or exercise. This is called stress incontinence.

Today you were fitted with a _____ pessary. Ideally, your pessary should be removed and cleaned every _____ day(s). It is important to follow your doctor's directions in caring for your pessary so it will last as long as possible. Remove and clean your pessary as instructed by your doctor today. You can use a mild soap and water to clean it. If you are not going to wear it, make sure to dry it completely and store it in a safe place. Your pessary can be worn even during your period, although it is very important to remove your pessary daily during your menses. Some women will leave their pessaries in for several days; however, if you do this, you may experience more discharge and odor.

Your doctor might have told you today that you do not need to remove your pessary yourself. If this is the case, your doctor will remove and check it for you at your follow-up appointment.

You will need to return for follow-up within 1 week to make sure the pessary fits well and is not causing any irritation in your vagina. Please call the doctor before your appointment if you experience any of the following: vaginal bleeding, vaginal pain, difficulty urinating, or having a bowel movement. Also, call if your pessary is falling out or falls out. After your first follow-up appointment, your doctor will schedule less frequent regular visits.

Many styles of pessaries can be worn during intercourse. Your doctor should have told you today if you can wear your pessary during intercourse.

You may have an increase in vaginal secretions/discharge or odor while using a pessary. Using Milex® Trimo-san cream or gel three times a week may be helpful in decreasing the discharge and odor.

Please call the office if you have any problems or questions.

References

1. Vierhout ME. The use of pessaries in vaginal prolapse. *Eur J Obstet Gynecol Reprod Biol* 2004;117:4–9.
2. Smilen SW, Weber AM. Pelvic organ prolapse. *ACOG Practice Bulletin* Feb 2007.
3. Olsen Al, Smith VJ, Bergstrom JO, Colling JC, Clark AL. Epidemiology of surgically managed pelvic organ prolapse and urinary incontinence. *Obstet Gynecol* 1997;89:501–506.
4. Clemons JL, Aguilar VC, Tillinghast TA, Jackson ND, Myers DL. Patient satisfaction and changes in prolapse and urinary symptoms in women who were fitted successfully with a pessary for pelvic organ prolapse. *Am J Obstet Gynecol* 2004;190:1025–1029.
5. Brown JS, Nyberg LM, Kusek JW, Burgio KL, Dioko AC, et al. Proceedings of the national institute of diabetes and digestive and kidney diseases international symposium on epidemiologic issues in urinary incontinence. *Am J Obstet Gynecol* 2003;188:S77–S88.
6. Baden WF, Walker T. Fundamentals, symptoms and classification. In Baden WF, Walker T (eds) *Surgical repair of vaginal defects*. Philadelphia: J.B. Lippincott, 1992, p 14.
7. Farrell SA. Continence pessaries in the management of urinary incontinence in women. *J Obstet Gynaecol Can* 2004;26:113–117.
8. Handa VL, Jones M. Do pessaries prevent the progression of pelvic organ prolapse? *Int Urogynecol J Pelvic Floor Dysfunct* 2004;13:349–352.
9. Maito JM, Quam ZA, Craig E, Danner KA, Rogers RG. Predictors of successful pessary fitting and continues use in a nurse-midwifery pessary clinic. *J Nurse Midwifery* 2006;51:78–84.
10. Mutone MF, Terry C, Hale DS, Benson JT. Factors which influence the short-term success of pessary management of pelvic organ prolapse. *Am J Obstet Gynecol* 2005;193:89–94.
11. Clemons JL, Aguilar VC, Sokol ER, Jackson ND, Myers DL. Patient characteristics that are associated with continued pessary use versus surgery after 1 year. *Am J Obstet Gynecol* 2004;190:1025–1029.
12. Fernando RJ, Thakar R, Sultan AH, Shah SM, Jones PW. Effect of vaginal pessaries on symptoms associated with pelvic organ prolapse. *Obstet Gynecol* 2006;108:93–99.
13. Clemons JL, Aguilar VC, Tillinghast TA, Jackson ND, Myers DL. Risk factors associated with an unsuccessful pessary fitting trial in women with pelvic organ prolapse. *Am J Obstet Gynecol* 2004;190:345–350.
14. Weber AM, Richter HE. Pelvic organ prolapse. *Obstet Gynecol* 2005;106(3):615–634.
15. Adams E, Thomson A, Maher C, Hager S. Mechanical devices for pelvic organ prolapse in women (review). *Cochrane Collaboration* 2007;1:1–8.
16. Viera AJ, Larkins-Pettigrew M. Practical use of the pessary. *Am Fam Physician* 2000;61: 2719–2726, 2729.
17. Nygaard I. Prevention of exercise incontinence with mechanical devices. *J Reprod Med* 1195;40:89–94.

Additional Resources

Articles

Anders K. Devices for continence and prolapse. *BJOG* 2004;111(Suppl 1):61–66.
Farrell SA. Practical advice for ring pessary fitting and management. *J Soc Obstet Gynaecol Can* 1997;19:625–632.
Martina MF, Terry C, Hale DS, Benson JT. Factors which influence the short-term success of pessary management of pelvic organ prolapse. *Am J Obstet Gynecol* 2005;193:89–94.
Miser WF. For want of a pessary, the life was lost. *J Am Board Fam Pract* 2002;15(3):249.

Urinary incontinence: guide to diagnosis and management. National Guideline Clearinghouse. March 2007.

Wheeler LD, Lazarus R, Torkington J, O'Mahoney MS, Woodhouse K. Lesson of the week: perils of pessaries. *Age Ageing* 2004;33:510–511.

Miscellaneous

Trimo-San vaginal cream or gel – Milex products, available over the counter.

Milex pessary fitting kit (Cooper Surgical, Trumbull, CT) 1-800-243-2974; http:\\www.coopersurgical.com\

or

pessary fitting kit from Mentor Corp 1-800-525-0245 http:\\www.mentorcorp.com

or

Monarch Medical Products 1-866-241-1625, http:\\www.monarchmedicalproducts.com

Chapter 17
Bartholin Gland Cysts and Abscesses

Janice E. Daugherty

Introduction

Bartholin gland cysts are caused when trauma or inflammation obstructs the duct of the Bartholin gland, which normally secretes mucus near the hymenal ring [1]. Often asymptomatic, intermittent obstruction of the duct can cause the cyst to fluctuate in size. If secondarily infected, the cyst can become an abscess.

Visual inspection of the vulva will show a soft, compressible mass at approximately 4 o'clock or 8 o'clock on either side of the hymenal ring [2] (Figs. 17-1 and 17-2). If not infected, Bartholin gland cysts are usually nontender. Abscesses are usually tender to palpation and may cause discomfort when walking or sitting [3]. Abscesses may rupture spontaneously and may have associated cellulitis. In addition to a drainage procedure with re-creation of a gland orifice, local heat to the area can provide relief of discomfort and enhance healing.

Bartholin gland cysts or abscesses are distinct from other vulvar masses in their location and cystic texture on palpation. Solid or vascular vulvar masses generally would not lie in the same anatomic position as a Bartholin gland cyst or abscess [4]. Bartholin glands are most active during the reproductive years, so masses occurring before puberty or beyond the menopausal period are not likely to be Bartholin cysts.

The Word catheter, placed inside the Bartholin gland cyst, is a small latex device with a balloon that allows it to function as a self-retaining drain. It can remain in place within the cyst from several days to up to 2 weeks to allow a new gland opening to epithelialize [5]. Alternatively, women may need marsupialization procedure; in a small study by Haider and colleagues, most women preferred the Word Catheter placement [6].

J.E. Daugherty (✉)
Department of Family Medicine, Brody School of Medicine, East Carolina University,
Brody 4N-78, 600 Moye Blvd., Greenville, NC 27834, USA
e-mail: rawlj@ecu.edu

S.M. Sulik and C.B. Heath (eds.), *Primary Care Procedures in Women's Health*,
DOI 10.1007/978-0-387-76604-1_17, © Springer Science+Business Media, LLC 2010

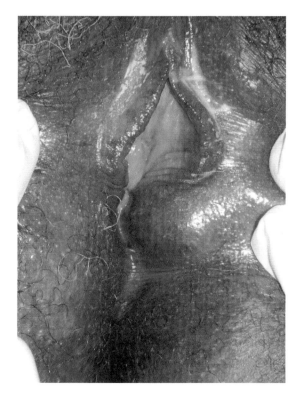

Fig. 17-1 Photograph of Bartholin gland cyst

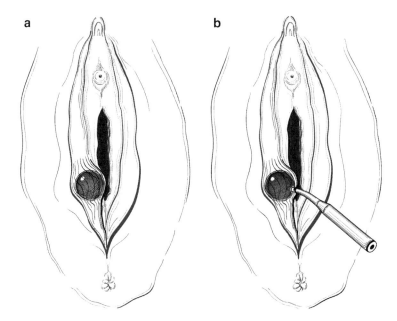

Fig. 17-2 Drawing of Bartholin gland (**a**) drawing of bartholin gland (**b**) word catheter in place within the bartholin cyst

Case Study

A 21-year-old woman presents for her annual health maintenance examination and states that she has for 6 months noted a swelling on the right side of her vulva near the vaginal opening. She is concerned because it gets larger at times, and she has had pain when she sits or has intercourse.

Diagnosis (Algorithm 17-1)

Bartholin gland cyst or abscess

Differential Diagnosis

- Hematoma
- Sebaceous cyst
- Hemangioma
- Lipoma
- Malignant neoplasm: primary or metastatic carcinoma
- Sarcoma

Indications (Algorithm 17-1)

Symptomatic cyst or abscess

- The purpose of the procedure is not only to drain the cyst fluid but also to reestablish a gland opening in good anatomical position.
- The procedure of first choice is usually incision and drainage of cyst or abscess with insertion of Word catheter.
- If prior drainage procedures have repeatedly failed, follow-up is unlikely to occur, or if a woman is not able to abstain from vaginal intercourse while the catheter is in place, marsupialization of the cyst may be the primary management [7].

Contraindications

- Bleeding disorders
- Sensitivity to latex, if use of Word catheter is intended

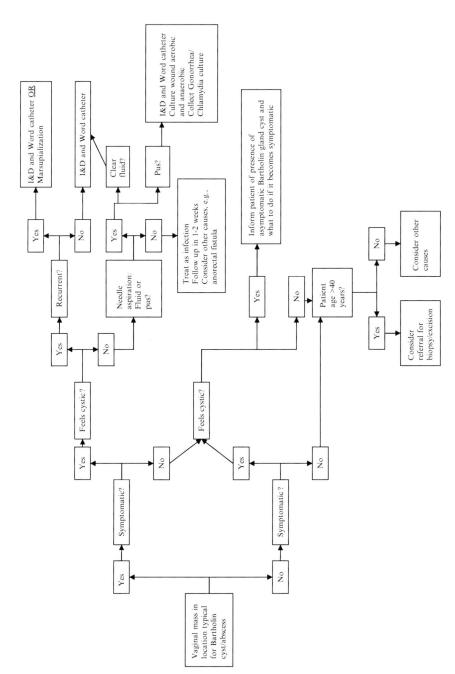

Algorithm 17-1 Decision tree for vaginal mass near hymenal ring

Equipment (Fig. 17-3)

- Word catheter
- Antiseptic solution
- No. 11 or 15 scalpel
- 1% lidocaine
- 22- or 25-gauge 1 in. needle for catheter inflation
- 30-gauge 1 in. needle for infiltration anesthesia
- 3 or 5 cc syringe
- Hemostat: curved mosquito
- Silver nitrate stick
- 4×4 sterile gauze pads
- Pickups with teeth
- Needle holder: small
- 3-0 or 4-0 absorbable suture on small cutting needle
- Scissors
- Eye protection
- Mask
- Gloves

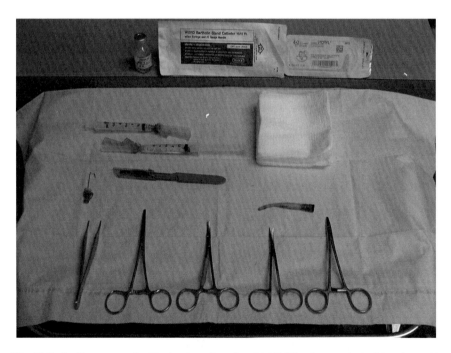

Fig. 17-3 Sterile setup tray for Word catheter insertion: (a) 1% lidocaine anesthetic; (b) syringe with 3 cc of 1% lidocaine; (c) Needle driver; (d) Hemostats; (e) Scissors; (f) Pickups; (g) Scalpel; (h) 4×4 inch gauze; (i) Word catheter; (j) 3 cc syringe with water; (k) add extra needle 1½" for a hook

Procedure

Procedure for Incision and Drainage with Word Catheter Placement

1. Remove Word catheter from the package. Attach a 22- or 25-gauge 1″ needle to a 3 cc syringe filled with tap water.
   - (Note: newer Word catheters are designed to be filled using a catheter-tip syringe rather than a needle.)
2. Carefully insert the needle into the center of the wider end of the catheter and test the balloon by filling it with approximately 3 cc of water (Fig. 17-4).
3. Aspirate the water from the catheter and leave the catheter in place on the needle.
   - The syringe will serve as a handle to make the catheter easier to insert into the cyst, and fewer punctures mean less likelihood that the water will leak out.
4. Place patient in lithotomy position.
5. Have assistant place traction on the vulvar skin to provide good exposure to the area.
6. Infiltrate the area over the cyst, just inside the hymenal ring, with local anesthetic in an area about 1.5 cm across.
7. Cleanse the area with antiseptic solution.
8. Stabilize the cyst with either your fingers or a needle-hook into the cyst (Fig. 17-5).
9. Make a stab incision approximately 1.5 cm deep and 0.5 cm long into the cyst (Fig. 17-6).

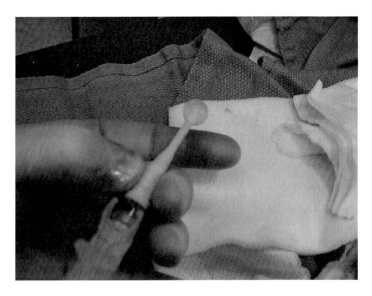

Fig. 17-4 Testing Word catheter balloon system

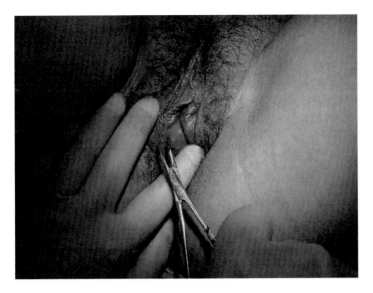

Fig. 17-5 Stabilization of Bartholin's cyst prior to incision and drainage

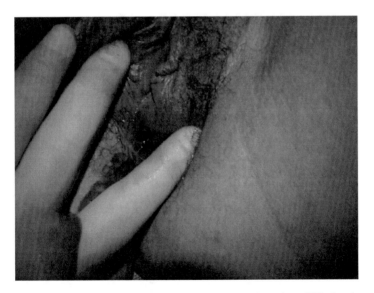

Fig. 17-6 Incision has been made into Bartholin's cyst prior to insertion of Word catheter

10. Insert a hemostat and spread the tips within the cyst or abscess to break up any loculation.
11. Insert the Word catheter into the cyst (Fig. 17-7) and fill the bulb with 2–3 cc of water. Remove the needle from the catheter (Fig. 17-8).

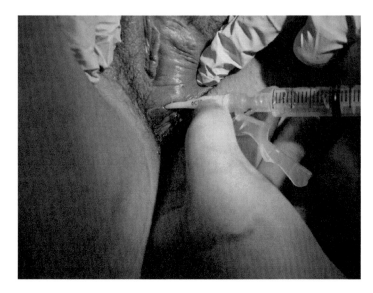

Fig. 17-7 Insertion of Word catheter

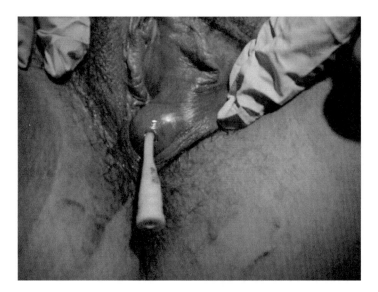

Fig. 17-8 Word catheter in place after insertion

12. If desired, place a small absorbable suture next to the incision, tie a knot, and then tie the suture around the catheter. Do not place a suture through the catheter.
13. Push the distal end of the Word catheter up through the hymenal ring into the vagina. Instruct the patient that she can push it back up when it slips out.

Procedure for Marsupialization

1. Place patient in lithotomy position.
2. Have assistant place traction on the vulvar skin to provide good exposure to the area.
3. Infiltrate the area over the cyst, just inside the hymenal ring, with local anesthetic in an area about 2.5 cm across.
4. Cleanse the area with antiseptic solution.
5. Stabilize the cyst with either your fingers or a needle-hook into the cyst (Fig. 17-9a).
6. Excise an ellipse of mucosa and its underlying cyst wall approximately 1–1.5 cm in diameter (Fig. 17-9b, c).
7. Insert a hemostat and spread the tips within the cyst or abscess to break up any loculation.
8. Suture the vulvar mucosa to the cyst wall around the circumference of the incision, using either running or simple interrupted absorbable sutures (Fig. 17-9d).

Complications and Risks

- Bleeding at the site
- Infection
- Reactions to local anesthetic
- Reactions to the latex of a Word catheter

Tricks and Helpful Hints

- Having an assistant to help with maintaining exposure to the area will make the procedure much easier.
- As the Word catheter is made of latex, its balloon is subject to weakness and rupture brought on by age and environmental exposure to petroleum products. Store Word catheters in a cool, dark location, away from petroleum products or vapors.
- Do not inflate the catheter with air: it will leak out too soon. Sterile water is not necessary for filling the catheter, as the area is not sterile.
- Take care when inserting the needle into the catheter not to pierce the side or end of the catheter.
- Stabilize the cyst wall by using either a curved hemostat or make a needle-hook by using a hemostat to bend a 25-gauge 1½″ needle attached to a small locking syringe. The syringe serves as a handle for the hook, which can be placed into the cyst to stabilize it, facilitate exposure, and make it less likely for the skin and the cyst wall to "eclipse" the incision, which makes proper insertion of the Word catheter difficult (see Fig. 17-10).
- A portable warm soak can be made by folding a washcloth in quarters and then once again to make a rectangle approximately the size of a sanitary pad (Fig. 17-11).

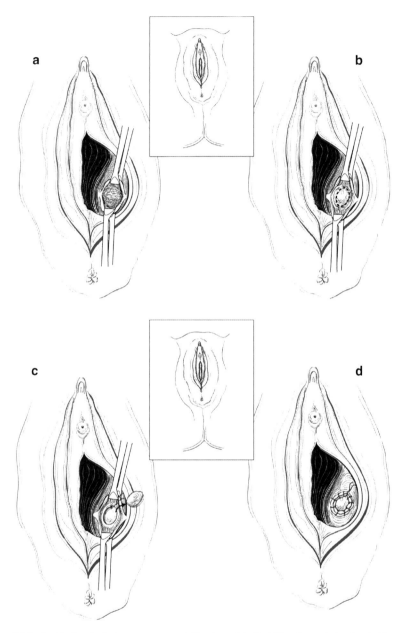

Fig. 17-9 (**a–d**) Bartholin's cyst marsupialization. (**a**) Stabilization of the bartholin cyst.
(**b**) An elliptical incision is made on the center of the cyst. (**c**) Excise an ellipse of mucosa and
its underlying cyst wall approximately 1–1.5 cm in diameter. (**d**) Suture the vulvar mucosa to
the cyst wall around the circumference of the incision, using either running or simple interrupted absorbable sutures

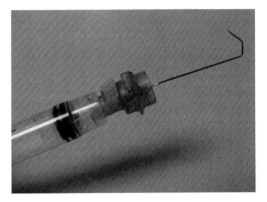

Fig. 17-10 Make a needle-hook by using a hemostat to bend a 25-gauge needle attached to a small Luer-tip syringe. The syringe serves as a handle for the hook, which can be placed into the cyst to stabilize it, facilitate exposure, and make it less likely for the skin and the cyst wall to "eclipse" the incision, making proper insertion of the Word catheter difficult

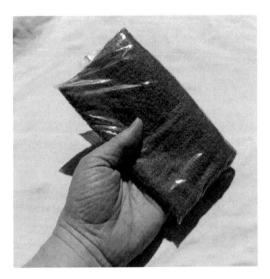

Fig. 17-11 Moist washcloth in a plastic sandwich bag can be microwaved and reused as a heat pack

Place the washcloth in a sandwich-size zipper-lock plastic bag, add enough water to soak the cloth, and seal the bag. Heat the bag and cloth in the microwave for a few seconds until it is warm but not hot to the touch. The woman can place this in her underclothing to provide moist heat without wetting her clothing. She can reheat the cloth as necessary without opening the bag.

Procedure Note

(Provider to customize as needed.)

Incision and Drainage with Word Catheter Placement

The procedure was discussed with the patient, including benefits of draining cyst fluid/pus and establishing a new gland opening, as well as the likely relief of discomfort. Risks, including bleeding, infection, early dislodging of the catheter, and possible recurrence of the cyst/abscess were discussed, as were alternative treatments for this condition. The patient states no known allergy to latex, iodine, or local anesthetics. Aftercare instructions were discussed. The patient signed a consent form for this procedure.

The patient was placed in the lithotomy position. The cyst was identified and palpated near the hymenal ring. Local anesthesia was achieved with 1–2 cc of 1% lidocaine by local infiltration. The area was cleansed with povidone–iodine and manually stabilized, and an incision was made into the cyst. A Word catheter that had been previously tested was placed into the cyst cavity and filled with water to allow retention of the balloon. (A retention suture of 4-0 absorbable suture was placed around the catheter.)

The patient tolerated the procedure well, and aftercare instructions were repeated. She is to return to the office in 2 weeks for follow-up.

Marsupialization of Bartholin Gland Cyst

The procedure was discussed with the patient, including benefits of draining cyst fluid/pus and establishing a new gland opening, as well as the likely relief of discomfort. Risks, including bleeding, infection, early dislodging of the catheter, and possible recurrence of the cyst/abscess were discussed, as were alternative treatments for this condition. The patient states no known allergy to iodine or local anesthetics. Aftercare instructions were discussed. The patient signed a consent form for this procedure.

The patient was placed in the lithotomy position. The cyst was identified and palpated near the hymenal ring. Local anesthesia was achieved with 1–2 cc of 1% plain lidocaine by local infiltration. The area was cleansed with povidone–iodine, manually stabilized and an ellipse of mucosa and cyst wall was removed. The edge of the mucosa was sutured to the cyst wall in a circumferential fashion with running absorbable suture.

The patient tolerated the procedure well, and aftercare instructions were repeated. She is to return to the office in 2 weeks for follow-up.

Coding

Incision and Drainage with Word Catheter Placement
CPT® Codes (Current Procedural Terminology, AMA, Chicago, IL)
Procedure: 56420
Supplies: 99070

ICD 9-CM-Diagnostic Codes (International Classification of Diseases, 9th Revision, Clinical Modification, Center for Disease Control and Prevention)
Bartholin gland cyst   616.2
Bartholin gland abscess   616.3
Marsupialization of Bartholin Gland Cyst
CPT® Codes (Current Procedural Terminology, AMA, Chicago, IL)
Procedure: Marsupialization of Bartholin gland cyst   56440
ICD 9-CM-Diagnostic Codes (International Classification of Diseases, 9th Revision, Clinical Modification, Center for Disease Control and Prevention)
Bartholin gland cyst   616.2
Bartholin gland abscess   616.3

Postprocedure Patient Instructions

Incision and Drainage with Word Catheter Placement

- It is best if the catheter can remain in place for 2 weeks. Intercourse may cause irritation of the surgical site or cause the catheter to come out too early, so it is best avoided while the catheter is in place.
- If using Word catheter, patient will need to tuck the end of the catheter back into the vagina when it comes out with straining, etc.
- Otherwise, the woman may resume her normal activities immediately after the procedure.
- Antibiotics are not necessary unless there is cellulitis, or systemic signs of infection associated with an abscess.
- Instruct the patient to report any heavy bleeding, apply moist heat as much as possible during the first few days after the procedure, and return for follow-up as scheduled.
- Keeping the abscess open is adequate to allow healing in most cases.
- Instruct the patient to avoid intercourse for 2 weeks, even if the catheter should fall out before then.

Marsupialization of Bartholin Gland Cyst

- Warm moist soaks will help ease the discomfort and speed healing

Case Study Outcome

At her follow-up visit 2 weeks after the procedure, the patient had good resolution of her symptoms and the tract around the Word catheter was well-healed. The balloon was deflated with a needle, and the catheter was removed. She was wished well and requested to follow-up as needed.

Postprocedure Patient Handout

(Provider to fill in blanks/circle applicable choice when given multiple choices and to customize as needed.)

What Is a Bartholin Gland Cyst or Abscess?

The Bartholin glands are small mucus-producing glands on either side of the vaginal opening. If a gland opening becomes blocked due to irritation or infection, the mucus can accumulate and form a cyst. If this fluid becomes infected, it can form an abscess.

How Is a Bartholin Gland Cyst or Abscess Treated?

The purpose of treatment is to drain the fluid and create a new opening for the gland. If the fluid is drained without creating a new opening, the cyst or abscess is more likely to come back. The usual treatment for Bartholin cysts is to drain the fluid and insert a small tube, called a Word catheter, which has a balloon that helps keep it in place within the cyst for about 2 weeks. Leaving the tube in place allows the body to heal with a new opening for the gland. The Word catheter procedure can be done in the office with local anesthesia.

What Can I Do at Home to Feel Better?

Applying a warm pack to the area can help with the swelling and discomfort. Sometimes an abscess will drain on its own, and moist heat can help it heal more quickly. Getting extra rest will also help your body heal more quickly.

Acetaminophen 650 mg taken every 4 h or Ibuprofen 400 mg every 4–6 h will help with your discomfort.

If you have a Word catheter in place, it is better to avoid sexual intercourse until the catheter is removed by your healthcare practitioner. You can bathe normally with the catheter in place.

What If the Cyst or Abscess Comes Back?

If a cyst or abscess has come back more than once after the Word catheter procedure, your healthcare practitioner may recommend a procedure that makes a larger opening in the cyst. This procedure can usually be done in the office.

When Should I Call My HealthCare Practitioner?

If you have:

- Discomfort that is increasing rather than decreasing
- Fever or chills
- Any questions or concerns

Remember to keep your appointment for follow-up in 2 weeks.
Your appointment date and time is _____.

References

1. Blumstein H. Bartholin gland diseases. emedicine 2003; available at: http://www.emedicine.com/emerg/topic54.htm.
2. Hill DA, Lense JJ. Office management of Bartholin gland cysts and abscesses. *Am Fam Physician* 1998;57:1611–1616.
3. Omole F, Simmons BJ, Hacker Y. Management of Bartholin's duct cyst and gland abscess. *Am Fam Physician* 2003;68:135–140.
4. Wilkinson EJ, Stone IK. *Atlas of vulvar disease*, 5th edn. Baltimore: Williams & Wilkins, 1995, pp 11–15.
5. Apgar B. Bartholin's cyst/abscess: Word catheter insertion. In Pfenninger JL, Fowler GC (eds) *Procedures for primary care physicians*. St. Louis, MO: Mosby, 1994, pp 596–600.
6. Haider Z, Condous G, Kirk E, Mukri F, Bourne T. The simple outpatient management of Bartholin's abscess using the Word catheter: a preliminary study. *Aust N Z J Obstet Gynaecol* 2007;47(2):137–140.
7. Cho JY, Ahn MO, Cha KS. Window operation: an alternative treatment method for Bartholin gland cysts and abscesses. *Obstet Gynecol* 1990;76(5 Pt 1):886–888.

Additional Resources

Articles

Marzano DA, Haefner HK. The Bartholin gland cyst: past, present, and future. *J Low Genit Tract Dis* 2004;8(3):195–204.

Websites

http://www.operationalmedicine.org/Videos/Bartholin1.mpg: a video of the procedure of Word catheter insertion.

Equipment Companies

Rusch Corporation, 1-800-553-5214, www.rusch.com
CooperSurgical, 1-800-243-2974, www.coopersurgical.com
Milex Products 1-800-621-1278 www.milexproducts.com

Chapter 18
Endometrial Biopsy

Kristen McNamara

Introduction

The endometrial biopsy is a safe, simple office procedure that can be used to diagnose most abnormal bleeding in women. The most common indication for the procedure is postmenopausal bleeding or dysfunctional uterine bleeding in younger women. Other uses include the workup of an Atypical Glandular Cells (AGC) Pap in women over 35, evaluation of endometrial cells on a Pap in post-menopausal women, evaluation of women at higher risk for endometrial cancer prior to instituting Hormone Replacement Therapy (HRT), evaluation of women bleeding on tamoxifen therapy, and, infrequently, as an evaluation for infertility. In most cases, the office endometrial biopsy has replaced Dilatation and Curettage (D&C) due to its ease of performance in the outpatient setting. This also allows for the evaluation of bleeding women who are poor candidates for general anesthesia.

Endometrial biopsy has a high overall accuracy when an adequate specimen is obtained. The overall sensitivity for detecting carcinoma is 99.6% in postmeno-pausal women and 91% in perimenopausal women. Endometrial sampling with a Pipelle® (Unimar, Wilton, CT) also detects atypical hyperplasia with a sensitivity of 81% and a specificity of 98% [1, 2]. Some practitioners also use uterine ultra-sound to assess endometrial lining thickness prior to the endometrial biopsy.

While no anesthesia is required for most endometrial biopsies, it is recommended that the patient take a dose of a Non-Steroidal Anti-Inflammatory medication (NSAID) such as ibuprofen prior to the procedure to decrease discomfort and cramping. In addition, use of local anesthesia with 1% lidocaine via a paracervical block and/or intramyometrially has been shown to decrease pain as well. Use of a paracervical block can also decrease the risk of vasovagal events postprocedure [3].

K. McNamara (✉)
Assistant Professor, Department of Family Medicine, St. Joseph's Hospital,
301 Prospect Avenue, Syracuse, NY 13203, USA
e-mail: kristen.mcnamara@sjhsyr.org

S.M. Sulik and C.B. Heath (eds.), *Primary Care Procedures in Women's Health*,
DOI 10.1007/978-0-387-76604-1_18, © Springer Science+Business Media, LLC 2010

Topical anesthesia can be used locally on the cervix for some reduction of discomfort caused by placement of the tenaculum [4].

Performing an endometrial biopsy on a woman with a stenotic os is difficult technically for clinicians and uncomfortable for the patient. Nulliparous, breastfeeding, postmenopausal women, or women using progestogen-only contraceptives are at greatest risk for cervical stenosis. Treatment for cervical stenosis prior to performing the endometrial biopsy may involve insertion of a laminaria several hours to 1 day prior to the procedure, use of 200 mg of misoprostol intravaginally or orally the day prior to the procedure, or premedication with Premarin® (Wyeth Pharmaceuticals Inc., Madison, NJ) cream vaginally for 2 weeks prior to the procedure.

Case Study

A 56-year-old postmenopausal female, LMP at age 54, presents to the office complaining of 2 days of vaginal bleeding last week that spontaneously resolved. She has not had any menses or vaginal bleeding in 2 years, and the episode was accompanied by abdominal cramping. She used two pads on the first day of bleeding and one pad on the second day of bleeding. The bleeding spontaneously resolved, and she is currently feeling well. A pelvic exam is essentially unremarkable, and she has no other health problems. She is on no medications. Her Pap smear is current and is normal.

Diagnosis (Algorithm 18-1)

Postmenopausal vaginal bleeding; rule out endometrial malignancy.

Indications (Algorithm 18-1)

- Postmenopausal vaginal bleeding
- Dysfunctional uterine bleeding
- AGC-US (Atypical Glandular Cells of uncertain significance) Pap in a woman over 35
- Evaluation of endometrial thickness >5 mm in a postmenopausal women
- Endometrial cells on Pap in a postmenopausal woman
- Endometrial dating in an infertility evaluation (used infrequently)
- Evaluation of endometrium prior to onset of HRT use in high-risk women
- Evaluate bleeding in women on tamoxifen

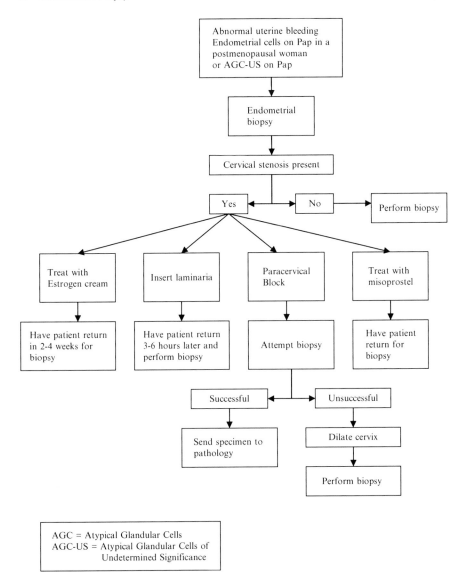

Algorithm 18-1 Decision tree for endometrial biopsy procedure

Contraindications

- Pregnancy
- Known cervical cancer

Relative Contraindications

- Acute cervicitis/pelvic infection
- Active uterine bleeding (may be difficult to obtain a core sample of endometrium adequate for analysis)
- Cervical stenosis
- Difficulty passing cannula secondary to cervical stenosis, large leiomyomas, marked uterine flexion, patient sensitivity

Equipment (Fig. 18-1)

- Antiseptic solution
- Tenaculum
- Hurricaine® gel (Beutlich LP Pharmaceuticals, Waukegan, IL) (topical anesthetic)
- Vaginal speculum

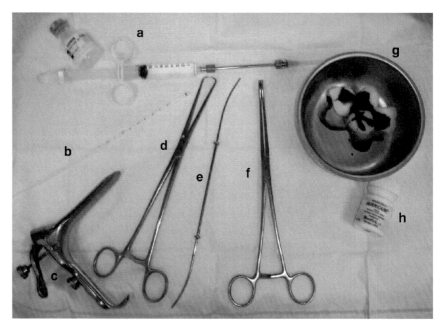

Fig. 18-1 Equipment set-up for endometrial biopsy: (a) 1% lidocaine with epinephrine anesthetic in 10 cc syringe with needle extender; (b) Endometrial sampler, sterile; (c) Sterile speculum; (d) Sterile cervical tenaculum; (e) Sterile uterine sound; (f) Sterile long-looped forceps; (g) Metal basin with betadine-soaked cotton swabs; (h) Hurricaine® gel (Beutlich LP Pharmaceuticals, Waukegan, IL) for topical anesthesia

- Formalin sample bottle with labels
- Endometrial biopsy sampler [Pipelle® (Unimar, Wilton, CT), Endocell™ Endometrial Sampler (Wallach surgical Devices, Orange, CT), or Endometrial Aspirator]

Optional Equipment

- Uterine sound (Endometrial sampler can be used to sound the uterus)
- 1% lidocaine with epinephrine
- Needle extender
- 10 cc syringe

Procedure

1. Obtain informed consent for the procedure, and obtain urine pregnancy test if the patient is not postmenopausal.
2. Place patient in dorsal lithotomy position.
3. Perform a bimanual examination to determine the position and size of the uterus
4. Insert vaginal speculum and visualize cervix.
5. Cleanse the cervix with the antiseptic solution.
6. Sound the uterus (determine depth of uterus to avoid perforation) and document the depth (usually 6–9 cm). This may be done using a uterine sound or the biopsy sampler itself inserted through the cervical os.
7. If there is difficulty inserting the sound, the cervical canal may be straightened and the cervix stabilized using a tenaculum. Hurricaine® anesthetic should be applied to the cervix prior to placing the tenaculum. The "teeth" of the tenaculum should be placed on the cervix horizontally, at 11 o'clock and 1 o'clock positions, approximately 1 cm from os (Fig. 18-2).
8. Insert the sampler through the cervical os. If resistance is encountered, use gentle pressure. If there is still resistance, terminate the procedure and follow steps below for stenotic cervical os (Fig. 18-3a).
9. Stabilize the sheath with one hand and draw the piston completely back in one continuous motion. This creates a vacuum, or negative pressure, within the uterus (Fig. 18-3b).
10. Rotate the sheath between the thumb and index finger and move it in and out between the fundus and the internal os three or four times until the sampler is full. These actions pass the sampler opening through a helical arc against the uterine walls. The negative pressure vacuum draws the endometrial tissue into the sampler. The tissue can be visualized in the lumen of the sampler (Fig. 18-3c).
11. Withdraw the device (with piston still drawn back).
12. Expel the sample into the formalin by advancing the piston back into the sheath. Do not put the tip of the sampler directly into the formalin in the container.

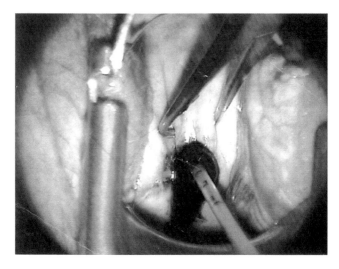

Fig. 18-2 Proper placement of tenaculum and insertion of endometrial sampler

Some clinicians use the sampler to repeat the procedure to obtain a second sample (Fig. 18-3d).
13. Some clinicians cut the tip of the sampler and send it with the specimen.
14. Remove the tenaculum, if applied.
15. Remove the speculum from the vagina and send the specimen to pathology.

Complications and Risks

- Missed lesion in biopsy sample (5–15% false negative rate)
- Uterine perforation (0.1–1.0%)
- Infection (0.4%)
- Excessive uterine bleeding
- Cramping (common and brief)
- Vasovagal syncope (10% of patients)

Tricks and Helpful Hints (Algorithm 18-1)

- Storing the sampling device in the freezer stiffens the plastic enough that a tenaculum may be unnecessary.
- For cervical stenosis:
    - Pretreat postmenopausal women or women who have not had vaginal deliveries with Premarin® cream one half-full applicator into the vagina every other night for 2–4 weeks prior to the procedure.

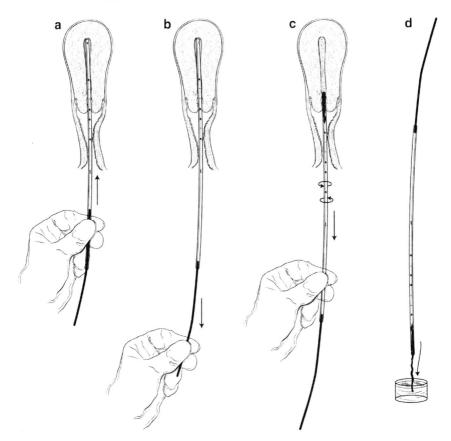

Fig. 18-3 (**a**) Endometrial sampler is inserted to the fundus of the uterus. (**b**) The sampler is stabilized and the piston is pulled entirely back to the stopper. (**c**) The endometrial sampler is moved in and out and rotated clockwise counter-clockwise to obtain the uterine sample. (**d**) The sample is placed in the formalin container to send to pathology

- Insert laminaria into the cervical os 1 day prior to procedure or in the morning and have the patient return later in the day for the procedure.
- Have the patient insert 200 µg of misoprostol into her vagina or take orally the day prior to procedure. (This may cause some mild cramping.)
• For uncomfortable patients:
  - Two to three days prior to the procedure, have the patient begin taking ibuprofen or other NSAID to decrease the discomfort felt during the procedure.
  - A paracervical block done just prior to the procedure can decrease the pain during the endometrial biopsy.
  - To perform a paracervical block:
    (a) Use 5–10 cc of 1% lidocaine with epinephrine.
    (b) Place a needle extender onto the syringe with a 26-gauge needle.
    (c) Stabilize the cervix by placing a tenaculum, as described previously.

   (d) Inject submucosally 1–2 cc of lidocaine into the cervix at the 12, 3, 6, and 9 o'clock positions. (Can use 2:00, 4:00, 8:00, and 10:00 positions if preferred.)
   (e) Proceed with the biopsy as described previously.
   (f) If also injecting intramyometrially, use the remaining lidocaine and inject through the cervical os using an angiocatheter or spinal needle, leave needle in place for approximately 3 min before withdrawing and starting the procedure [5, 6].

Interpretation of Results [7, 8] (Algorithm 18-2)

- *Insufficient Tissue*: Follow-up will depend on reason biopsy was done. If need to repeat, consider mid-cycle sample rather than at the end of menses.
- *Proliferative or secretory endometrium*: Normal findings, no follow-up required, and confirms ovulation.
- *Atrophic endometrium*: No treatment needed.
- *Hyperplasia*:
   - Simple (cystic)
      (a) 0–2% progress to cancer
      (b) If bleeding persists, treat with progesterone.
      (c) No follow-up biopsy is needed.
   - Complex (adenomatous) *without* atypia
      (a) 12% progress to cancer – close follow-up is required.
      (b) Treatment with progesterone and follow up biopsy to confirm resolution is necessary.
   - Complex (adenomatous) *with* atypia
      (a) 30% progress to cancer
      (b) If child bearing *not* completed:
         - Progesterone treatment for 3–6 months
         - Regular endometrial sampling every 6 months
      (c) If child bearing complete, simple hysterectomy is recommended.
- *Carcinoma*: Refer to gynecology oncology for staging and hysterectomy.
- *Endometritis*: Multiple causes
   - Acute: infection, necrosing endometrial polyp
   - Chronic: infection, sarcoidosis, radiation effects, carcinoma, retained IUD, retained products of conception (postmiscarriage or termination)

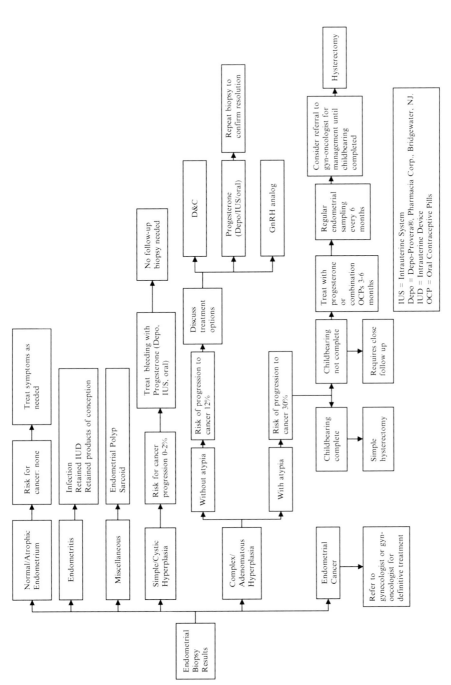

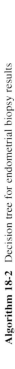

Algorithm 18-2 Decision tree for endometrial biopsy results

Procedure Note

(Provider to customize as needed.)

After the patient gave informed consent, she was placed in the dorsal lithotomy position. Bimanual exam was performed, revealing a mobile anteverted uterus. A speculum was inserted, and the cervix was visualized. Cervix was cleaned with an iodine solution. There was difficulty sounding the uterus with the endometrial sampler. Hurricaine® gel was applied, and a tenaculum was placed in the 11:00–1:00 position. The uterus was sounded to ___ cm using the endometrial sampler. The sampler piston was drawn back, and multiple passes were made in the uterine cavity to obtain a sample. Two endometrial samples were placed in a sterile container of formalin. The tenaculum was removed and the patient had no bleeding from the os or the tenaculum site. The speculum was removed. The patient tolerated the procedure well, and the sample was sent to pathology.

Coding

CPT® Codes (Current Procedural Terminology, AMA, Chicago, IL)

58100	Endometrial sampling (with or without endocervical sampling, without cervical dilatation, any method)
57800	Dilation of cervical canal, instrumental
59200	Insertion of cervical dilator, laminaria

ICD 9-CM-Diagnostic Codes (International Classification of Diseases, 9th Revision, Clinical Modification, Center for Disease Control and Prevention)

182.0	Cancer uterus
219.1	Benign neoplasm, uterus
233.2	Cancer in situ, uterus
621.2	Enlarged uterus
621.3	Endometrial hyperplasia
625.9	Pelvic pain
626.5	Functional vaginal bleeding
626.8	Dysfunctional uterine bleeding
626.9	Abnormal uterine bleeding
627.0	Premenopausal menorrhagia
627.1	Postmenopausal bleeding
622.1	Atypical glandular cells
V07.4	Postmenopausal HRT
10.42	Personal cancer uterus

Postprocedure Patient Instructions

- Patient may experience dizziness/syncope after the procedure: Have the patient sit up slowly on the exam table postprocedure.
- Mild cramping is expected: The patient may take ibuprofen.
- Vaginal bleeding/spotting is common postprocedure. Patient can resume sexual activity after her bleeding has stopped.
- Postprocedure infection is uncommon. Instruct the patient to call the office if a fever, foul smelling vaginal discharge, or abdominal pain develops.
- Have patient return in 1 week to discuss results of the biopsy.

Case Study Outcome

The patient's biopsy showed secretory endometrium. The she was reassured that she did not have cancer or precancerous cells. She will continue to be monitored by her physician.

Patient Handout

(Provider to customize as needed.)

An endometrial biopsy evaluates the tissue inside of the uterus and is used to check for cancerous or precancerous cells. This procedure involves passing a small tube into your uterus and removing part of the endometrium (lining) of your uterus. Your clinician may be doing this test to evaluate any abnormal vaginal bleeding, check on the lining of the uterus if you are on hormones, or check for endometrial cancer.

The endometrial biopsy can be uncomfortable, and we recommend you start taking ibuprofen, three 200 mg tablets three times daily, with food for 2 days prior to the procedure. This will help alleviate the discomfort during the procedure.

The procedure takes less than 10 min, and after the procedure the sample from your uterus will be sent for microscopic evaluation by a pathologist. You will return to the office in 1 week to discuss those results.

After the procedure, you may have some mild cramping. If this happens, you may take ibuprofen, three 200-mg tablets three times a day with food. Some vaginal bleeding or spotting is common after your procedure. If you have heavy vaginal bleeding, more than one pad every 2 h, please call your clinician. Infection following this procedure is also uncommon. If you develop fever, foul smelling vaginal discharge, or lower abdominal pain, please contact the office.

References

1. Huang GS, Gebb J, Einstein M, Shahabi S, Novetsky A, Goldberg G. Accuracy of preoperative endometrial sampling for detection of high grade endometrial tumors. *Am J Obstet Gynecol* 2007;196(3):243.e1–243.e5.
2. Dijkhuizen FP, Mol BWJ, Brölmann HAM, Heintz APM. The accuracy of endometrial sampling in the diagnosis of patients with endometrial carcinoma and hyperplasia: a meta-analysis. *Cancer* 2000;89(8):1765–1772.
3. Cincelli E, Didonna T, Schonauer LM, Stragapede S, Falco N, Pansini N. Paracervical anesthesia for hysteroscopy and endometrial biopsy in postmenopausal women: a randomized, double-blind, placebo-controlled study. *J Reprod Med* 1998;43:1014–1018.
4. Leclair C. Anesthesia for office endometrial procedures: a review of the literature. *Curr Womens Health Rep* 2002;2(6):429–433.
5. Zullo F, Pellicano M, Stigliano CM, Di Carlo C, Fabrizio A, Nappi C. Topical anesthesia for office hysteroscopy a prospective randomized study comparing two modalities. *J Reprod Med* 1999;44(10):865–869.
6. Trolice MP, Fishburne C Jr, McGrady S. Anesthetic efficacy of intrauterine lidocaine for endometrial biopsy: a randomized double-masked trial. *Obstet Gynecol* 2000;95: 345–347.
7. Zuber T. Endometrial biopsy. *Am Fam Physician* 2001;63(6):1131–1135, 1137–1141.
8. Dunn TS, Stamm CA, Delorit M, Goldberg G. Clinical pathway for evaluating women with abnormal uterine bleeding. *Obstet Gynecol Surv* 2002;57(1):22–24.

Additional Resources

Articles

Tanriverdi HA, Barut A, Gun BD, Kaya E. Is pipelle biopsy really adequate for diagnosing endometrial disease? *Med Sci Monit* 2004;10(6):CR271–CR274.
Clark TJ, Mann CH, Shah N, Khan KS, Song F, Gupta JK. Accuracy of outpatient endometrial biopsy in the diagnosis of endometrial cancer: a systematic quantitative review. *BJOG* 2002;109(3):313–321.
Barnhart KT, Gracia CR, Reindl B, Wheeler JE. Usefulness of pipelle endometrial biopsy in the diagnosis of women at risk for ectopic pregnancy. *Am J Obstet Gynecol* 2003; 188(4):906–909.
Cooper JM, Erickson ML. Endometrial sampling techniques in the diagnosis of abnormal uterine bleeding. *Obstet Gynecol Clin North Am* 2000;27(2):235–244.
Apgar BS, Newkirk GR. Office procedures. Endometrial biopsy. *Prim Care* 1997;24(2):303–326.
Barik S. Topical anesthesia for diagnostic hysteroscopy and endometrial biopsy for postmenopausal women: a randomized placebo-controlled double blind study. *Br J Obstet Gynaecol* 1997;104(11):1326–1327.
Apgar B. Dysmenorrhea and dysfunctional uterine bleeding. *Prim Care* 1997;24(11):161–178.

Chapter 19
Breast Cyst Aspiration

Cathryn B. Heath

Introduction

A breast mass is a common presenting symptom in a primary care office setting, at times accompanied by symptoms of pain and tenderness. It is also frequently found on a well woman examination and is a concern to both clinician and patient due to the fear of malignancy. Most breast masses are caused by fibrocystic changes of the breast, but these must be differentiated from breast cancer. Over half of the women in the United States will have fibrocystic changes sometime during their reproductive life; these changes are most common between the ages of 30 and 50. Seven percent of women in the Western world will have palpable breast cysts [1]. Fibrocystic changes consist of two different forms: fibroadenomas, which are solid, and cysts, which are liquid-filled sacs. Most fibrocystic changes fluctuate with hormonal cycles, worsening just prior to menses and improving after the initiation of menses. If a mass is noted by the clinician or the patient, consideration of returning after the patient's menses for a reevaluation may be appropriate. If the mass is still present, a diagnostic mammogram and sonogram should be ordered. If the breast cyst shows a thickened cyst wall, intramural tumor, multiple septae, or is eccentric on ultrasound, it has a higher likelihood of being malignant [2]. A breast mass must be evaluated even if the mammogram is read as normal, as breast cancer can present in a similar fashion.

Breast cysts are often uncomfortable, and patients may prefer drainage by aspiration for relief of symptoms. Breast cyst aspiration is a very easy office procedure that can be performed with minimal risks or complications. If the mass is not completely resolved with aspiration, referral to a breast surgeon for further evaluation is recommended. Follow-up in 2 weeks is recommended, as many breast cysts recur [3].

C.B. Heath (✉)
Department of Family Medicine, University of Medicine and Dentistry of New Jersey, Robert Wood Johnson Medical School, 317 George Street, New Brunswick, NJ 08901 USA
e-mail: cheath1965@aol.com

S.M. Sulik and C.B. Heath (eds.), *Primary Care Procedures in Women's Health*,
DOI 10.1007/978-0-387-76604-1_19, © Springer Science+Business Media, LLC 2010

The technique for Fine Needle Aspiration (FNA) is similar to that of breast cyst aspiration, although the number of passes through a lesion are higher. FNA can have an accuracy rate of up to 99%, with as few as 0.4% false positives [4], and is considered (with physical examination and mammogram) part of the "triple test" for diagnosis of breast masses.

With an FNA, most clinicians use a 23 G or 25 G needle, either with or without anesthetic, as larger-gauge needles tend to increase discomfort with the same clinical yield [5]. Some clinicians use a plain syringe, while others use a pistol grip syringe mechanism, which allows a one-handed method of applying negative pressure to the syringe. A newer pencil grip syringe holder also facilitates a one-handed method of applying negative pressure to the syringe.

Fine needle aspirations require sending adequate cytopathological specimens to pathology. If performing FNAs in the office, it is imperative to check with the pathology laboratory for the optimal method of specimen presentation and transportation.

Case Study

A 36-year-old female presents to the office for her routine gynecologic evaluation. She is a G2P2 whose last menses were 1 week ago. She has a past history of fibrocystic breast disease. Her family history is positive for breast cancer in her mother at the age of 55. During the examination, a 2×2 cm mass is palpated in the upper outer quadrant of the left breast. She has been doing regular breast examinations and does not remember feeling this particular mass within the last 3 months. The mammogram shows a mass; and ultrasound shows it is cystic. She is uncomfortable due to its size and is requesting an aspiration.

Diagnosis (Algorithm 19-1)

Unilocular breast cyst

Indications (Algorithm 19-1)

Uncomfortable breast mass documented to be cystic by ultrasound

Contraindications

- Previous history of breast cancer
- Mass lying too close to the chest wall
- Ultrasound shows noncystic lesion

Algorithm 19-1 Decision tree for breast mass aspiration and/or FNA

Equipment (Fig. 19-1)

- 23 G or 25 G needle or butterfly with tubing (Fig. 19-2a, b)
- 5–10 cc syringe (Fig. 19-2a)
- Needle holder: pistol or pencil grip (optional) (Fig. 19-3)
- Hemostat
- Red top tube
- Antiseptic solution, such as chlorahexidine
- Ultrasound, if available
- Surface anesthetic (EMLA™ cream (AstraZeneca, London, England), spray freezant (i.e., ethyl glycol))
- Bandage
- 2 × 2 gauze pads (for use for pressure under bandage if needed)
- Gloves
- Glass microscope slides with fixative (for FNA)

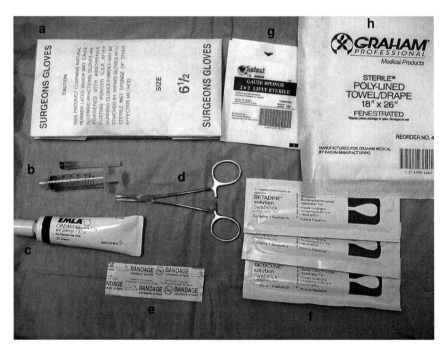

Fig. 19-1 Sterile tray set up for breast cyst aspiration. (a) Sterile gloves; (b) 5 cc Luer lock syringe with 23 gauge 1½ in. needle; (c) EMLA™ (AstraZeneca, London, England) cream (topical anesthetic); (d) Straight hemostat; (e) Adhesive bandage; (f) Betadine® Solution Swabsticks (Purdue Pharma, Stamford, CT); (g) 2 × 2 in. gauze pads (Select Medical Products); (h) Fenestrated sterile drape (Graham® Professional Medical Products, Green Bay, WI)

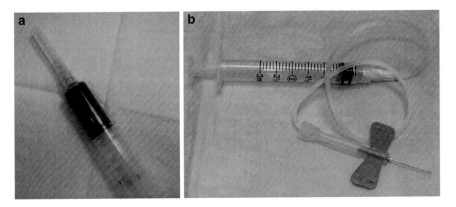

Fig. 19-2 (**a**) Syringe and needle, this one with grey green fluid from breast cyst. (**b**) Butterfly with tubing

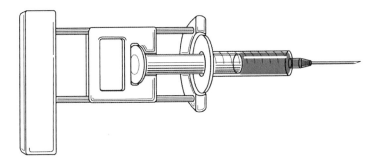

Fig. 19-3 Pistol grip syringe

Procedure

Breast Cyst Aspiration

1. Clean area with antiseptic solution three times in an outward circular fashion.
2. Apply topical anesthesia or ethyl chloride. If applying EMLA™, you must wait for 40 min prior to doing procedure. Local anesthesia may be used instead, but may distort architecture.
3. "Juice" the syringe (slide it back and forth a couple of times to ease aspiration later) and then leave 0.1–0.2 cc of air to the syringe prior to insertion. Put needle on end of the syringe.
4. Using gloves on both hands, grasp breast mass in nondominant hand, cupping the mass within fingertips and applying some tension to remove it from the

chest wall (Fig. 19-4). Alternatively, some practitioners capture the lesion between the second and third finger of the nondominant hand and pin the lesion above one of the patient's ribs (Fig. 19-5).

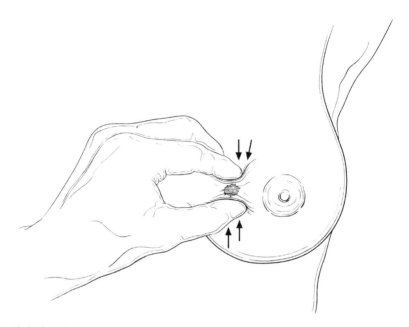

Fig. 19-4 Cupping lesion between first and second finger of nondominant hand

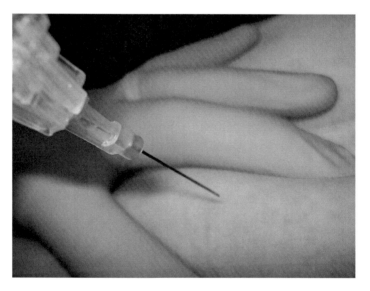

Fig. 19-5 Breast mass localization with nondominant hand

5. If ultrasound is available, ask assistant to place ultrasound lateral to lesion, aiming toward lesion.

6. Hold the syringe like a pencil during insertion, keeping the needle bevel up.

7. After insertion into the lesion, apply suction. This can be accomplished by placing thumb under the plunger or inching one's fingers up the syringe to the plunger. Alternatively, you can have an associate withdraw the plunger to create the suction. With a pistol grip syringe holder, the syringe is held by the handle, with suction being applied after insertion by pulling back on the handle (Fig. 19-6).

8. Milk the mass (gently squeeze) until it is totally gone. If there is too much fluid for the selected syringe, use the hemostat to twist the needle off the syringe, remove the fluid, and reinsert syringe onto needle again. It is not necessary to remove the needle from the patient.

9. When the mass is gone, stop applying suction and remove the needle. There is usually minimal bleeding involved. Apply pressure with the 2×2 gauze and then apply the bandage, if needed.

10. If the fluid is a clear grayish-green color (Fig. 19-2a), it is not necessary to send to the lab. If there is any blood or if the fluid is any other color, put the fluid into the red top tube for transport [3]. Use as many red top tubes as necessary to send fluid.

11. If available, use the ultrasound to document that the cyst is gone.

12. Document whether the mass is entirely gone or still present. If still present, refer for surgical evaluation [6].

If the mass is solid and nothing is coming through the needle, follow the steps for Fine Needle Aspiration.

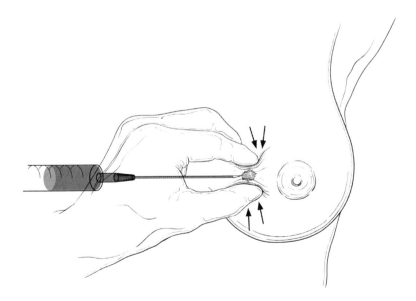

Fig. 19-6 Aspiration and "milking" of breast cyst

Fine Needle Aspiration Technique

Use steps 1–7 of breast cyst aspiration. If no fluid advances, then proceed to step 1 of Fine needle aspiration technique as listed below.

1. While applying suction, use a gentle pumping motion to the syringe, passing up and down through the lesion, changing the angle of the direction with each pass.
2. Discontinue negative pressure by removing the thumb from the plunger on regular syringe, or with a syringe holder by discontinuing the pressure.
3. Withdraw the needle from the patient.
4. Place specimen onto a glass slide by pushing plunger fully down the barrel of the syringe, thereby emptying syringe entirely (Fig. 19-7). The small amount of air that was left in the syringe prior to the procedure will force the specimen out of the needle onto the slide. Rolling the bevel of the needle over the slide may permit some of the solid specimen to be placed on the slide. The specimen may be quite small, as little as a drop of liquid.
5. Place another glass slide directly on top of the first slide, applying slight pressure. Wipe the slides laterally from each other, which will disperse the specimen on both the slides (Fig. 19-8). If the specimen looks too thick, use another microscopic slide to smear a third specimen. Repeat procedure until all specimen sent are thinly placed across multiple slides.
6. Use fixative on slides. This can be either Pap smear fixative or hair spray.
7. Send specimen to pathology.
8. Repeat procedure up to four times, or recommend referral to surgery as most surgeons will do multiple biopsy specimens.

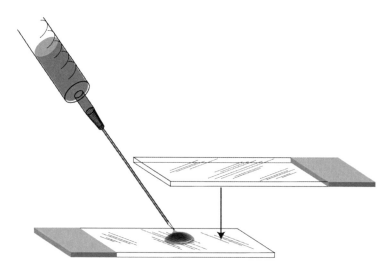

Fig. 19-7 Insertion of specimen on microscopic slide for FNA

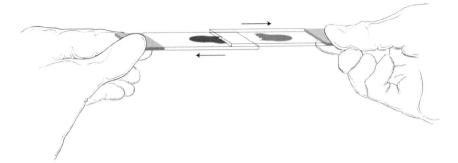

Fig. 19-8 Spreading specimen across microscopic slides

Complications and Risks

- Pneumothorax (rare)
- Bleeding (rare)
- Infection
- Inadequate specimen (for FNA)
- Further work up if mass is not totally gone with aspiration

Tricks and Helpful Hints

- *Do not* let go of the mass or allow your associate to hold the mass while attempting to aspirate. This increases the likelihood of inadvertently causing a needle stick to yourself or your assistant.
- "Juice" the syringe by sliding the barrel up and down several times within the syringe prior to using on the patient. This facilitates easier withdrawal of the plunger during the aspiration.
- If possible, avoid the use of injectable anesthesia, as it distorts the skin above the mass and may make the mass more difficult to palpate. If necessary for patient comfort, consider using ethyl chloride or EMLA™.

Interpretation of Results (Algorithm 19-1)

- Grey green fluid from a breast cyst is considered benign and can be discarded.
- Any bloody fluid should be sent to pathology for evaluation.
- Any solid lesion should have at least one specimen sent to pathology. Multiple specimens are necessary to improve statistical odds that lesion is benign. Consider surgical or interventional radiology consultation.

Procedure Note

(Provider to fill in blanks/circle applicable choice when given multiple choices and customize as needed.)

Breast Cyst Aspiration

Risks, benefits, and complications of breast mass evaluation discussed; consent signed. Patient placed in supine position; mass localized. (Topical anesthetic applied.) Area prepped and draped in a sterile fashion. Mass located and held with nondominant hand; breast mass aspirated with a 25 gauge needle on a 10 cc syringe. _____ccs of fluid obtained with complete resolution of breast cyst. Bandage applied. Patient tolerated procedure well.

Fine Needle Aspiration

Risks, benefits, and complications of breast mass evaluation discussed; consent signed. Patient placed in supine position; mass localized. (Topical anesthetic applied.) Area prepped and draped in a sterile fashion. Mass located and held with nondominant hand; breast mass aspirated with a 25 gauge needle on a 10 cc syringe.
Needle passed through mass with no fluid obtained with suction.
OR
Multiple passes through breast mass with suction applied; suction removed and specimen placed on microscope slide.
OR
Multiple passes done through breast mass with additional specimens sent to lab.

Bandage applied; patient tolerated procedure well.

Coding

CPT® Codes (Current Procedural Terminology, AMA, Chicago, IL)

88170	Breast mass evaluation and recommendations for breast cancer screening
19000	Aspiration and drainage of one breast cyst
19001	Aspiration and drainage of breast cyst – each additional
10021	FNA without imaging guidance

ICD 9-CM-Diagnostic Codes (International Classification of Diseases, 9th Revision, Clinical Modification, Center for Disease Control and Prevention)

217	Benign lesion breast
610.0	Solitary cyst of breast
610.1	Fibrocystic breast disease
610.2	Fibroadenosis of breast
611.72	Breast lump
174.1	Cancer breast central
174.0	Cancer breast areola
174.4	Cancer breast, upper/outer quadrant
174.6	Cancer breast, axillary fold

Case Study Outcome

Breast cyst successfully aspirated in the office under local anesthesia. Grey green fluid obtained and mass completely resolved. No recurrence when reexamined in 1 month.

Patient Handout

(Provider to customize as needed.)

Breast cyst aspiration is an office procedure that involves putting a needle into the cyst and removing all the fluid. If you choose to have this done, plan on taking three 200 mg ibuprofen 1 h before coming to the office. The area will be cleaned with an antibacterial disinfectant. The clinician will insert a needle to remove the fluid. After the procedure is done, a bandage will be applied.

Fine needle aspiration is a process that takes a small amount of a solid lump and sends it to pathology for evaluation. It generally takes up to 2 weeks to get a reading from the pathologist.

Call your clinician's office if you are experiencing any warmth, swelling, bleeding, or shortness of breath after the procedure. Please make a follow-up appointment in 2 weeks to reevaluate your mass and discuss the results.

References

1. Dixon JM, McDonald C, Elton RA, Miller WR. Risk of breast cancer in women with palpable breast cysts: a prospective study. *Lancet* 1999;353(9166):1742–1745.
2. Vargas HI, Vargas MP, Gonzalez KD, Eldrageely K, Khalkhaliet I. Outcomes of sonography-based management of breast cysts. *Am J Surg* 2004;188(4):443–447.
3. Hamed H, Coady A, Chaudary MA, Fentiman IS. Follow-up of patients with aspirated breast cysts is necessary. *Arch Surg* 1989;124(2):253–255.
4. Lau SK, McKee GT, Weir MM, Tambouret RH, Eichhorn JH, Pitman MB. The negative predictive value of breast fine needle aspiration biopsy: The Massachusetts General Hospital experience. *Breast J* 2004;10:487–491.
5. Daltrey IR, Kissin MW. Randomized clinical trial of the effect of needle gauge and local anesthetic on the pain of breast fine-needle aspiration cytology. *Br J Surg* 2000;87:777–779.
6. Bhate RD, Chakravorty A, Ebbs SR. Management of breast cysts revisited. *Int J Clin Pract* 2007;61(2):195–199.

Additional Resources

Articles

Lucas JH, Cone DL. Breast cyst aspiration. *Am Fam Physician* 2003;68(10):1983–1986.
Marchant DJ. Benign breast disease. *Obstet Gynecol Clin North Am* 2002;29(1):1–20.

Equipment

Cameco pistol syringe holder syringe: http://www.belpro.ca/cameco.htm
Tao pencil grip syringe holder:http://www.taoaspirator.com/

Chapter 20
Vulvar Skin Biopsy

Matthew L. Picone

Introduction

Vulvar lesions consist of a wide array of benign, premalignant, and malignant lesions that involve the vulva (Fig. 20-1). The decision to biopsy is determined by many factors including the time course of the lesion, uncertainty of diagnosis, symmetry of the lesion, irregularity of the borders, bleeding tendencies of the lesion, family history of vulvar malignancy, and patient concerns. All of these factors independently play a role in the decision to biopsy.

Cancer of the vulva is statistically the fourth most common gynecologic malignancy (following cancer of the endometrium, ovary, and cervix) and comprises 5% of malignancies of the female genital tract [1]. Vulvar carcinoma presents most commonly in the postmenopausal female. Risk factors include cigarette smoking, history of lichen sclerosis or any vulvar dystrophy, cervical cancer, immunodeficiency syndromes, and Human Papilloma Virus (HPV).

As always, a thorough history (before patient undresses) and complete gynecologic exam are necessary to make the diagnosis and to determine the appropriate treatment plan. Hygiene habits and personal care products used (including detergents, fabric softeners, soaps, feminine hygiene sprays, sanitary napkins, and habits of douching) should be evaluated. Soaps, shaving products, hair removal techniques, and spermicides are all irritants that cause a number of dermatoses in the vulvar area. Hormonal status can be determined based on the physical exam of the vulva to assess for hypoestrogenism. A discussion of the potential "home cures" that the patient has tried should be explored, as these remedies can often make visual diagnosis difficult. Finally, patient concerns for cancer should be elicited.

M.L. Picone (✉)
Assistant Professor, Department of Family Medicine, St. Joseph's Hospital Family Medicine Residency, Syracuse, New York, NY 13066, USA
e-mail: piconem@pol.net

S.M. Sulik and C.B. Heath (eds.), *Primary Care Procedures in Women's Health*, DOI 10.1007/978-0-387-76604-1_20, © Springer Science+Business Media, LLC 2010

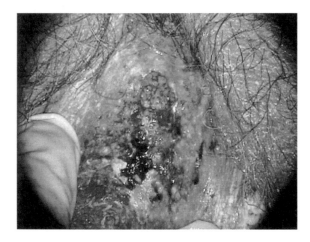

Fig. 20-1 Paget's skin lesion of the vulva

Often asymptomatic, vulvar lesions present in a variety of ways to the physician. Pruritis is usually the most common symptom complaint. Physicians are often the first to see these lesions and bring them to the patient's attention.

Case Study

A 65-year-old presents to your office for her annual physical exam and Pap smear. Review of systems reveals that the patient has been postmenopausal for the past 13 years with no history of hormone replacement therapy. During the physical exam, an irregularly shaped, nonulcerated, raised, flesh-toned plaque measuring approximately 1.5×1.5 cm in diameter is noted. Patient was unaware that the lesion was present. Biopsy was suggested based upon the uncertainty of diagnosis.

Diagnosis

Vulvar lesion, Not Otherwise Specified (NOS)

Differential Diagnosis [2, 3] (Algorithm 20-1)

- Vulvar intraepithelial neoplasia
- Cancer: most common is squamous cell carcinoma
- Condyloma Acumulata: genital warts
- Lichen Sclerosis

- Vestibular papillae
- Acrochordon: skin tags
- Cysts: bartholin, pilonidal, dermoid, mucous cysts
- Molluscum contagiosum: immunosuppressed disorders
- Hyperkeratosis or lichen simplex: white patches
- Vitiligo: depigmenting autoimmune disorder
- Acanthosis Nigricans: pigmented macules/plaques
- Junctional nevi: common
- Seborrheic keratosis
- Dermatofibroma
- Extramammary breast: found along the nipple line
- Fox-Fordyce disease
- Kaposi's sarcoma: immunodeficiency syndromes
- Dysplastic nevi

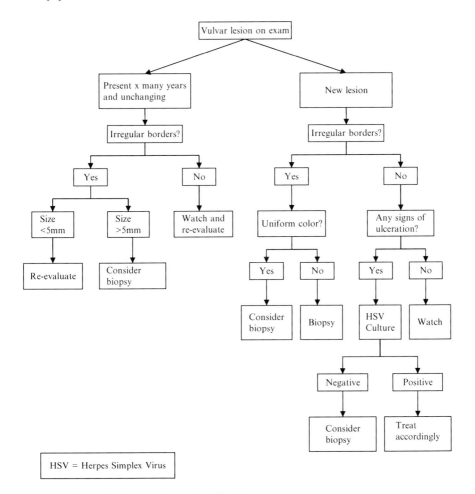

Algorithm 20-1 Decision tree for vulvar skin lesion

- Melanoma: family history sometimes present
- Dermatitis: chemical or allergic
- Psoriasis
- Infection

Indications

Diagnostic

Contraindications

- Bleeding or Coagulation Disorders
- Uncooperative patient

Equipment (Fig. 20-2)

Nonsterile tray for anesthesia:

- Nonsterile Gloves
- 4×4 inch gauze pads
- 3-cc syringe filled with 1% lidocaine with epinephrine and 25–27-gauge needle
- Labeled formalin container(s) for the number of biopsies

Sterile tray for the procedure:

- Sterile gloves
- Desired punch biopsy instrument (2–6 mm)
- Scalpel with blade if preferred
- Needle holder for suturing if needed
- Desired size of suture usually 4-0 or 5-0 nylon
- Iris scissors
- Small-gauge needle

Procedure

1. Sign consent for the procedure.
2. Clean the skin with povidine–iodine solution after determining the selection of site.
3. Pick the site for biopsy at the center of the lesion and not at the periphery [4] (Fig. 20-3).

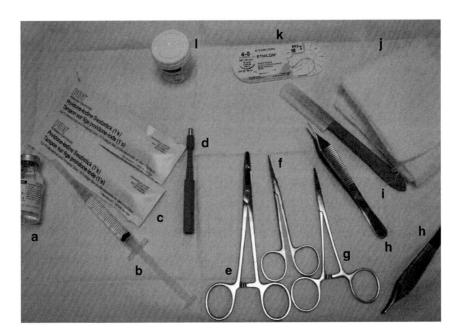

Fig. 20-2 Equipment tray for vulvar skin biopsy. (a) lidocaine; (b) 1% lidocaine in 5 cc syringe; (c) PDI® Povidone-Iodine Swabsticks (Orangeburg, NY); (d) Punch biopsy; (e) Needle driver/holder; (f) Fine scissors; (g) Hemostat; (h) Needle nose pick-ups; (i) Scalpel; (j) Gauze; (k) Ethilon™ 4-0 Nylon Absorbable Suture (Ethicon Inc., West Somerville, NJ); (l) Formalin specimen container

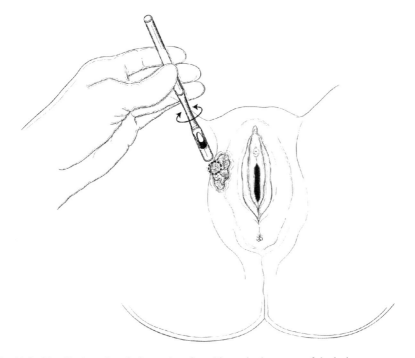

Fig. 20-3 Identify the vulvar lesion and perform biopsy in the center of the lesion

4. Use generous local anesthesia to surround the lesion. Allow 3–5 min for anesthesia to be fully absorbed.
5. Identify the lines of least skin tension (the lines vertical to the vulva).
6. Stretch the skin around the site perpendicular to the skin lines with the opposite hand (Fig. 20-4a).
7. Hold the punch biopsy vertical to the skin and rotate downward between the first and second fingers in a clockwise and counterclockwise fashion, penetrating the dermis and subcutaneous tissues.
8. Lift the lesion with a small-gauge needle and cut the base with iris scissors, and place in formalin. Properly label the specimen and send to pathology with identification of biopsy, any pertinent history, and presumed diagnosis (Fig. 20-4b).
9. Place sutures perpendicular to the tension lines for the vulva that were identified earlier using 4-5.0 nylon suture.
10. Apply antibiotic ointment and a bandage.
11. If preferred, the entire lesion can be removed. Follow the steps previously delineated. Once the area is anesthetized, make a fusiform incision with the scalpel that encompasses the entire lesion. The blade should be pressed firmly to penetrate the entire thickness of the dermis.
12. Grasp the corner of the incision with a pair of forceps and cut the lesion free with the scalpel or iris scissors.
13. Close the incision as above.

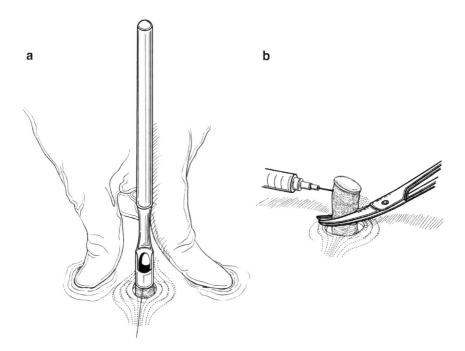

a

b

Fig. 20-4 (a) Stretch the skin at the biopsy site perpendicular to the skin lines with the non-dominant hand. (b) Lift the punch biopsy with a needle and cut the base to avoid crushing the tissue

Complications and Risks

- Bleeding
- Recurrence
- Scarring/Keloids
- Infection: rare
- Pain

Tricks and Helpful Hints

- Use a small-guage needle instead of forceps to avoid crushing the lesion and interfering with pathology interpretation.
- If 6 mm punch is required, it may be better to perform an fusiform incisional removal.
- Consider delaying submission for payment until pathology returns, as payment is higher for cancerous lesions.

Interpretation of Results

Treatment is determined by the final pathology. If cancerous, then referral to specialist is indicated. See Algorithm 20-1.

Procedure Note

(Provider to customize as needed.)

The patient was placed in the lithotomy position. The area was cleansed, and sterile technique was utilized. After local anesthesia was administered, a 4 mm punch to the region of concern was performed. The lesion was placed in formalin and sent to pathology. Hemostasis and closure of the wound was obtained by placing two 5-0 interrupted sutures. The patient tolerated the procedure well and will return in 10 days for pathology report and suture removal.

Coding

CPT® Codes (Current Procedural Terminology, AMA, Chicago, IL)
56605	Biopsy of vulva or perineum [one lesion]
56606	Biopsy of each additional vulvar or perineal lesion

ICD 9-CM-Diagnostic Codes (International Classification of Diseases, 9th Revision, Clinical Modification, Center for Disease Control and Prevention) [non-comprehensive]
624.9	Unspecified noninflammatory lesion of vulva
701.9	Skin Tag
221.2	Benign Vulvar Neoplasm
078.11	Condyloma Acumulata

Postprocedure Patient Instructions

- Instruct the patient to keep the bandage in place for the next 24–36 hours followed by air drying the area and keeping it clean and dry until the follow-up appointment.
- Have the patient call the office for signs of infection, pain, redness, fever, discharge, or wound opening.
- Tell the patient to return to the office in 10 days for suture removal and pathology report.

Case Study Outcome

The biopsy was successfully obtained and sutures were removed 10 days post biopsy with excellent approximation of the site. Pathology report revealed a Vulvar Intraepithelial Neoplasm (VIN) 3. The patient was referred to a specialist for complete excision. She will follow up 2 months after surgery has been performed.

Patient Handout

(Provider to customize as needed.)

A vulvar biopsy is a procedure done to take a small piece of an abnormal area that is found on the vulva, which many call "the lips." The procedure is done in the office to help determine or clarify what type of growth is present.

You may want to take Tylenol (650 mg) or Ibuprofen (600 mg) 1 hour prior to the visit for some mild discomfort that may occur. There will be a local anesthesia given to the area before a biopsy is performed; this may cause mild pain and possibly burning. After the area is numb, you may experience nothing at all or a pressure sensation.

After the procedure is performed, the lesion will be sent out to a lab that will help us determine the cause of the abnormal growth. At the follow-up visit, we will have the report and will discuss any future treatment plans.

There is a small risk for bleeding, infection, and possibly excessive scar formation or discoloration that persists at the biopsy site. You should call the office if signs of infection should occur, such as redness, swelling, increased pain, or discharges from the biopsy site.

References

1. Jemel A, Siegel R, Ward E, Murray T, Xu J, Smigal C, Thun MJ. Cancer statistics, 2006. *CA Cancer J Clin* 2006;56:106–130.
2. Fischer GO. The commonest causes of symptomatic vulvar disease: a dermatologist's perspective. *Australas J Dermatol* 1996;37:12–18.
3. Foster DC. Vulvar disease. *Obstet Gynecol* 2002;100:145–163.
4. Pariser RJ. Skin biopsy: lesion selection and optimal technique. *Mod Med* 1989;57:82–90.

Chapter 21
Treatment of Genital Warts

Cathryn B. Heath

Introduction

Genital warts caused by Human Papilloma Virus are the most common viral sexually transmitted disease in the United States. Over 24 million Americans are infected with Human Papilloma Virus (HPV), with the current prevalence among adolescents up to 15% and college-aged women up to 26.8% [1]. An increased prevalence has been correlated with earlier onset of sexual activity, multiple sex partners, and a higher frequency of casual relationships [2]. Approximately 500,000 to 1 million new cases of genital warts are believed to occur annually, which accounts for greater than 1,000,000 provider visits per year [2].

Genital warts are soft, moist, fleshy colored lesions on the genital area. Warts can also be flat, cauliflower-like, papular or rounded, keratotic with a thick horny surface, multiple or single lesions on the labia, vulva, vagina, cervix, penis, scrotum, glans, urethra, perianal area, or rectum [3]. There is a broad spectrum of disease presentation ranging from asymptomatic external lesions to invasive carcinoma. Lesions may appear within weeks or months of initial contact. Two-thirds of individuals who have had sexual contact with a partner with genital warts will develop lesions within 3 months. In the anogenital area, warts, dysplasia, and carcinoma are all indistinguishable. There should be a higher index of suspicion in patients older than 40, immunocompromised patients, women with lesions refractory to treatment, and patients with any large atypical appearing lesions. A biopsy should be performed whenever the clinician is unsure of the diagnosis or when lesions do not respond to treatment.

The expression of anogenital warts varies considerably, although most individuals have a subclinical infection that is cleared spontaneously by the host immune response. Anogenital HPV types are divided based on their oncogenic response into low- and high-risk types. Almost all cervical cancers and over 50–80% of vulvar,

C.B. Heath (✉)
Department of Family Medicine, University of Medicine and Dentistry of New Jersey, Robert Wood Johnson Medical School, 317 George St, New Brunswick, NJ 08901, USA
e-mail: cheath1965@aol.com

S.M. Sulik and C.B. Heath (eds.), *Primary Care Procedures in Women's Health,*
DOI 10.1007/978-0-387-76604-1_21, © Springer Science+Business Media, LLC 2010

vaginal, and anal carcinomas are due to high-risk types of HPV. Over 90% of genital warts, however, are due to the low-risk oncogenic types 6 and 11, and do not become cancerous [4]. However, individuals who have one type of HPV may harbor other types of HPV and other types of sexually transmitted infections (STIs); therefore, it is important to perform a Pap smear and STI screening on all women with genital warts.

Genital warts develop anywhere in the anogenital tract and over half the patients who are infected have multiple sites of infection. Many warts are asymptomatic and are found only on physical examination; however, there is a wide variety of symptoms also described. These include burning, anogenital pruritis, vaginal discharge, bleeding, and, rarely, dyspareunia. The vulva is the most common site for genital warts in women, but up to 25% will also have perianal warts. Most warts are visible with the naked eye, but a magnifying glass or colposcope can aid in identifying additional or smaller lesions. Use of acetic acid on the vulva for diagnosis of genital warts is not useful as acetowhite changes on the vulva are not specific for HPV [3].

Warts are considered highly contagious, yet may resolve on their own. Ten of the 30 known types of anogenital HPV can cause cervical cancer. In 2006, the HPV vaccine Gardasil® (Merck & Co., Inc., Whitehouse Station, NJ) became available to immunize women against HPV types 6, 11, 16, and 18. Types 6 and 11 are responsible for most anogenital warts, and types 16 and 18 account for over 80% of cervical cancer types worldwide. In the phase III trial of this medication, the rate of vulvar, vaginal, and anogenital lesions of the vaccinated population decreased by a rate of 34%, while the rate of cervical lesions decreased by 20% [5]. Vaccination has been approved in women aged 9–26 years, and is considered most effective prior to exposure to the HPV virus. The vaccine requires a series of three immunizations and is given at the interval of 2 months after initial vaccine and then 6 months after first vaccination.

A variety of treatments exist for anogenital warts, both patient-administered (podofilox, 5% imiquimod cream, and 15% sinecatechins) and provider-administered (podophyllin resin, Trichloroacetic Acid (TCA), cryotherapy, laser vaporization, or intralesional interferon [6]). Patient preference and affordability are important in choosing a regimen for each patient. There are no treatments that are 100% effective, recurrence is common, and up to 70% of patients have been treated more than once for their warts. A number of therapies are contraindicated in pregnancy, and therefore the patient's pregnancy status and method of contraception must also be considered.

The patient administered therapies allow for privacy of treatment, which helps reduce the psychological discomfort and stress associated with this condition. Available treatments have been: 0.5% podofilox (Condolox® Gel, Corona, CA) and 5% imiquimod cream (Aldara™, 3M Company, St. Paul, MN); sinecatechin (Veregen®, MediGene, Germany) became available in 2008. For women who prefer treatment in an office setting, podofilox is an antimitotic agent that works by arresting the formation of the mitotic spindle in metaphase, preventing cell division. Podophyllin resin (10–25%, less stable formulation than podofilox) is available in tincture of benzoin. With podofilox and podophyllin resin, the surface area treated must not exceed 10 cm^2 and no more than 0.5 cc should be used at any one application [7]. Clearance rates vary from 45% to 88%, with recurrences common. Podofilox and podophyllin resin should not be used during pregnancy and cannot be used in the vagina or rectum.

Five percent topical imiquimod (Aldara®) cream is a local immune modulator that induces interferon and cytokine release, stimulating both innate and cell-mediated immune responses. The cream is applied to the individual lesions three times per week for 12–16 weeks [3]. There is no limit to the amount of cream used at each treatment, and a single sachet packet can cover most areas effectively. Local erythema and some swelling are the most common side effects and are reported in over 50% of patients. Clearance rates range from 72% to 84% in women with higher clearance rates reported in women compared to men. Up to 81% of patients report at least a reduction in the wart area if not completely resolved. Recurrence rates are reported from 5% to 19%, which is less than rates reported by cytodestructive methods. There is currently no data available on intra-vaginal use, although there are several case reports noted with successful treatment. Imiquimod is category B and is safe for use in pregnancy, although its safety has not been firmly established.

A new ointment derived from a water extract of green tea was approved by the Federal Drug Administration (FDA) in late 2007 for use on external and perianal warts. Sinecatechins ointment (Veregen®) is composed of eight catechins, which may act to inhibit proinflammatory enzymes and proteases found in HPV. It is approved for immunocompetent patients above the age of 18. In the phase III trials of the medication, 56.8% of women cleared the virus versus 34.1% of the placebo patients. Men had a clearance rate of 60.1% versus 40.5% who cleared with placebo [8]. The most common side effects of the ointment were redness (70%), itching (69%), burning (67%), pain (56%), and erosions/ulcerations (49%) [9] Sexual contact needs to be avoided while undergoing treatment. In addition, sinecatechin ointment was found to weaken condoms and diaphragms; use of these contraceptives with Veregen® is not recommended. Sinecatechin ointment is pregnancy category C.

The provider-administered treatment modalities depend on expertise and equipment availability of the provider. Chemical agents that can be applied in the provider office include podofilox, podophyllin resin, and Trichloroacetic Acid (TCA). Bichloroacetic acid is no longer available.

TCA is used in concentrations of 80–90% and can be used on both skin and mucosal surfaces. They are not systemically absorbed and can be used during pregnancy. Application causes burning and this is reduced by applying petroleum jelly to the surrounding skin before application of the acid. Multiple applications are usually necessary and clearance rates approach 80%. Recurrence rates are similar to other treatment modalities.

Cryotherapy can be used to treat genital warts. Both nitrous oxide and liquid nitrogen may be used. The freeze thaw cycle with cryotherapy causes cell lysis and is cytodestructive. The ice ball should extend 2–3 mm past external lesions.

Both nitrous oxide and liquid nitrogen can be used for anogenital and vulvar warts; however, cryotherapy of the cervix should be done only with nitrous oxide as liquid nitrogen is not cold enough to produce adequate freezing of the area. With weekly treatments until clear, approximately 90% resolve with recurrence rates up to 40%. Cryotherapy may be used safely during pregnancy.

Surgical removal of condyloma can be accomplished with scissors, scalpel, electrocautery, or loop excision. These methods are appropriate as first line therapy for large or obstructing lesions. Excision with scissors or a scalpel is best for smaller lesions or when a biopsy is needed to rule out cancer or dysplasia. Clearance rates approach 70% with recurrence often at the surgical margins. Large condyloma are very vascular and may require a surgical setting where bleeding can be easily controlled and better anesthesia can be used.

Laser vaporization can also be used for treatment although this requires extensive expertise of the provider and costly equipment. Clearance rates approach 87% with recurrence rates also at the margins of approximately 50%. Laser is especially effective in the vagina and for extensive eternal genital and perianal warts. There has been some concern about the virus being transmitted through the vaporization fumes. Therefore, it is important for all practitioners to use filtered masks [10]. Intralesional interferon has also been used with success rates up to 60%; however, it is costly, painful, and has multiple systemic side effects.

Due to the extensive recurrence rates with individual treatment modalities, combination therapies have been proposed, but there are no established guidelines for their use.

Case Study

A 25-year-old G0P0 presents for a well woman's examination. During the course of the history, she relates that she has been sexually active with one partner having just started a relationship within the last 3 months. She wants to be checked for sexually transmitted diseases and notes that she has noticed some "bumps" on her genital area in the last month. On physical examination, five lesions are found scattered on the patient's introitus.

Differential Diagnosis (Algorithm 21-1)

- Microglandular papillomatosis (normal papillary tissue in the vestibule of the female-single base for each projection versus multiple projections with papilloma)
- Hymenal remnants
- Condyloma lata
- Bowenoid papulosis
- Buschke–Lowenstein tumors
- Nevi
- Seborrheic keratosis

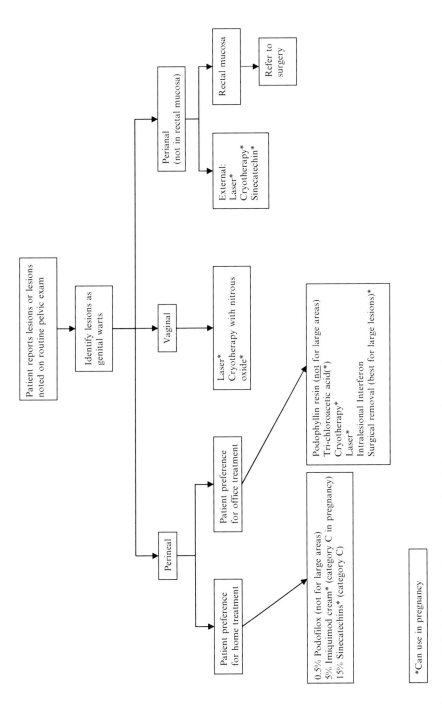

Algorithm 21-1 Decision tree for treatment of genital warts based on location

- Molluscum contageosum
- Cancer

Indications (Algorithm 21-1)

- Noted lesions present on examination
- Symptomatic lesions
- Patient desire for treatment
- Lesions that obstruct the vaginal opening

Contraindications (Algorithm 21-1)

- Some methods should not be used during pregnancy (podophyllox, podophyllin, or imiquimod)
- Some methods are not for use with vaginal lesions (podophyllox, podophyllin)
- Lesions in rectal mucosa or in urethra should be referred to a specialist

Equipment

Equipment is variable depending on method chosen:

- Cryotherapy: liquid nitrogen or nitrous oxide, water-based gel, cryoprobe, cotton-tipped applicator, or handheld cryogen
- Podophyllin: 10–25% podophyllin resin, pregnancy test, cotton-tipped applicator, and petroleum jelly
- TCA: TCA, cotton-tipped applicator, talc or baking soda, petroleum jelly
- Surgical excision: EMLA® (AstraZenaca, London, UK) or 1% xylocaine, iris scissors, scapel, electrocautery or aluminum chloride solution

Procedure

Patient Directed Methods (Suggest First Time Use in Office)

Podophyllox 0.5 mg Solution or Gel

1. Gently wash and dry application area.
2. Apply with cotton swab or on finger directly on the lesion.
3. Apply twice daily for 3 days to each lesion; then do not apply for 4 days. Repeat this cycle up to four times.
4. Patient should wash hands after application.

Imiquimod 5% Cream

1. Gently wash and dry application area.
2. Rub cream on each lesion until cream is no longer visible.
3. Wash hands after application.
4. Remove all cream by washing the area 6–10 h posttreatment.
5. Apply a thin layer over each lesion for on alternate days, either according to a Monday, Wednesday, Friday regimen, or a Tuesday, Thursday, Saturday regimen.
6. May be repeated for a total of four cycles.

Sinecatechins 15% Ointment

1. Is approved for external genital and perianal warts in immunocompetent women and men 18 years or older.
2. Ointment should be applied after bathing or showering.
3. Hands should be washed prior to and after application.
4. Up to 250 mg per application applied topically three times a day (TID).
5. Itching and burning frequently occur; continuation of application until side effects are intolerable or until warts disappear is recommended.
6. Applied up to 16 weeks or until complete clearance of warts.
7. Medication to be refrigerated or kept up to 77°F.

Physician-Directed Methods

Cryotherapy

1. Place patient in dorsal lithotomy position.
2. Cotton-tipped application or Cryoprobe method or Cryogun (Fig. 21-1).
   Cotton-tipped application:

   - Apply liquid nitrogen on lesion with large cotton-tipped applicator until ice ball extends 3 mm beyond perimeter of lesion.
   - May need to exchange applicators as liquid nitrogen will evaporate in less than 15 s.

   Cryoprobe method or Cryogun (Fig. 21-1):

   - Apply water-based gel solution to tip of cryoprobe.
   - Put cryoprobe on wart and apply freezant until ice ball covers wart and 2–3 mm beyond wart, approximately 10–20 s.
   - Consider "freeze–thaw–freeze" method on recalcitrant lesions.
   - Patients may return every 1–2 weeks for repeat treatment.

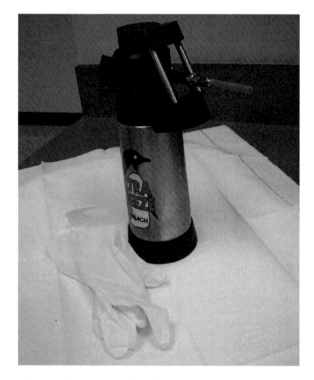

Fig. 21-1 Set-up for cryotherapy (e.g., Ultrafreeze™ Liquid Nitrogen Cryosurgical System, Wallach Surgical Devices, Orange, CT)

Podophyllin Resin: 10–25% Podophyllin

- Pregnancy test should be done prior to start of treatment.
- Place patient in dorsal lithotomy position.
- Apply petroleum jelly around each lesion to protect skin.
- Apply podophyllin with a small cotton-tipped applicator.
- Air dry.
- Use no more than 0.5 ml of podophyllin or on 10 cm² area.
- Instruct patient to wash off in 1–4 h.
- May be reapplied weekly until lesion is gone.

TCA (Trichloroacetic Acid) (Fig. 21-2)

- Place patient in dorsal lithotomy position.
- Apply petroleum jelly around each lesion to protect skin.
- Apply TCA with small cotton-tipped applicator; need to apply with care as TCA is runny and can easily destroy surrounding tissue.
- Allow to air-dry. A whitish frost should appear on lesion after application.

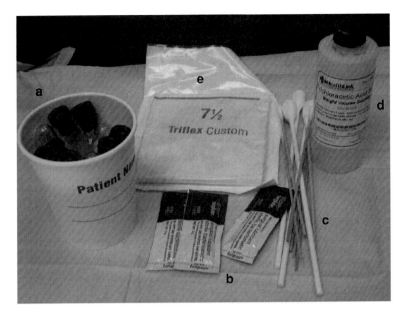

Fig. 21-2 Set-up for trichloroacetic acid. (a) Small test tubes for acid solution; (b) Surgilube®
(Fougera, Melville, NY) lubricant for protecting surrounding skin; (c) Cotton-tipped applicators;
(d) Trichloroacetic acid (e.g., HealthLink®, Jacksonville, FL); (e) Surgical nonlatex gloves

- Apply talc or baking soda to absorb any remaining acid.
- May be reapplied weekly up to 6 weeks.

Laser Treatment

- Carbon dioxide laser can be used.
- Suggest local anesthetic, such as xylocaine 1% (injected) or topical EMLA®
  cream, be used prior to procedure.
- Surgeon to use mask during application as HPV virus is present in flume of
  smoke created by laser.

Surgical Removal

- Anesthetize patient with xylocaine 1% subcutaneously, or EMLA® cream to be
  applied topically 45 min prior to procedure.
- May use electrocautery or scalpel.
- Alternatively may use tangential scissors technique by cutting off exophytic lesion.
- May need electrocautery or aluminum chloride solution to create hemostasis.

Complications and Risks

- Erythema and pain at treatment site
- Blistering (uncommon)
- Severe side effects from absorption of podophyllin include:
  – Nausea
  – Vomiting
  – Renal failure
  – Fetal death

Tricks and Helpful Hints (Algorithm 21-1)

- Recommend patient takes a Nonsteroidal Anti-Inflammatory (NSAID) 1 h prior to appointment time.
- Vaginal lesions: use laser, cryotherapy with cotton applicator only or TCA.
- Pregnancy: use cryotherapy, TCA, or surgical removal.
  – Important as want to minimize exposure of neonate to HPV lesions as may get laryngopapillomatosis (risk 0.04%).
- Anal warts: use cryotherapy, TCA, or surgical removal.
  – If there are anal warts, check patient by anoscopy for rectal mucosal warts.
  – Do *not* treat warts in the rectal mucosa; these are best treated by a surgeon.
- Genital or anal lesions in prepubescent girls may be associated with sexual abuse.
- Persons with immunodeficiency may have particularly difficult warts to treat; Imiquimod may be most effective.
- Patients should be warned to be vigilant for the next 3 months and check for recurrence of warts.
- While most subtypes of external warts are low risk, patients should have a current Pap smear or one should be obtained at the time of treatment.
- For imiquimod: treatment can be stopped for several days and then restarted if a significant erythematous reaction occurs.
- For any self-applied creams or ointments: If a woman wishes to use tampons, it is recommended that she do so prior to application of antiviral topical medications.
- Cryoprobes should be avoided in the vagina and rectum as there is a higher risk of fistula formation in these areas secondary to the greater depth of freezing.
  – For podoflox: Redness and itching may occur after use.

Procedure Note (Depends on treatment used)

(Provider to fill in blanks/circle applicable choice when given multiple choices and customize as needed.)

> *Patient placed in dorsal lithotomy position. Petroleum jelly applied/Local anesthetic applied. _____*
> *method was used to treat _____number of condylomata. Patient instructed to wash off podophyllin/TCA within 6 h of treatment. Patient tolerated procedure well. Follow-up appointment for retreatment was made.*

Coding

CPT® Codes (Current Procedural Terminology, AMA, Chicago, IL)
Per lesion: same coding is used for all treatments

17110	1–14 lesions
17111	15 or more lesions

ICD 9-CM-Diagnostic Codes (International Classification of Diseases, 9th Revision, Clinical Modification, Center for Disease Control and Prevention)

078.11	Condyloma acuminata
078.19	Penile warts
078.1	Viral warts

Postprocedure Patient Instructions

Patients should be instructed to wash off the podophyllin or TCA within 6 h of treatment. Some burning or swelling may be experienced and can be relieved with additional NSAIDs and a warm bath. They should be encouraged to use condoms while being treated for their genital warts.

Case Study Outcome

Patient treated in the office with cryotherapy. Subsequent follow-up revealed no lesions.

Postprocedure Patient Handout

(Provider to customize as needed.)

You have just been treated for genital warts. Warts are caused by a highly infective virus. It is important that you refrain from having sexual relations until these lesions are gone as they commonly spread to sexual partners. Even skin to skin contact with the wart without actually having sex will spread external genital warts. It is especially important to avoid pregnancy while undergoing treatment for genital warts. Your partner should see a physician and be checked for genital warts as well.

A nonsteroidal antiinflammatory (ibuprofen or naproxen) can help with the pain of treatment 1 h prior to the treatment and the evening after the treatment. If you have been treated by a liquid, cream, or gel, be sure to follow the instructions for when you should remove the compound. If you have severe pain or swelling, be sure to wash the medication off immediately. Most lesions need to be rechecked by a physician. If your doctor treated you with cryotherapy or TCA, please make a follow-up appointment within 1–2 weeks for a recheck.

References

1. Gunter J. Genital and perianal warts: new treatment opportunities for human papillomavirus infection. *Am J Obstet Gynecol* 2003;89(3S):S3–S11.
2. Cates W. Reproductive tract infections. In Hatcher RA (ed) *Contraceptive technology*, 18th edn. New York: Ardent Media, 2004, pp 207–208.
3. Atkins D, Workowski KA, et al. Center for Disease Control and Prevention; sexually transmitted diseases treatment guidelines for 2006. Reviewed April 2007; Available at: http://www.cdc.gov/std/treatment/2006/genital-warts.htm. Accessed November 4, 2007.
4. Henderson Z, Irwin KL, Montano DE, Kasprzyk D, Carlin L, Greek A, Freeman C, Barnes R, Jain R, Jain N. Anogenital warts knowledge and counseling practices of US clinicians: results from a national survey. *Sex Transm Dis* 2007;34(9):644–652.
5. Garland SM, Hernandez-Avila M, Wheeler CM, Perez G, Harper DM, Leodolter S, Tang GWK, Ferris DG, Steben M, Bryan J, Taddeo FJ, Railkar R, Esser MT, Sings HL, Nelson M, Boslego J, Sattler C, Barr E, Koutsky LA. Quadrivalent vaccine against human papillomavirus to prevent anogenital diseases. *N Engl J Med* 2007;356(19):1928–1943.
6. Kodner CM, Nasraty S. Management of genital warts. *Am Fam Physician* 2004;70(12): 2335–2342.
7. Lipke M. An armamentarium of wart treatments. *Clin Med Res* 2006;4(4):273–279.
8. Gross G, Meyer K-G, Pres H, Thielert C, Tawfik H, Mescheder A. A randomized, double-blind, four-arm parallel-group, placebo-controlled Phase II/III study to investigate the clinical efficacy of two galenic formulations of Polyphenon® E in the treatment of external genital warts. *J Eur Acad Dermatol Venereol* 2007;21(10):1404–1412.
9. Veregen description; Rxlist:the internet drug Index.2007. Available at: http://www.rxlist.com/cgi/generic/veregen.htm. Accessed November 11, 2007.
10. Garden JM, O'Banion MK, Shelnitz LS, Pinski KS, Bakus AD, Reichmann ME, Sundberg JP. Papillomavirus in the vapor of carbon dioxide laser treated verrucae. *JAMA* 1988;259(8): 1199–1202.

Chapter 22
Colposcopy

Laurie Turenne-Kolpan

Introduction

Colposcopy is a procedure used to evaluate the abnormal Pap smear as well as to visualize abnormalities noted anywhere along the lower female reproductive tract. The colposcope is a binocular microscope that enables the provider to examine the vulva, vagina, and cervix under magnified view. The goal of colposcopy is to identify areas of abnormal epithelium and perform directed biopsies, which will allow for a histological evaluation of abnormal cytological results.

The procedure is simple and can be performed in the outpatient office; however, recognition of the normal verses abnormal cervix requires a certain level of expertise. Practitioners performing colposcopy should be adequately trained. Such training can be found from a number of sources such as courses offered by the American Society for Colposcopy and Cervical Pathology (ASCCP), the American Academy of Family Physicians (AAFP), and the National Procedures Institute (NPI).

Case Study

A 23-year-old female presents to your office for her annual exam and Papanicolaou (Pap) smear. She is sexually active and using oral contraceptives. She has never had a Pap smear and has no history of any sexually transmitted disease. She smokes one pack of cigarettes per day. Her exam is normal. Pap smear results return as Low-Grade Squamous Intraepithelial Lesion (LSIL).

L. Turenne-Kolpan (✉)
Department of Family Practice, Hunterdon Medical Center, Flemington, NJ, USA
e-mail: turenne-kolpan.laurie@hunterdonhealthcare.org

S.M. Sulik and C.B. Heath (eds.), *Primary Care Procedures in Women's Health*,
DOI 10.1007/978-0-387-76604-1_22, © Springer Science+Business Media, LLC 2010

Diagnosis

Abnormal Pap Smear with LSIL.

Indications (Algorithms 22-1, 22-2)

- Atypical Squamous Cell of Undetermined Significance (ASC-US) with HPV positive for high-risk types.
- Two or more ASC-US Pap smear results.
- Atypical Squamous Cells, cannot rule out high-grade lesion (ASC–H).
- Low-Grade Squamous Intraepithelial Lesion (LSIL).
- High-Grade Squamous Intraepithelial Lesion (HSIL).
- Atypical Glandular Cells of Undetermined Significance (AGC-US).
- History of intrauterine DES exposure.

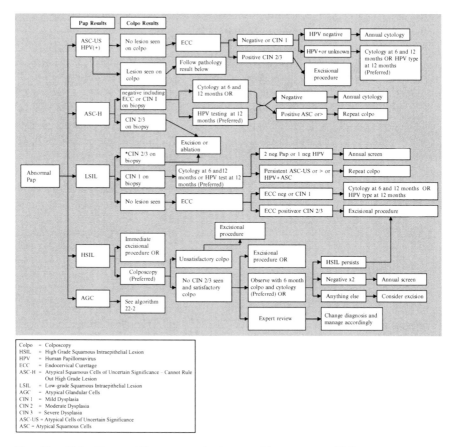

Algorithm 22-1   Abnormal Pap smear and colposcopy biopsy report guidelines

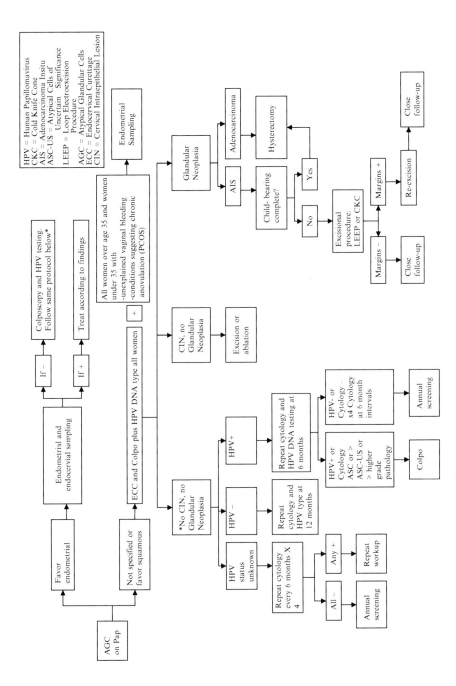

Algorithm 22-2 Atypical glandular cells algorithm

- Suspicious lesion seen or palpated on exam.
- Leukoplakia.

Contraindications

- Pregnancy is only a contraindication for Endocervical Curettage (ECC); biopsies are performed for suspicion of cancer only.
- Heavy menses.
- Uncooperative patient.
- Active cervicitis.

Equipment (Fig. 22-1)

- Vaginal speculum (metal or plastic)
- Small and large cotton-tipped applicators
- 3–5% acetic acid (vinegar)
- Lugol's solution

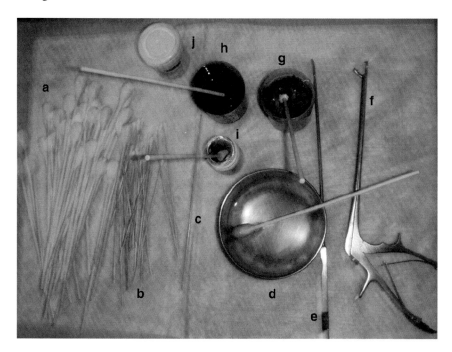

Fig. 22-1 Set-up tray for colposcopy: (a) Large cotton swab applicators; (b) Small cotton swab applicators; (c) Endocervical brush; (d) Basin with acetic acid; (e) Sterile Endocervical curette; (f) Sterile Kevorkian punch biopsy; (g) Monsel's solution; (h) Lugol's solution; (i) topical anesthetic; (j) Formalin specimen container

- Specimen containers
- Kogan endocervical speculum
- Endocervical curette with or without basket
- Tischler or Kevorkian biopsy forceps
- Cervical hook
- Monsel's solution
- Silver nitrate sticks
- Toothpicks
- Papanicolaou smear supplies

Optional Equipment

Cytobrush with a straw, ring forceps or long kelly, Telfa® (Covidien, Dublin, Ireland) pads cut into small squares.

Procedure

1. Check a urine pregnancy test prior to procedure, and obtain surgical consent.
2. Place the patient in the dorsal lithotomy position.
3. Insert the speculum into the vagina and visualize the cervix under medium magnification (12–15X). Ensure the entire cervix can be visualized.
4. Wipe off excess mucus with large cotton swab and identify landmarks. The squamocolumnar junction is the area of delineation between squamous and columnar epithelium (Fig. 22-2). The active transformation zone is the area

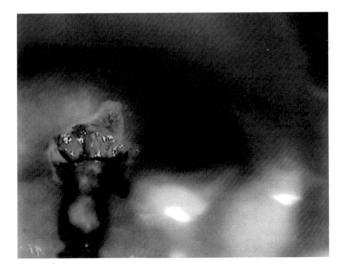

Fig. 22-2 Colposcopic view of squamocolumnar junction

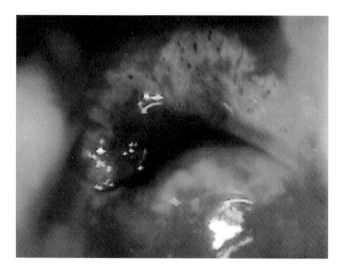

Fig. 22-3 Higher magnification view of cervix with green filter

where prior columnar epithelium has been changed or is in the process of changing into squamous epithelium, and thus is the area where dysplasia is most likely to occur. Gland openings, crypts, or nabothian cysts are usually seen in this area. An adequate colposcopy requires that the entire transformation zone and squamo-columnar junction be seen.

5. Perform Pap smear if desired. Recent evidence shows this practice is rarely useful even if the first cytology was obtained by a conventional smear [1, 2].

6. Use the green filter and higher magnification (25–40X) to identify any abnormal vessels (Fig. 22-3).
   - Normal saline can be used with the green filter if preferred.
   - Abnormal vascular patterns include the presence of mosaicism, which is caused by vessels lying along the superficial area of the cervix forming a pattern similar to mosaic tiles (Fig. 22-4), punctuation, which is caused by vessels lying perpendicular to the cervical surface and creates an appearance of the cervix being dotted with a red marker (Fig. 22-5), and atypical vessels, which are evidence of the presence of a blood vessel lying on top of the cervical surface (Fig. 22-6). The presence of larger or more coarse vessels in any of these vascular patterns is associated with higher-grade dysplasia.

7. Return to white light, medium magnification, and apply 3–5% acetic acid with large cotton swabs or cotton balls (Fig. 22-7).
   - These need to be held against cervix for at least 1 minute (min). Acetic acid may cause minor stinging, which will quickly abate.
   - Identify any areas of whitened epithelium (acetowhite). Look for all borders of the lesion.

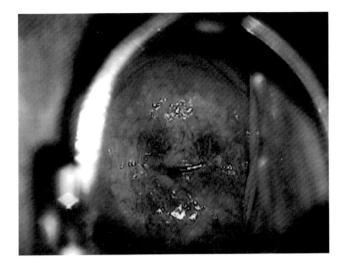

Fig. 22-4 Cervix with mosaic tile pattern

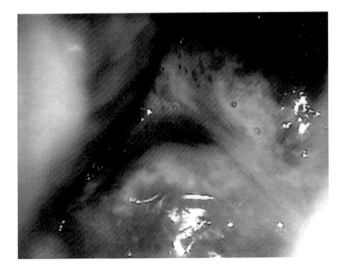

Fig. 22-5 Cervix with coarse punctation

- Identify which areas are the most densely white. High-grade dysplasia is typically associated with thick, well-demarcated areas of acetowhite. The acetowhite reaction will fade quickly (especially in low-grade disease) and more acetic acid may need to be applied (Fig. 22-8).
8. If the entire squamocolumnar junction is not seen or if an acetowhite area enters into the cervical canal, place the Kogan speculum into the cervical os and open slowly and gently.

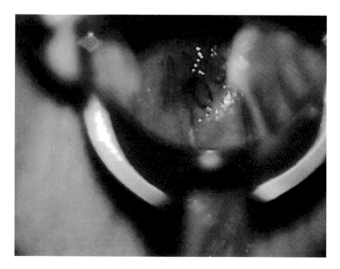

Fig. 22-6 Cervix with green filter showing superficial horizontal abnormal blood vessels

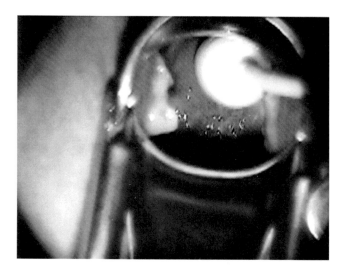

Fig. 22-7 Application of acetic acid under medium magnification

- If you are still unable to see the entire squamocolumnar junction or acetowhite area, or if you cannot get the Kogan speculum through the os, the colposcopy is considered unsatisfactory.
- Remove the endocervical speculum.
9. Apply Lugol's solution if desired (Fig. 22-9).
   - Abnormal epithelium has low levels of glycogen and does not take up iodine well; therefore, abnormal areas will remain light (mustard yellow in color) or "Lugol's Negative." Normal epithelium remains a deep dark brown stain.
   - Be aware that glandular epithelium will also not take up Lugol's solution.

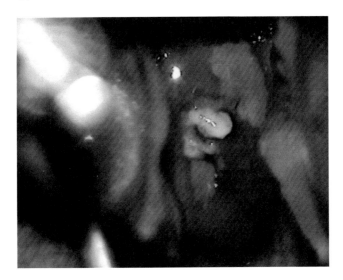

Fig. 22-8 Thick, well-demarcated lesions with acetowhite reaction indicating potential high grade lesion

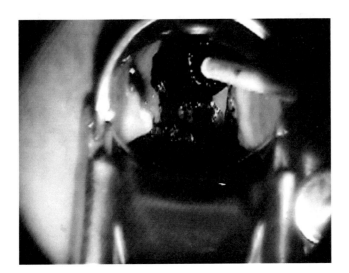

Fig. 22-9 Application of Lugol's solution to cervix with large cotton-tipped applicator

10. Perform the Endocervical Curettage (ECC) by inserting the curette through the external os, and, with firm pressure, scrape the sides of the canal using downward strokes around the entire canal (360° × two rotations) (Fig. 22-10).
11. Place the specimen from the curette into a formalin container. This can be facilitated by using a small square of Telfa® to wipe the curette, and then place the telfa in the container. If additional sample is seen at the os, it can be grasped with a ring forceps or a long Kelly forceps.

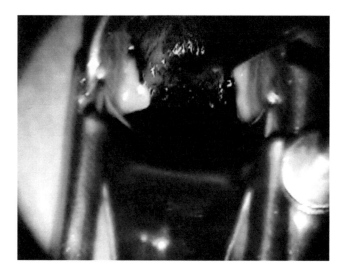

Fig. 22-10 Endocervical curettage performed after application of Lugol's solution

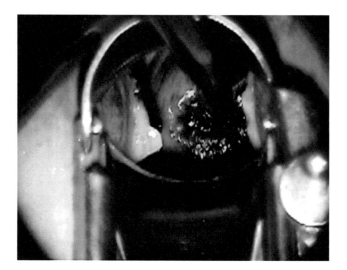

Fig. 22-11 Cervical biopsy with Tischler forceps

- Alternatively, a cytobrush can be used to obtain any residual sample from the os, and the tip of the brush can be cut off into the container.
12. Use the Tischler forceps to biopsy the most abnormal areas of the cervix. Start with the abnormal area most posterior on the cervix so as to avoid bleeding into the next area for biopsy (Fig. 22-11).

  - Recent evidence has shown that even in the hands of the most expert colposcopists, taking more than one biopsy increases the sensitivity of detecting CIN 3 [3]. Therefore, it is recommended that liberal biopsies be taken of the abnormal cervix. It is *not currently recommended*, however, that random biopsies be taken of the normal cervix.

13. Place biopsies in a formalin jar. A toothpick or broken stem of a wooden cotton-tipped applicator can be used to remove the biopsy from the forceps. Do not place the forceps directly into the formalin.
    - Although all biopsies can be sent in the same specimen container, the more common approach is to use a separate container for each specimen, allowing the provider to compare the histology results obtained with the visual abnormality seen.
14. Remove excess blood/clot from the vagina.
    - Apply pressure to all bleeding sites with large cotton-tipped applicators.
    - Apply Monsel's solution to all bleeding areas by using firm pressure over the bleeding site. Silver nitrate sticks may also be used (occasionally will stain the cervix).
    - Visualize the cervix under medium magnification to ensure hemostasis.
15. Remove the speculum and have the patient return to a sitting position slowly. Rapid sitting can cause a vasovagal response.

Complications and Risks

- Discomfort
- Bleeding
- Infection
- Missed disease

Tricks and Helpful Hints

- An alternate way of performing the ECC is to use intensive cytobrushing. A cytobrush is inserted through a straw and into the os. It is rotated 360° five times and then removed through the straw. The purpose of the straw is to prevent contamination of the endocervical sample with ectocervical disease. A recent study has shown this method to be more sensitive and less painful than the traditional ECC [4].
- Some colposcopists prefer to perform the ECC after the biopsies as this is the most uncomfortable part of the procedure. The concern with this method is contamination of the endocervical specimen with ectocervical disease. Care must be taken to avoid this.
- If a colposcopy is unsatisfactory because the os is stenotic, the patient may be given intravaginal estrogen 2 g inserted nightly for 2 weeks, or 200–400 µg of misoprostel inserted intravaginally 6 hours (h) before the procedure. The colposcopy is repeated. Either of these techniques has been shown to open the os, often enough to allow for an adequate exam.

Interpretation of Results (Algorithms 22-1, 22-2)

It is important to relate the histological results with the colposcopic and cytologic results. If significant discrepancies are present, further evaluation needs to occur. This can initially be accomplished by having the pathologist review the slides from both the Pap smear and histological samples obtained at colposcopy. If the discrepancy is not resolved, the patient warrants referral to a provider who can perform a diagnostic excisional procedure (Loop Electrode Excisional Procedure or cold knife cone biopsy).

Unsatisfactory Colposcopy

The colposcopy is considered unsatisfactory if the cervix cannot be fully visualized, the entire squamocolumnar junction cannot be fully visualized, or the limits of the lesion cannot be seen. If the initial cytology was HSIL, or histology is shown to be CIN-2 or CIN-3, the patient should undergo a diagnostic excisional procedure. If the cytology was less severe than HSIL and the colposcopy and histology were normal, the patient may be followed up either by a Pap at 6 and 12 months, HPV testing at 1 year (preferred method), or repeat Pap and colposcopy at 1 year [5].

Normal Colposcopy

See Algorithm 22-1.

CIN 1

See Algorithms 22-1 and 22-2.

CIN 2/3

Treatment is required for most cases of CIN 2 and 3. This can be performed by either ablative (cryotherapy, laser ablation, cold coagulation, or electrofulguration) or excisional (LEEP, cold knife cone, or laser excision) methods and should include treatment of the entire transformation zone. If the patient has disease within the canal, an excisional procedure is required. Most current guidelines do allow for an option to observe CIN 2 and 3 in adolescents with a combination of cytology and colposcopy performed at 6-month intervals. If both are normal for two consecutive exams, the patient may return to normal screening [6]. See Algorithms 22-1 and 22-2.

Procedure Note

(Provider to fill in blanks/circle applicable choice when given multiple choices and to customize as needed.)

Name:_____ Date:_____

Chart #: _____

Dae of Birth:_____ Contraception:

_____ HCG_____

G_____ P_____ A———— Pap Smear History:

_____

Reason for Colposcopy:

–

_____

_____

_____

_Smoking: _____

Colposcopic Exam   () Satisfactory () Unsatisfactory **12**

TZ= Transformation Zone

Go= Gland Openings

NC= Nabothian cysts

CO= Condylomy

WE= White Epithelium   **9**

MO = Mosaic punction

LK = Leukoplakia

AV = Atypical Vessels

X = Biopsy Site

SCJ SEEN: (X)Y   N   **6**

ECC DONE: (X)Y   N

Impression:

_____

Disposition:

_____

Suggest subsequent examination and/or follow-up: _____

_____
Physician's Signature

Coding

CPT® Codes (Current Procedural Terminology, AMA, Chicago, IL)

57452	Colposcopy of the upper vagina and cervix
57454	Colposcopy with biopsy(ies) and ECC
57455	Colposcopy with biopsy(ies)
57456	Colposcopy with ECC
57450	Colposcopy of the entire vagina and cervix

ICD 9-CM-Diagnostic Codes (International Classification of Diseases, 9th Revision, Clinical Modification, Center for Disease Control and Prevention)

795.0	Abnormal Pap Smear of cervix and cervical HPV
795.00	Abnormal Pap Smear, glandular
622.10	Dysplasia, cervix, unspecified
622.11	Dysplasia, cervix, mild (CIN 1)
622.13	Dysplasia, cervix, moderate (CIN 2)
233.1	Dysplasia, cervix, severe (CIN 3)

Postprocedure Patient Instructions

Explain to the patient that menstrual like cramps are common and can be treated with ibuprofen 600 mg every 6 h as needed. Spotting will occur, but bleeding should not persist beyond a week and should not be heavier than a menstrual period. If Monsel's solution or iodine was used, inform the patient that her vaginal discharge may be brown or black over the next several days. The patient should be instructed not to put anything in the vagina until all bleeding has resolved for 24 h to reduce the likelihood of infection. She should be counseled on the signs of infection and should be told to call for any abdominal pain beyond cramping and for fevers, shaking chills, and foul smelling vaginal discharge. A follow-up visit should be scheduled with the patient to review her results and make a definitive treatment plan.

Case Study Outcome

The patient was found to have CIN 2 (moderate dysplasia) on biopsy. She was referred for a LEEP procedure.

Patient Handout

(Provider to customize as needed.)

A colposcopy is a procedure by which your doctor can examine your vulva, vagina, and cervix more closely to evaluate for any possible abnormalities. Most patients are requested to have a colposcopy for further evaluation of an abnormal Pap smear. The procedure is done similarly to a Pap smear in that a speculum is placed into the vagina while you lie on the exam table. The provider will then use a colposcope, which is an instrument that shines light on the cervix and magnifies the view. A vinegar solution, and perhaps an iodine solution, will be applied to your cervix to better identify any areas of potential concern. If such areas are noted, your doctor will take a biopsy, which is the removal of a small amount of tissue, and this will be examined in a lab. If you are not pregnant at the time of your colposcopy, a scraping of the inside of your cervix will also be performed and sent to the lab.

The cervix does not have the same kind of nerve endings as your skin, so while you may feel some pinching with a biopsy, it will not be severe. More likely you will feel menstrual-like cramps. These can be reduced by taking three tablets (600 mg) of over-the-counter ibuprofen 1 hour (h) prior to the procedure. Do NOT take this if you are pregnant or allergic to aspirin, ibuprofen, or naproxen.

We ask that you do not douche, do not use tampons or vaginal medications, and do not have sexual intercourse for 24 h prior to your procedure.

After the procedure, you may have some brownish/black vaginal discharge from the medicines used to stop any bleeding. You may also have some spotting for 1–3 days and some menstrual-like cramps. These should improve with additional doses of ibuprofen. Do not put anything in the vagina (douches, tampons, etc.) and do not have intercourse until all spotting has stopped for 24 h.

Risks to the procedure are very minimal, but please call us if you have heavy vaginal bleeding (more than your normal menstrual period), significant abdominal pain, fevers, chills, or foul smelling vaginal discharge.

References

1. Mao C, Balasubramanian A, Koutsky L. Should liquid-based cytology be repeated at the time of colposcopy? *J Low Genit Tract Dis* 2005;9(2):82–88.
2. Rieck G, Bhaumik J, Beer H, Leeson S. Repeating cytology at initial colposcopy does not improve detection of high-grade abnormalities: a retrospective cohort study of 6595 women. *Gynecol Oncol* 2006;101(20):228–233.
3. Gage J, Hanson V, Abbey K, Dippery S, Gardner S, Kubota J, Schiffman M, Solomons D, Jeronimo J. Number of cervical biopsies and sensitivity of colposcopy. *Obstet Gynecol* 2006;108(2):264–272.
4. Maksem J. Endocervical curetting vs. endocervical brushing as case finding methods. *Diagn Cytopathol* 2006;54(5):313–316.
5. Dresang L. Colposcopy: an evidence-based update. *J Am Board Fam Pract* 2005;18(5):383–392.
6. Wright T, Massad S, Dunton C, Spitzer M, Wilkinson E, Solomon D. 2006 concencus guidelines for the management of women with cervical intraepithelial neoplasia or adenocarcinoma in situ. *Am J Obstet Gynecol* 2007;197(4):340–345.

Additional Resources

Articles

Wright T, Massad S, Dunton C, Spitzer M, Wilkinson E, Solomon D. 2006 Consensus guidelines for the management of women with abnormal cervical cancer screening tests. *Am J Obstet Gynecol* 2007;197(4):346–355.

Wright T, Cox T, Massad L, Twiggs L, Wilkinson E. 2001 Consensus guidelines for the management of women with cervical cytological abnormalities. *JAMA* 2002;287:2120–2129.

Wright T, Cox T, Massad L, Carlson J, Twiggs L, Wilkinson E. 2001 Consensus guidelines on the management of women with cervical intraepithelial neoplasia. *Am J Obstet Gynecol* 2003;189(1):295–304.

Aggarwal R, Suneja A, Agarwal N, Mirshra K. Role of misoprostol in overcoming an unsatisfactory colposcopy: a randomized double-blind placebo-controlled clinical trial. *Gynecol Obstet Invest* 2006;62(2):115–120.

Books

Apgar B, Brotzman G, Spitzer M. *Colposcopy principles and practice: an integrated textbook and atlas.* Philadelphia: W.B. Saunders, 2002.

Chapter 23
Cervical Cryotherapy

Laurie Turenne-Kolpan

Introduction

Cryotherapy is an ablative technique that has been used to treat all grades of cervical dysplasia for more than 50 years. It is a preferred method of many primary care providers because of its cost-effectiveness, safety, and ease in performance. Cryotherapy causes destruction of cells by producing a rapid freezing of tissue followed by a slow thaw. This causes intracellular ice crystals to form, followed by expansion of intracellular material, leading to rupture of the cells [1]. The depth of freezing is directly proportional to the length of ice ball formation around the side of the probe, so that an ice ball 7-mm thick around the probe will yield a depth of freezing equal to 7 mm [2]. It is important to note that the temperature of the tissue in the distal 2 mm of the ice ball is insufficient to cause cell death, so the level of actual tissue destruction is generally 2 mm less than the thickness of the ice ball [1].

Treatment in properly selected patients with cryotherapy for Cervical Intraepithelial Neoplasia (CIN) and CIN 2 can be as high as 95% effective; however, for larger CIN 2 (or moderate dysplasia) and CIN 3 (or severe dysplasia) lesions, the effectiveness may be significantly reduced. This is not due to the severity of the lesion but to the depth of dysplasia that occurs with more severe lesions [1, 3]. Cervical crypts have a depth up to 7 mm. Most mild and moderate dysplasia will be confined to an area above 5 mm, making cryotherapy a good choice for treatment. Crypt involvement, however, is a characteristic of high-grade lesions such as CIN 3; therefore, treatment of these lesions should be managed with excision rather than cryotherapy [1]. Large lesions that are greater than 3 cm in diameter or involve more than two quadrants can be associated with a lower cure rate with cryotherapy [2].

L. Turenne-Kolpan (✉)
Department of Family Practice, Hunterdon Medical Center, Flemington, NJ, USA
e-mail: turenne-kolpan.laurie@hunterdonhealthcare.org

S.M. Sulik and C.B. Heath (eds.), *Primary Care Procedures in Women's Health*,
DOI 10.1007/978-0-387-76604-1_23, © Springer Science+Business Media, LLC 2010

Cryotherapy is indicated for treatment of both low-grade and small high-grade biopsy-proven squamous dysplasia. As this therapy is ablative and does not allow for tissue exam, it is essential that the colposcopy performed is adequate and that the histology does not differ more than 1 degree of severity from the cytology on the Pap smear [2, 3]. If these conditions are not met, a diagnostic excisional procedure must be performed [4]. Because the majority of cases of CIN 1 will spontaneously regress, the consensus guidelines set forth by the American Society for Colposcopy and Cervical Pathology (ASCCP) recommend observation without treatment, although immediate treatment is an acceptable option [4]. If observation is elected and the patient continues to have CIN 1, treatment verses further observation can be offered at that point. Treatment failures do occur; however, in properly selected patients, similar success rates have been shown with cryotherapy, laser ablation, fulguration, cold coagulation, LEEP, laser conization, and cold knife conization [4].

Studies comparing the flat and shallow conical probe tips show no difference in effectiveness for eradicating CIN, but they do show a slight increase in posttreatment migration of the squamocolumnar junction into the canal with the conical tip [5].

Cryotherapy may also be used to treat external genital warts; however, a different freezing regimen is employed.

Case Study

A 27-year-old G2P2 had a colposcopy performed in your office for a Pap smear result of Low-Grade Intraepithelial Lesion (LSIL). The histology report returns as CIN 1, and an Endocervical Curettage (ECC) shows benign endocervical cells. You review her chart and see that her colposcopy was adequate and showed an acetowhite lesion approximately 1 cm in length at the 12 o'clock position. This is her third colposcopy, and prior histology reports have also revealed CIN 1. She does not smoke and is on oral contraceptives. At this point, she is requesting definitive treatment.

Diagnosis

Persistent low-grade dysplasia

Indications (Algorithm 23-1)

- Persistent low-grade squamous intraepithelial lesion.
- Moderate dysplasia with a small lesion encompassing less than two quadrants of the cervix confirmed by adequate colposcopy.
- External genital warts (see Chap. 21 on genital warts).

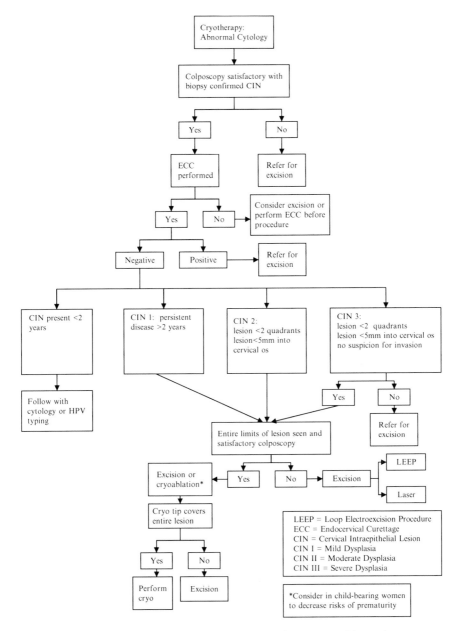

Algorithm 23-1 Decision tree for treatment of an abnormal pap smear with cryotherapy

Contraindications (Algorithm 23-1)

- Large lesions that do not fit entirely under the probe tip
- Inadequate colposcopy
- Positive endocervical curettage

- Histology that differs more than 1° from the cytology of the Pap smear
- Lesions that extend more than 2–3 mm into the canal
- Current heavy menses or within 1 week of expected menses
- Pregnancy
- Active cervicitis
- High-grade lesions with a noncompliant patient
- Invasive lesions

Equipment (Fig. 23-1)

- Nitrous oxide 20-lb tank
- Flexible tubing from the tank to probe
- Probe tips either flat or slightly coned. Sizes include 19 and 25 mm
- Vaginal speculum
- Water-soluble lubricant
- Colposcope (Some clinicians repeat the colposcopic exam at the time of the cyrotherapy procedure.)
- 5% acetic acid

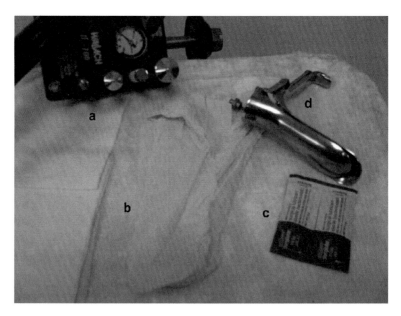

Fig. 23-1 Equipment tray for cervical cryotherapy: (a) Cryo tips with cryo tank and attachments (Wallach LL100 Cryosurgical System, Wallach Surgical Devices, Orange, CT); (b) gloves; (c) water-based lubricant Surgilube® (Fougera, Melville, NY); (d) speculum

Optional Equipment

- Vaginal sidewall retractors
- Condom or glove finger for retraction of vaginal wall

Procedure

1. Check urine pregnancy test prior to procedure.
2. Ensure the tank pressure is adequate and open the valve on the tank (Fig. 23-2). (The needle will be in the green zone on the pressure gauge.)
3. Place the patient in the dorsal lithotomy position.
4. Insert the speculum into vagina.
5. Apply 5% acetic acid to identify the location and size of the lesion, with or without magnification from a colposcope.
6. Select the appropriate probe size.
7. Apply water-soluble lubricant to the tip of the probe to achieve an even freeze.
8. Apply the probe over the cervix, ensuring the entire lesion and transformation zone are completely covered.

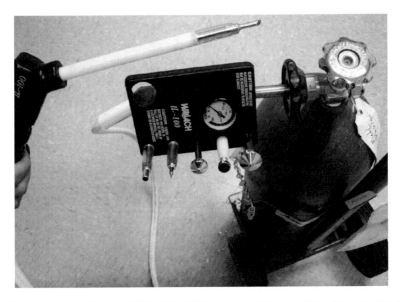

Fig. 23-2 Cryo tank with probe (Wallach LL100 Cryosurgical System, Wallach Surgical Devices, Orange, CT)

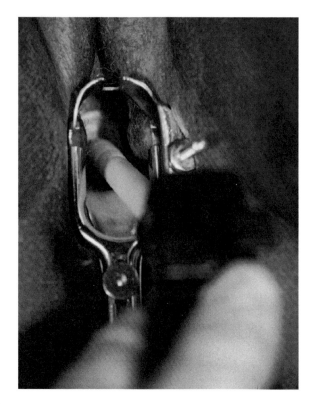

Fig. 23-3 Place probe onto the cervix after lubricant has been applied to the probe tip and pull trigger on the probe gun

9. Pull the trigger on the probe gun. The probe should adhere within a few seconds. Pull back slightly on the gun so the cervix is slightly forward, decreasing the likelihood of freezing the vaginal sidewalls (Fig. 23-3).
10. Continue freezing until a 7–10 mm ice ball is noted around the entire probe. This usually takes about 3 min, although the duration of application is less important than the size of the resultant ice ball formation.
11. Defrost the probe by releasing the trigger or pushing the defrost button, depending on your unit. The probe will detach shortly. Do not pull on the probe until it is visibly defrosted to avoid pain and cervical laceration.
12. Wait for the cervix to completely thaw, evidenced by a return of its pink color.
13. Repeat the freeze–thaw cycle. Once the probe is disengaged the second time, the speculum can be removed.
14. Have the patient return to a sitting position slowly to avoid vasovagal symptoms.
15. Close the value on the tank and discharge the remaining freezant.

Complications and Risks

- Treatment failure.
- Cervical stenosis.
- Difficulty with subsequent colposcopic exams as a result of the squamocolumnar junction retreating into the canal [6].
- Skip lesions (lesions further in the cervical canal behind the stenosis).
- Pelvic cramping typically lasts no more than a few days.
- Freezing of the vaginal wall.
- Profuse watery discharge, often malodorous lasting 2–4 weeks.
  - This occurs as a result of necrotic tissue and exudate being sloughed from the treatment site.
- Bleeding and infection: very rare.

Tricks and Helpful Hints

- The optimal time to perform this procedure is 1 week after the start of the menstrual cycle. If a patient starts her cycle shortly after the procedure is performed, the subsequent edema of the cervix can cause stenosis of the os, retained menses, and significant pain and cramping. If this happens, the cervix can be probed with a cotton swab or cervical dilator, which will usually initiate the flow.
- Do not use "nipple-tipped" probes as they increase the rates of cervical stenosis and subsequent inadequate colposcopic exams.
- If vaginal side walls collapse into the canal and obscure full cervical visualization, the finger from a glove or a condom with the tip cut can be placed over the speculum blades, or vaginal sidewall retractors can be used to displace the redundant tissue and protect it from accidental freezing.
- The most common complaint about the procedure is the profuse watery discharge which occurs afterward. Amino-Cerv® Vaginal Cream (CooperSurgical, Trumbull, CT) 1 applicatorful into the vagina nightly for 14 days may help reduce this.
- Having the patient take 600 mg of ibuprofen 30–45 min prior to the procedure and every 6 h as needed over the next few days can reduce cramping.

Procedure Note

(Provider to fill in blanks/circle applicable choice when given multiple choices and to customize as needed.)

Date of Birth:_____contraception_____HCG_____
G_____P_____A___Pap Smear History_____
Reason for Cryotherapy:

_____
_____Smoking_____
Time Out Done a
(Final Verification of patient/procedure/site)

Colposcopy performed () yes () no

Finding:_____

Cryotherapy:

A_____cm flat/conical tipped probe was applied over the cervix with full coverage of the transformation zone and squamous lesion. The cervix was frozen yielding a _____mm ice ball. A full thaw was completes. The cervix was frozen a second time yielding a _____ mm ice ball. the speculum was removed and the patient slowly returned to a sitting position.

Complications:_____

Impression:_____

Suggest subsequent examination and/or follow-up:_____
_____

Amnio Cerv prescribed intravagionally nightly for 14 days ()yes ()no

_____
                                                                 Physician's Signature

---

Coding

CPT® Codes (Current Procedural Terminology, AMA, Chicago, IL)
57511   Cryocautery of the cervix, initial, or repeat

ICD 9-CM-Diagnostic Codes (International Classification of Diseases, 9th Revision, Clinical Modification, Center for Disease Control and Prevention)
622.11   Dysplasia, cervix, mild (CIN 1)
622.13   Dysplasia, cervix, moderate (CIN 2)
233.1   Dysplasia, cervix, severe (CIN 3)

Postprocedure Patient Instructions

The patient should be advised of the watery discharge that will ensue and persist for 2–4 weeks. This discharge is often malodorous as it is a result of the sloughing of the dead cervical tissue. Prescribing Amino-Cerv® for 14 days may help reduce this. Cramping is common and should be relieved with ibuprofen, 600 mg every 6 hours. A small percentage will need stronger pain management. These patients should be reexamined to rule out an infection or retained menstrual flow prior to prescribing additional medication. The patient may have a small amount of spotting, but should not have significant bleeding. Infection is uncommon and can be greatly reduced by having nothing inserted in the vagina for 3 weeks following the procedure. Patients should call for any fevers, shaking chills, or pain unrelieved by nonsteroidals. Follow-up is essential after cryotherapy as failure of treatment does happen. Options for follow-up include repeating Pap smears every 6 months for a total of three negative screens; this should then be followed by annual screening. A cytology report of Atypical Squamous Cells of Undetermined Significance (ASC-US) or higher should prompt a repeat evaluation with colposcopy. A second option for follow-up includes high risk HPV DNA testing no sooner than 6 months and up to 12 months after treatment. If the patient is negative for high-risk types of HPV, she can return to annual cytologic screening. If positive, a repeat colposcospy needs to be performed [4]. See Algorithm 23-2.

Case Study Outcome

The patient had cervical cryotherapy performed without complications. A follow-up Pap smear at 6 months was normal. She will continue to have cytological screening every 6 months for the next year, and, if both remain normal, she will have annual screening thereafter for at least 20 years.

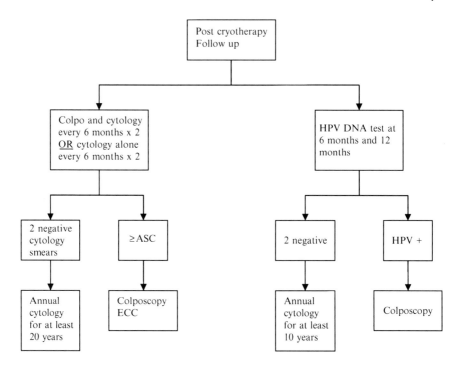

Algorithm 23-2 Postcryotherapy follow-up algorithm

Patient Handout

(Provider to customize as needed.)

Cryotherapy is a method of treatment for cervical dysplasia (abnormal cells on your cervix that are precancerous) that involves destroying abnormal tissue in the cervix by freezing it. This is performed right in our office. The best time to have the procedure done is the week after your period has started, and this can be done even if you are still having a small amount of spotting.

The procedure starts like a Pap smear, with you lying on your back and you feet in the footrests (stirrups). A speculum will be placed in the vagina to visualize the cervix. A metal probe is put against the cervix and gets very cold, allowing for the freezing. It is normal to hear a hissing sound as the procedure begins, and then you may feel some cramping similar to menstrual cramps. There is generally no pain beyond the cramps. Taking three ibuprofen tablets (600 mg) 30 minutes (min) prior to the procedure will help minimize this. You may also feel a little warm and flushed. This goes away within a few minutes after the procedure ends. The freezing will take about 3 min, and then the cervix will be allowed to thaw for about 5 min. This process is repeated once.

Cryotherapy is generally very safe and effective. The possible complications include the cramping as mentioned previously, infection, and narrowing of the cervical canal, which can very rarely be significant enough to cause difficulties letting menstrual flow out. This can be repaired. Finally, while cryotherapy is 85–95% effective in treating cervical abnormalities, failures can and do occur. Therefore, it is very important that you get your follow-up Pap smears as directed by your clinician.

After cryotherapy, you can expect a profuse watery vaginal discharge that may have an odor and can last for 2–4 weeks. Your doctor may prescribe Amino Cerv® cream to be used intravaginally every night for 14 days in an attempt to decrease this. To decrease the risk of infection, we recommend that nothing be placed in the vagina (douching, tampons etc.) and that you abstain from intercourse for 3 weeks. Typically, cramping may last for 1–2 days and can be minimized with ibuprofen, three tablets (600 mg) taken every 6–8 h as needed with food.

Please call us if you have any fever, bleeding heavier than a period, or abdominal pain not relieved with ibuprofen.

References

1. Apgar B, Brotzman G, Spitzer M. *Colposcopy principles and practice: an integrated textbook and atlas.* Philadelphia: W.B. Saunders, 2002.
2. Pfenninger J, Fowler G. *Procedures for primary care.* St. Louis, MO: Mosby, 2003.
3. Mayeaux E. Cryotherapy of the uterine cervix. *J Fam Pract* 1998;47:99–102.
4. Spitzer M, Apgar B, Brotzman G. Management of histologic abnormalities of the cervix. *Am Fam Physician* 2006;173(1):105–112.
5. Sienstra K, Brewer B, Franklin L>A comparison of flat and shallow conical tips for cervical cryotherapy. *J Am Board Fam Pract* 1999;12(5):360–366.
6. Sparks R, Scheid D, Oemker V, Stader E, Reilly K, Hamm R, McCarthy L. Association of cervical cryotherapy with inadequate follow-up colposcopy. *J Fam Pract* 2002;51:526–529.

Chapter 24
LEEP: Loop Electrosurgical Excision Procedure

Sandra M. Sulik

Introduction

Loop Electrosurgical Excision Procedure (LEEP) uses alternating electrical current to remove abnormal cervical tissue, which provides a specimen for pathological review. Historically, physicians have used high frequency current for lesion removal as early as the 1940s. The introduction of the large loop with an insulated cross bar in 1989 by Prendeville revolutionized the treatment of cervical dysplasia. Other methods, such as cryotherapy and laser vaporization evaporated tissue, did not allow for pathologic review. LEEP confers the advantage over cryotherapy and laser by providing tissue for histopathological review, thus allowing for prediction of recurrence of disease [1].

LEEP and Loop Electrosurgery remain the most common terms for this procedure although Diathermy Loop Treatment, Loop Excision of the Transformation Zone (LETZ), and Large Loop Excision of the Transformation Zone (LLETZ) are other terms noted in the literature.

LEEP uses low-voltage high-frequency alternating current to produce an uninterrupted sine wave. As the loop is introduced into the tissue, an arc of current occurs causing the tissue cells to be rapidly heated and to explode into steam. The steam envelope allows for a continuous arc, thus allowing for a clean cut through the tissue and producing minimal thermal artifact. Once the tissue has been removed, the coagulation mode can be used with a ball electrode to fulgurate the tissue and cause hemostasis. With the more modern units, the coagulation and cut modes can be combined into a blend mode that produces less bleeding while minimizing the thermal artifact. The current is dispersed through a grounding pad with a large surface area to prevent burns.

S.M. Sulik (✉)
Department of Family Medicine, St. Joseph's Family Medicine Residency,
SUNY Upstate Medical Center, Fayetteville, NY, USA
e-mail: smsulik@aol.com

S.M. Sulik and C.B. Heath (eds.), *Primary Care Procedures in Women's Health*,
DOI 10.1007/978-0-387-76604-1_24, © Springer Science+Business Media, LLC 2010

The type of generator used for the LEEP procedure (Fig. 24-1) is similar to any electrosurgical generator used in either urological or laparoscopic surgery. The alternating current output ranges from 100 to 4,000 KHz and comes with a variety of features. These features may include isolated circuitry and Return Electrode Monitoring (REM). Isolated circuitry helps prevent alternate site burns by automatically deactivating the electrical surgical generator if any current transmitted through the active electrode is not returned through the patient electrode. The REM emits a warning sound and/or light if the return circuit is interrupted. Most generators will allow for combining of the cut and coagulation modes into a blend mode. Blend 1 provides 75% cut with 25% coagulation, which helps decrease bleeding during the procedure. Higher blend modes, while available, can increase the amount of thermal artifact in the tissue and make pathological diagnosis of the margins more difficult [2].

Most loops have an insulated cross bar and shaft to prevent thermal injuries. The ball electrodes (Fig. 24-2) range in sizes from 3 to 5 mm, and both the ball electrodes

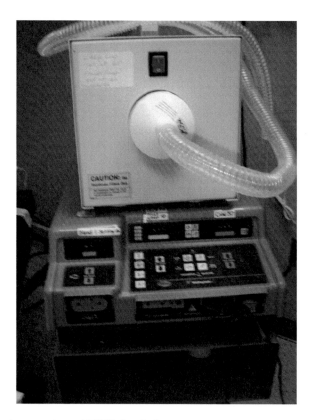

Fig. 24-1 Smoke evacuator and LEEP electrical generator

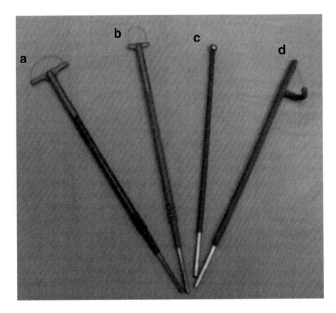

Fig. 24-2 Samples of loops and ball cautery tools. (a) 0.8 × 2.0 cm loop; (b) 1.0 × 1.0 cm loop; (c) Ball electrode; (d) Fischer cone loop

and the loops are connected to a probe with a monopolar output. (The grounding electrode is usually an adhesive gel pad, or a solid "antenna" may be used.) The grounding pad should be applied near the operative site, usually the upper thigh or buttocks. The pad wire should be connected to the generator and tested prior to the procedure to ensure the system is functioning properly.

A smoke evacuator is essential to remove the smoke plume during the procedure in order to provide adequate visualization. The smoke evacuator will filter any airborne particles and coexisting microorganisms into the plume and out of the air in the procedure room. Generally, the smoke evacuator is turned on prior to the generator and is a separate unit; however, there are a number of manufacturers that combine the smoke evacuator with the generator so that both turn on at the same time.

An insulated speculum is recommended for this procedure, and most have an attachment site for the smoke evacuator. This helps prevent secondary burns from the speculum to the vagina or vulvar areas. Special coated vaginal/lateral wall retractors are also available. Human Papilloma Virus has been isolated from laser plumes: thus, clinicians are encouraged to wear micropore or sub-micron surgical masks during the procedure.

Efficacy and patient acceptance of the LEEP procedure compares positively to other modes of treatment for cervical dysplasia. Studies indicate that LEEP is

91–98% effective in treating cervical intraepithelial lesions compared to 81–95% efficacy for cryotherapy and 83–94% efficacy for laser treatment of the cervix. Most patients report the degree of discomfort with the procedure to be minor, with 85% of patients reporting no discomfort at all [3].

The morbidity associated with the LEEP is related to the volume of tissue removed and the depth of excision into the endocervical canal. This has direct implications in younger women who have not completed childbearing. The overall rate of preterm delivery or spontaneous preterm Premature Rupture of Membranes (pPROM) postLEEP is directly related to the increased depth of the cervical tissue removed during LEEP, with women who have >1.7 cm removed having a greater than threefold increased risk of pPROM compared to untreated women [4]. Women who have had LEEP are more likely to deliver preterm overall and to have more low birth weight babies; however, there are no differences in maternal or neonatal outcomes [5].

Posttreatment follow up for the LEEP patient should include an office visit to discuss the pathology results. If margins of the specimen are negative, follow-up recommendations include either repeat Pap smears every 6 months×2 followed by annual cytology, or HPV typing in 6–12 months, and, if negative, annual cytology thereafter. If either Pap or HPV testing is positive, a repeat colposcopy with ECC is recommended. If testing is negative, a return to annual cytologic screening for at least 20 years is appropriate [6]. If there are positive margins, follow-up should occur more often. Studies have found using high-risk HPV detection via Hybrid Capture II (Digene, Gaithersburg, MD) testing to be more sensitive than cytology, although less specific, and follow up using both HPV testing and cytology together detected all patients with recurrent/residual disease with 100% sensitivity and 100% negative predictive value [7]. Women with positive margins have a higher incidence of recurrent dysplasia usually within 2 years and a higher incidence of cervical carcinoma for at least 20 years posttreatment [6].

Case Study

The patient returns to your office after receiving a phone call from your nurse stating that you would like to talk with her about her abnormal Pap smear. You inform her that her pap has returned as High Grade Intraepithelial Lesion (HSIL) and that she needs to have further evaluation with a colposcopy. Colposcopy was performed and biopsies were taken. She returns to your office for her results, which show severe dysplasia at the 4:00 and 6:00 biopsies with a negative Endocervical Curettage (ECC). You discuss the risks and benefits of the LEEP procedure for definitive treatment and she elects to schedule the procedure.

Diagnosis

Severe dysplasia with negative ECC

Indications

- Any biopsy proven CIN lesion with adequate colposcopy
- Diagnostic purposes for inadequate colposcopy
- LEEP preferred over cryotherapy for the following:
    a. High-grade lesions that encompass greater than 2 quadrants of the cervix
    b. Large lesions not covered by the cryoprobe
    c. Irregularly shaped cervix
    d. Recurrent CIN after previous therapy
    e. If "See and Treat" at a single visit is necessary (not preferred method)

Contraindications

- Bleeding or coagulopathy
- Less than 12 weeks postpartum
- Clinically apparent invasive carcinoma of the cervix
- Heavy menses (relative)
- Active/severe cervicitis (relative)
- Pregnancy (relative): should be performed only by experienced specialist when carcinoma suspected.

Advantages

- Allows for histologic audit of colposcopic diagnosis with histopathologic examination to rule out microinvasion
- Allows for excision of the dysplastic lesion and transformation zone
- Can treat lesions of all sizes involving all four quadrants of the cervix
- Easily learned technique
- Uses inexpensive readily available equipment with relatively low operating costs
- Is office or outpatient procedure
- Can be performed with initial colposcopy ("See and treat," although this is not the preferred method of treatment)

Equipment (Fig. 24-3)

- Electrical generator
- Smoke evacuator and tubing
- Grounding pad

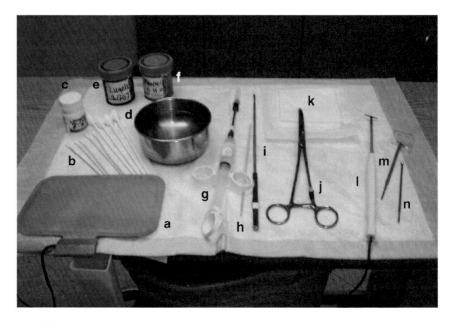

Fig. 24-3 Equipment set up for LEEP. (a) Grounding pad; (b) Large and small cotton swabs; (c) Hurricaine® gel (Beutlich LP Pharmaceuticals, Waukegan, IL); (d) Metal basin with acetic acid; (e) Lugol's solution; (f) Monsel's solution; (g) 10 cc syringe with 1% lidocaine with epinephrine with needle extender; (h) Endocervical brush; (i) Sterile Endocervical curette; (j) Sterile Long Kelly forceps; (k) Gauze; (l) Monopolar probe with 0.8×2 cm loop attached; (m) 1.0×1.0 cm loop; (n) Ball electrode

- Insulated speculum
- Lateral wall spreaders: insulated (optional)
- Loops: range in sizes from 1.0×1.0 cm to 2.0×1.5 cm
- Ball electrode: sizes range from 3 to 5 mm
- 20% Benzocaine (Hurricaine® gel, Beutlich LP Pharmaceuticals, Waukegan, IL)
- 1% lidocaine with epinephrine: 5–10 cc
- Needle extender
- 25- or 28-gauge needle
- Colposcope
- Acetic Acid
- Lugol's solution
- Monsel's solution
- Specimen jar
- Endocervical Curette (ECC) (optional)
- Large cotton swabs (Scopettes®, Birchwood Laboratories Inc., Eden Prairie, MN)
- Small cotton swabs
- Long Kelly or ring forceps
- Face mask: micropore or submicro surgical face mask

Optional Equipment

- Suture material: chromic or vicryl 3.0 absorbable
- Long-handled needle holder and scissors
- Vasopressin for bleeding

Procedure

1. Obtain informed consent and sign permit.
2. Check pregnancy test.
3. Place patient in lithotomy position; apply grounding pad.
4. Check equipment to make sure all functioning appropriately.
5. Insert insulated speculum and visualize cervix.
   (a) Adequate visualization of the entire cervix is key to a simple procedure.
   (b) Use the vaginal/lateral wall spreaders if necessary to provide adequate visualization.
6. Perform colposcopy and apply Lugol's solution.
7. Anesthetize the cervix.
   (a) Use 20% benzocaine (Hurricaine®) gel prior to lidocaine (Fig. 24-4).
   (b) Inject at 12:00, 3:00, 6:00, 9:00 positions around the cervix with up to 0.5–1 cc of lidocaine per site locally (Fig. 24-5). (Alternatively, you can inject at 2:00, 4:00, 8:00, and 10:00.)

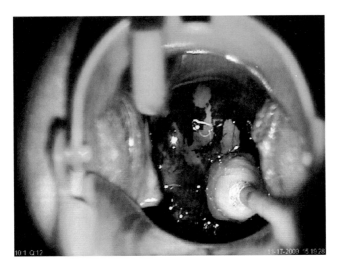

Fig. 24-4 Apply topical benzocaine to the cervix with a large swab prior to injecting the local anesthetic

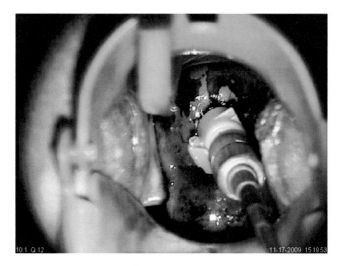

Fig. 24-5 Injection of lidocaine anesthetic at the 12:00 position on the cervix

    (c) Use depth of 1–2 mm only (submucosal).

    (d) Allow several minutes to pass, and check to see if area is anesthetized.

  8. Choose appropriate loop, and attach to the monopolar probe.

    (a) Check settings to ensure appropriate for chosen loop.

    (b) Smaller loops require less current (i.e., 1.0 × 1.0 set at approximately 40 MHz, varies machine to machine).

    (c) Check to make sure setting is on Blend 1.

  9. Make dummy pass over the cervix with generator on stand-by to ensure adequate removal of the lesion.

10. Turn on smoke evacuator and generator, and recheck settings.

11. Pass loop into tissue, and remove entire transformation zone around lesion (Fig. 24-6).

    (a) If necessary, make additional passes with loop to remove the entire lesion.

    (b) Start the flow of current by either using the index finger to press the cut button on the hand-held tool or by using the foot pedal.

    (c) Start excision approximately 5 mm lateral to the lesion, and place loop just at but not touching the cervix. Start the flow of current prior to touching the cervix.

    (d) The cut should be made with a continuous flow of current, passing the loop to a depth of at least 8 mm – maximal crypt involvement of CIN reaches a depth of 5 mm. Stopping the flow of current can increase thermal artifact and may damage the loop.

    (e) Push the loop into the tissue and slowly draw the loop across the transformation zone with equal pressure until 5 mm past the lesion edge, then remove the loop from the tissue perpendicularly (Fig. 24-7).

12. Remove specimen (Fig. 24-8) with long Kelly, after generator is placed on stand-by.

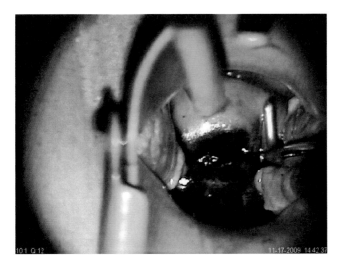

Fig. 24-6 Pass the loop through the tissue in a perpendicular fashion

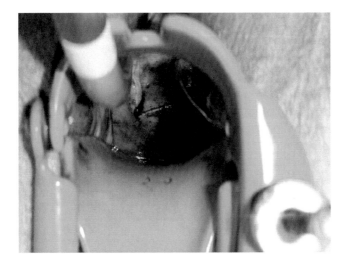

Fig. 24-7 Cervix with excision completed prior to hemostasis with ball cautery

13. Perform ECC if not done during colposcopy or if desired.
14. Use ball electrode to fulgurate the base of the tissue crater and achieve hemostasis. Press the coagulation button on the hand held tool or with the foot pedal. *Do not fulgurate the cervical os* (Fig. 24-9).
15. Apply Monsel's solution to crater.
16. Remove speculum and grounding pad.
17. Mark specimen as per your pathology department's recommendations and place in sterile container (Fig. 24-10).

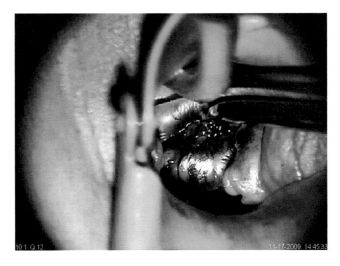

Fig. 24-8 Remove the cut specimen with a long Kelly

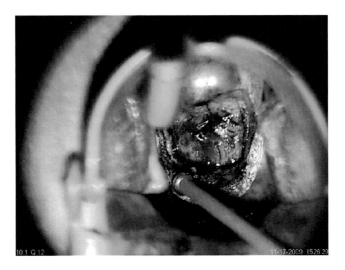

Fig. 24-9 Use the ball electrode to fulgurate the base of the excised cervix to achieve hemostasis

18. LEEP Cone Procedure: looks like a reverse "cowboy hat" when completed
    (a) Can be used when the lesion extends into the cervical canal.
    (b) Anesthetize the cervix in the same fashion, but use an additional 0.5–2 cc of lidocaine into the cervix to a depth of 1 cm at the 12 and 6:00 positions.
    (c) Use a 1.0 × 1.0 or a square loop to excise a 9–10 mm portion of the endocervical canal. If doing this first, the specimen does not need to be marked, but if performing after the LEEP on the ectocervix, mark the endocervical

Fig. 24-10 LEEP tissue sample to be sent to pathology

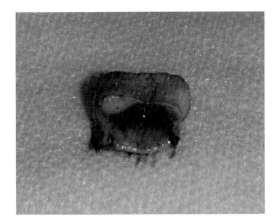

edge of the specimen so that the pathologist can assess if the margins are negative for disease.

(d) The remaining transformation zone is excised in the usual manner as described previously.

19. Have the patient sit up slowly after procedure to ensure vasovagal response does not occur.

20. Observe patient for 15–20 min postprocedure before discharging to home.

Complications and Risks

- Burns to vaginal walls, usually due to poor visualization or operator experience.
- Bleeding: immediate bleeding 0.5–1%, late bleeding 1–8.5%. Perioperative bleeding is uncommon with the use of the Blend mode fulguration and Monsel's. Excessive bleeding can be controlled by use of vasopressin. Rarely, a figure of eight suture is necessary to control the bleeding.
- Posttreatment cervical stenosis: more common with postmenopausal women, women on Depo-Provera® (Pfizer, New York, NY) or Implanon® (Schering Corporation, Kenilworth, NJ), or in breastfeeding women postpartum.
- Consider treatment with estrogen vaginal cream for several weeks postLEEP.
- Infection: rare.
- Cervical incompetence.
- Positive margins or recurrent disease.

Tricks and Helpful Hints

- When using the lateral wall spreaders, a larger speculum is usually necessary: use a Graves or a long Graves.

- A cartridge system (Campion syringe or dental syringe) can be used for anesthesia. A thumb syringe with a dental extender, a spinal needle, or a Potochy Needle® (CooperSurgical, Trumbull, CT) can also be used.
- Consider adding 8.3% sodium bicarbonate solution 1:1 or 1:4 to decrease pain with the injection.
- Excessive bleeding can be controlled with use of vasopressin.
  - Draw up 1 cc (20 units/cc) of vasopressin.
  - Withdraw 40 cc of saline from 100 cc mini bag, and inject 1 cc vasopressin into mini bag. Draw up 10 cc of solution, and inject directly into the cervix into the bleeding areas.
- Cone LEEP can also be done using a Fischer cone loop.

Interpretation of Results (Algorithm 24-1)

- Review pathology report to determine if entire lesion removed. Assess margins.
- If margins positive, closer follow-up usually necessary.
- If margins negative, follow-up as noted previously.

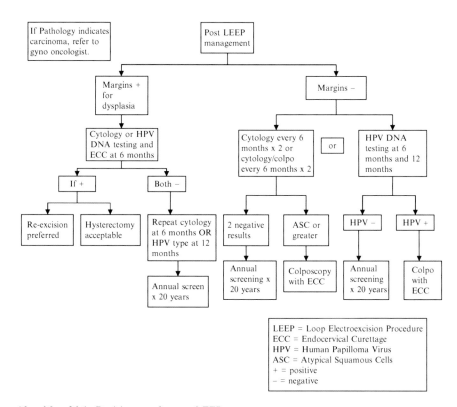

Algorithm 24-1 Decision tree for post-LEEP management

Procedure Note

(Provider to customize as needed.)

> *The permit was signed, and the pregnancy test was performed and is negative. The patient was placed in the lithotomy position, and the speculum was inserted. The cervix was visualized, and colposcopy was performed. The cervix was anesthetized with ___ cc of 1% lidocaine with epinephrine in the 3, 6, 9, 12:00 positions infused locally. One pass with the 0.8 × 2.0 cm loop was made to remove the transformation zone in its entirety. Hemostasis with the ball cautery and Monsel's was done. The specimen was marked with suture at the _____ position and sent to pathology. The patient tolerated the procedure well and will follow up in 2 weeks for results.*

Coding

CPT® Codes (Current Procedural Terminology, AMA, Chicago, IL)

57460	Colposcopy with loop electrosurgical excision or LEEP excision of the cervix
57500	Cervical biopsy
57520	Cervical conization with or without fulguration
57522	Cervical conization using loop technique
57505	Endocervical curettage
99070	Supplies and materials for kits and electrodes: A surgical tray charge is generally allowed for an office LEEP

ICD 9-CM-Diagnostic Codes (International Classification of Diseases, 9th Revision, Clinical Modification, Center for Disease Control and Prevention)

180.9	Cervical cancer
622.1	CIN 1 and 2 (mild to moderate dysplasia)
233.1	CIN 3 (severe dysplasia, carcinoma in situ)

Postprocedure Patient Instructions

- Instruct the patient to refrain from intercourse, tampons, or douching for 2–4 weeks postprocedure, until all bleeding has stopped.
- Discharge is common for 2–3 weeks but may last up to 6 weeks.
- The patient should report any excessive bleeding (heavier than a normal period, or soaking a pad per hour) or any malodorous discharge.
- Instruct the patient to make a follow up appointment to review pathology results within 2–4 weeks.

- Follow up with Pap smears every 6 months and/or colposcopy until two negative. Then follow up with annual cytology for at least 20 years *or* HPV typing at 6–12 months (12 months preferred); if negative, return to annual cytology for 20 years. If HPV-positive at follow-up, repeat colposcopy with ECC as per current 2006 ASCCP guidelines.

Case Study Outcome

The patient returned to your office for her LEEP, which was done without complications. She comes in today for results, and you review with her the pathology results. It contained severe dysplasia with negative margins. She will follow up in 12 months for HPV typing.

Postprocedure Patient Handout

You have just had a LEEP (Loop Electrosurgical Excision Procedure). This involves removing small pieces of abnormal cervical tissue that are then sent for pathologic evaluation. Most women tolerate LEEP well, as the procedure generally causes little bleeding. However, in order to make sure that you heal well, we ask that you avoid putting anything in your vagina for the next 2–4 weeks until the bleeding has stopped. This means:

- No douching
- No tampon use
- No vaginal sex

You should call your provider if any of the following occur:

- Increase in bleeding or heavy bleeding (more than a pad per hour)
- Fever, above 101°F.
- Pelvic pain
- Smelly discharge

Discharge, even dark brown discharge, is common after LEEP.

Please make a follow-up appointment to discuss your results in 2–4 weeks. You will also need to discuss frequency of Pap smears and follow up plans at this appointment.

References

1. Prendiville W. Large loop excision of the transformation zone. *Clin Obstet Gynecol* 1995;38(3):622–639.
2. Mayeaux EJ Jr, Harper MB. Loop electrosurgical excisional procedure. *J Fam Pract*1993; 36(2):214–219.
3. Sadler L, Saftlas A, Wang W, Exeter M, Whittaker J, McCowan L. Treatment for cervical intra-epithelial neoplasia and risk of preterm delivery. *JAMA* 2004 May 5;291(17):2100–2106.
4. Samson SL, Bentley JR, Fahey TJ, Fahey TJ, McKay DJ, Gill GH. The effect of loop electrosurgical excision procedure on future pregnancy outcome. *Obstet Gynecol* 2005;105(2):325–332.
5. Wright TC, Massad LS, Dunton CJ, Spitzer M, Wilkinson EJ., Solomon D. 2006 consensus guidelines for the management of women with cervical intraepithelial neoplasia or adenocarcinoma in-situ. *Am J Obstet Gynecol* 2007;197:340–345.
6. Alonso I, Torné A, Puig-Tintoré LM, Esteve R, Quinto L, Campo E, Pahisa J, Ordi J. Pre and postconization high-risk HPV testing predicts residual/recurrent disease in patients treated for CIN 2-3. *Gynecol Oncol* 2006;103(2):631–636. Epub 2006 Jun 14.

Additional Resource

Article

Wright TC, Massad LS, Dunton CJ, Spitzer M, Wilkinson EJ., Solomon D. 2006 consensus guidelines for the management of women with abnormal cervical cancer screening tests. *Am J Obstet Gynecol* 2007;197:346–355.

Web Site

www.asccp.org

Chapter 25
Hysterosalpingography/Hysterosalpingogram (HSG)

Sandra M. Sulik

Introduction

Hysterosalpingography (HSG) is a dye-based radiologic evaluation of the uterus and fallopian tubes. It is used primarily for the workup of infertility as well as for the evaluation of tubal patency post Essure® (Conceptus, Mountain View, CA) procedures. Other indications include the evaluation of women with a history of recurrent spontaneous abortions, postoperative evaluations for women who have undergone reversal of tubal ligation, and assessment of women prior to undergoing myomectomy. The primary role of the procedure is to evaluate the patency of the fallopian tubes [1]. The optimal time for the study to be performed is day 7–12 of the menstrual cycle. This ensures that there is not a pregnancy present and allows for optimal visualization of the endometrium in the proliferative phase.

Case Study

A 34-year-old woman presents to your office with the concern that she is unable to get pregnant. She and her husband have been trying for the past year without success. She has had no other pregnancies, denies history of any sexually transmitted infections, and has regular menses. Her husband has a child from a previous marriage. You discuss the infertility workup and suggest an evaluation with a hysterosalpingogram.

S.M. Sulik (✉)
Department of Family Medicine, St. Joseph's Family Medicine Residency, SUNY Upstate Medical Center, Fayetteville, NY, USA
e-mail: smsulik@aol.com

S.M. Sulik and C.B. Heath (eds.), *Primary Care Procedures in Women's Health*, DOI 10.1007/978-0-387-76604-1_25, © Springer Science+Business Media, LLC 2010

Diagnosis (Algorithm 25-1)

Infertility investigation

Indications (Algorithm 25-1)

- Infertility
- Recurrent spontaneous abortions
- Preoperative evaluation prior to myomectomy

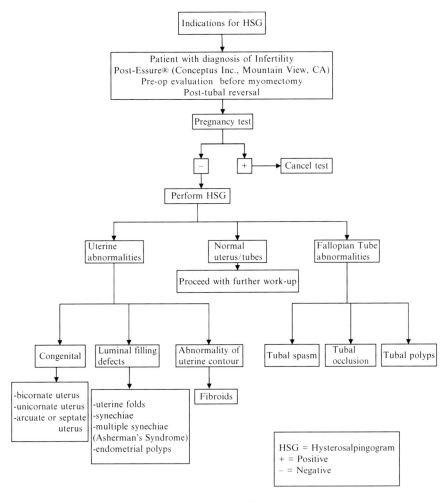

Algorithm 25-1 Indications and interpretations of HSG

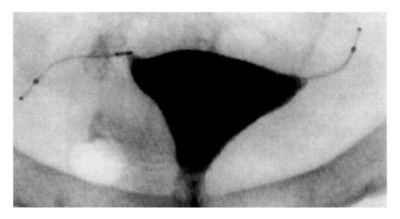

Fig. 25-1 HSG after Essure® (Conceptus, Mountain View, CA) placement (courtesy of James E. Brown, MD, Past President of Associates for Womens Medicine, PLLC, Attending Physician at St. Joseph's Hospital, Syracuse, New York)

- Postoperative evaluation following Essure® (hysteroscopically inserted permanent sterilization device) (Fig. 25-1)
- Postoperative evaluation following tubal ligation reversal

Contraindications [1] (Algorithm 25-1)

- Pregnancy
- Active pelvic infection
- Active vaginal bleeding
- Allergy to contrast dye

Equipment (Fig. 25-2)

- Radiologic shields for provider, radiologist, and technician
- Sterile tray with the following:
  - Sterile gloves
  - Sterile speculum
  - Small cup for antiseptic solution
  - Antiseptic solution
  - 3 cc syringe to test catheter balloon
  - 10 cc syringe to inject dye
  - HSG catheter
  - Tenaculum
  - Contrast medium
  - Menstrual pad

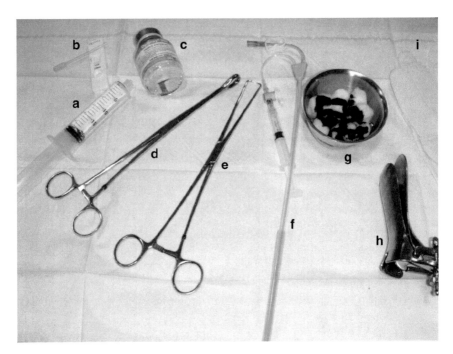

Fig. 25-2 Sterile tray set up for HSG: (a) 20 cc syringe filled with contrast dye; (b) Pregnancy test; (c) Contrast dye (e.g., Optiray®, Mallinckrodt Inc., St. Louis, MO); (d) Ring forceps; (e) Tenaculum; (f) Hysterosalpingogram catheter; with 3 cc syringe attached (g) Metal basin with cotton balls soaked in iodine; (h) Graves speculum; (i) Sterile gloves

Procedure

1. Perform pregnancy test.
   - The patient should be instructed to abstain from unprotected intercourse from the onset of the menses until after the procedure is completed.
2. Patient is placed in the lithotomy position, supine on the fluoroscopy table.
3. Check the HSG catheter, and flush the catheter with contrast material before insertion (Fig. 25-3).
4. Insert the speculum, visualize the cervix, and clean with antiseptic solution.
   - Insert the HSG catheter through the cervix into the endometrial cavity, and inflate the balloon using 3 cc of air. If necessary, use the tenaculum to help stabilize the cervix to insert the catheter.
5. Turn the stopcock to keep the balloon inflated.
6. Obtain a scout radiograph to check position of the catheter.
7. Inject contrast material slowly into the uterine cavity, until adequate fluoroscopic images are obtained.

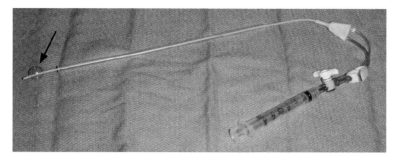

Fig. 25-3 Hysterosalpingogram catheter: check catheter balloon prior to start of the procedure

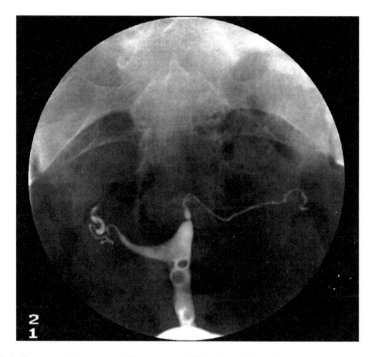

Fig. 25-4 Hysterosalpingogram with contrast spilling from both tubes

- Watch for spill of contrast medium into the fallopian tubes and then into the intraperitoneal area (Fig. 25-4).
- Observe for filling defects and contour abnormalities as early filling occurs.
- The shape of the uterus is best evaluated as the uterus is fully distended (Fig. 25-5).
- Additional spot radiographs may be obtained to evaluate any abnormality that is seen.
- Oblique views of the fallopian tubes may be needed and are obtained by having the patient roll from side to side (Fig. 25-6).

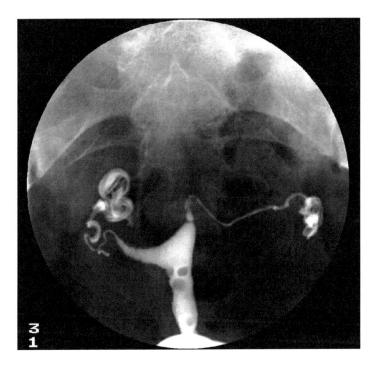

Fig. 25-5 The shape of the uterus is best visualized when fully distended

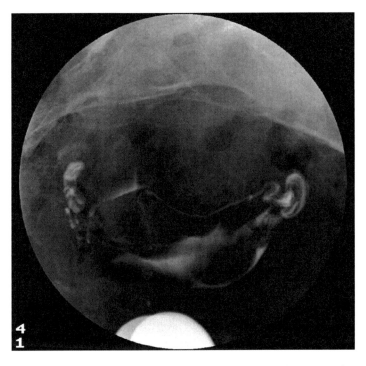

Fig. 25-6 Oblique views obtained by having the patient rotate side to side to asses for spill from both tubes

- A radiograph can be obtained once the balloon is deflated to evaluate the lower uterine segment.
8. Once the radiographs are obtained, deflate the balloon, and remove the catheter.

Complications and Risks

Spotting

Rare Complications

- Heavy vaginal bleeding
- Infection
- Reaction to contrast medium
- Perforation of the uterus or fallopian tube
- Potential for irradiation of an early, unsuspected pregnancy
- Severe cramping causing need to terminate the study before completion

Tricks and Helpful Hints

- Use an inverted bedpan or a pillow, or have the patient place her hands under her hips, in order to raise the pelvis; this will facilitate insertion of the speculum and better visualization of the cervix.
- If unable to easily pass the catheter, use the tenaculum to straighten the cervical canal.
- Have patient pretreat with a non-steroidal anti-inflammatory (NSAID) prior to procedure.
- If cervical stenosis is present, use a small dilator to open the cervical os prior for insertion of the HSG catheter.
- Removing the speculum prior to the dye injection allows for better visualization of the lower uterine segment.
- Excessive injection of dye prevents proper evaluation of the uterine cavity [2].
- Use of intrauterine lidocaine is not effective in reducing pain during the HSG [3].

Interpretation of Results [1, 2, 4] (Algorithm 25-1)

Uterus

- Should look like an inverted triangle with well-defined smooth contours.

- Uterine anomalies – three types:
  1. Congenital abnormalities of shape:
     a. Unicornuateuterus.
     b. Bicornuate uterus: demonstrates a cleft in the outer contour of the fundus.
     c. Arcuate or septate: shows a depression of the uterine fundus but a normal outer uterine contour.
  2. Luminal filling defects (common):
     a. Uterine folds: normal variants, parallel the long axis of the uterus and can extend into the uterine horns
     b. Synechiae (intrauterine adhesions) due to scarring/infection are seen as irregular filling defects; usually linear arising from one of the uterine walls.
     c. Multiple synechiae = Asherman syndrome.
     d. Endometrial polyps: well-defined filling defects best seen during the early filling stage. Sonohysterography is the preferred method of imaging endometrial polyps.
  3. Abnormalities of Uterine Contour:
     a. Leiomyomas most common, well-defined filling defects; only seen if submucosal. Seen best during early contrast filling of the uterus.
     b. Large myomas can distort the size of the uterus.

Fallopian Tubes

- Tubes should appear as thin, smooth lines that widen in the ampullary portion.
- Vary in length (approx. 10–12 cm) and tortuosity.
- There should be free spillage of contrast material into the peritoneal cavity.
- Tubal spasm can occur rarely and is difficult to distinguish from tubal occlusion.
- Tubal polyps: Rare; appear as smooth rounded filling defects without tube dilatation or occlusion; less than 1 cm in diameter and can be unilateral or bilateral.

Procedure Note

(Provider to customize as needed.)

> *Informed consent was obtained. Pregnancy test was done and is negative. The patient was placed in the lithotomy position on the fluoroscopy table, and the speculum was inserted. The cervix was visualized and cleaned with iodine solution. The HSG catheter was gently inserted through the cervix, and the balloon was filled with air. Position of the catheter was confirmed with fluoroscopy. The radiologist was called and, when ready, the dye was instilled via the catheter into the uterus. Spillage from both tubes was noted; no uterine abnormalities were seen. The study was completed, and the catheter was easily removed. The patient tolerated the procedure well.*

Coding

CPT® Codes (Current Procedural Terminology, AMA, Chicago, IL)

58340	Hysterosalpingography
74740	Hysterosalpingography, radiologic supervision, and interpretation
99070	Supplies and materials

ICD 9-CM-Diagnostic Codes (International Classification of Diseases, 9th Revision, Clinical Modification, Center for Disease Control and Prevention)

218.	Uterine leiomyoma
628.	Infertility, female (626.2 of tubal origin)
622.5	Incompetence of cervix
629.9	Unspecified disorder of female genital organs (habitual aborter without current pregnancy)

Patient Instructions

- The patient should be instructed to take an NSAID, i.e., ibuprofen 800 mg, three times daily for 1–2 days prior to the procedure and the morning of the procedure (at least 30 min prior).
- She should call the provider when her menses are due so that the test can be scheduled at the end of the menstrual cycle, ideally days 7–12 of the cycle.
- She should be instructed to abstain from unprotected intercourse from the start of her menses until the procedure is completed.

- The patient should be told to expect some cramping and flushing with instillation of the dye as well as with insertion of the catheter. Some cramping can continue post procedure but usually subsides shortly after the procedure is completed.
- The patient should expect sticky vaginal discharge after the procedure for several hours. Some spotting is also normal, but she should report any heavy vaginal bleeding or foul smelling discharge.

Case Study Outcome

HSG was performed without difficulty, both tubes were patent, and the uterus appeared normal in contour. Results were reviewed with the patient and her husband, and the infertility workup was continued.

Patient Handout

(Provider to customize as needed.)

Your provider has ordered a hystersalpingogram. This is an X-ray test done to look at the shape, size, and location of your uterus, fallopian tubes, and ovaries. Usually, this test is done to determine if the fallopian tubes are open and will allow an egg from your ovary to pass through the tube. This test is done as part of the work up for infertility. The test is also done after sterilization with the Essure®.

Before this test, your provider will perform a pregnancy test. A radiology technician or nurse will assist your provider and radiologist with the procedure. They will ask you for the dates of your last menstrual period and if you have any allergies. Before the test is done, you will be asked to empty your bladder and put on a hospital gown.

Once ready, you will lie down on the X-ray table, and an X-ray of your pelvis will be taken. The speculum will be inserted into your vagina, and your cervix will be cleaned with an antiseptic solution. The catheter will then be threaded through your cervix into your uterus, and a small balloon will be filled with air. This will keep the catheter in the proper position for the test. Once the catheter is in place, the radiologist will be called in, the dye will be injected through the catheter, and the X-ray pictures will be taken. You may be asked to turn onto one or both sides in order to see both fallopian tubes. When the dye is injected, you may experience a warm flush and some cramping.

When the test is completed, the catheter and the speculum will be removed. You will be given a menstrual pad to wear. You may have some spotting and a sticky discharge for the rest of the day of the test. If you have cramping, you can take ibuprofen.

The radiologist will review the X-rays and will send a report to your provider. Your provider will schedule a follow-up appointment with you to review the test results and discuss a treatment plan.

References

1. Simpson WL, Beitia LG, Mester J. Hysterosalpingography: a reemerging study. *RadioGraphics* 2006;26:419–431.
2. Lindheim ST, Sprague C, Winter III TC. Hysterosalpingography and sonohysterography: lessons in technique. *AJR Am J Roentgenol* 2006;186:24–29.
3. Frishman GN, Spencer PK, Weitzen S, Plosker S, Shafi F. The use of intrauterine lidocaine to minimize pain during hysterosalpingography: a randomized trial. *Obstet Gynecol* 2004; 103(6):1261–1266.
4. Baramki TA. Hysterosalpingography. *Fertil Steril* 2005;83(6):1595–1606.

Additional Resource

Article

Eng CW, Tang PH, Ong CL. Hysterosalpingography: current applications. *Singapore Med J* 2007;48(4):368–374.

Chapter 26
Medication Abortion Using Mifepristone and Misoprostol

Justine Wu

Introduction

Half of all pregnancies in the United States are unintended, and half of these pregnancies end in elective termination [1]. At current abortion rates, a woman has a 43% chance of having an abortion by the age of 45 [2]. Despite the demand for abortion services, 87% of all counties in the United States have no abortion provider [3]. Furthermore, the majority of women seek abortion services at nonprimary care sites, disrupting continuity of care for those who would prefer to access abortion service from their primary care provider. Almost 90% of all abortions occur in the first trimester, when safe, simple, and highly effective abortion services can be provided in the primary care setting [3]. If primary care clinicians were to offer abortion care, they could greatly improve timely access to safe abortion and relevant reproductive health services, particularly in rural and underserved settings.

Offering medication abortion in the office setting does not require expensive equipment or specialized procedural training, thus facilitating its incorporation into primary care. Medication abortion offers an important alternative to surgical abortion from a patient perspective (see Table 27-1 in Chap. 27 on MVA Abortion.). Women's reasons for choosing a medication abortion include a desire for privacy, a preference for a more "natural" method, and avoidance of an invasive procedure.

In September 2000, the U.S. Food and Drug Administration (FDA) approved mifepristone (also known as RU486 or Mifeprex®, Danco Laboratories, New York, NY) to be used with misoprostol (a prostaglandin) for medication abortion up to 49 days gestational age. This process first involves the administration of mifepristone (an anti-progestin), which effectively detaches the pregnancy from the endometrial lining and sensitizes the myometrium to prostaglandins. Misoprostol is administered

J. Wu (✉)

Department of Family Medicine, University of Medicine and Dentistry of New Jersey, Robert Wood Johnson Medical School, New Brunswick, NJ, USA
e-mail: drwuj1@yahoo.com

S.M. Sulik and C.B. Heath (eds.), *Primary Care Procedures in Women's Health*,
DOI 10.1007/978-0-387-76604-1_26, © Springer Science+Business Media, LLC 2010

approximately 6–72 hours (h) later and stimulates uterine contractions, thus causing expulsion of the pregnancy tissue (Fig. 26-1).

Researchers have developed alternative regimens for medication abortion using mifepristone and misoprostol that are associated with higher efficacy, less cost, more convenience, and fewer side effects than the FDA-approved regimen [4–10]. Clinicians need to consider many variables when selecting a regimen, including patient preferences, cost, and efficacy. Table 26-1 compares the most commonly used mifepristone regimens in the United States. Though less often used, medication abortion can also be accomplished using methotrexate and misoprostol. Advantages of using methotrexate include its relatively cheap cost and wide availability, and the fact that it can medically treat ectopic pregnancy under certain circumstances. However, given that methotrexate (used with misoprostol) can take a longer period of time for abortion completion (up to 4 weeks), it is not typically the regimen of choice for most US providers and patients.

Many states have laws regulating the provision of abortion services, including mandatory waiting periods, parental consent for minors, physician-only laws, and/ or mandatory health department reporting. Clinicians should be familiar with state regulations prior to introducing medication abortion in their practice.

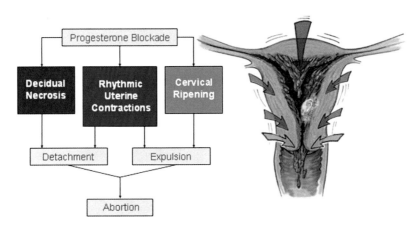

Fig. 26-1 Mifepristone (RU486) and Misoprostol Mechanism of Action. Mifepristone binds to progesterone receptors, causing decidual necrosis and detachment of the pregnancy from the endometrium. In addition, mifepristone induces uterine contractility and sensitizes the myometrium to prostaglandins. Misoprostol administration then promotes cervical ripening and further uterine contractions. The synergistic action of mifepristone and misoprostol ultimately causes pregnancy detachment and expulsion (reprinted with the permission of the National Abortion Federation. Early Options: A Provider's Guide to Medical Abortion. Medical Education Series. "Overview of Medical Abortion: Clinical and Practice Issues." 2005)

Table 26-1 A comparison of medication abortion regimens using mifepristone (RU486) and misoprostol

Regimen	Food and Drug Administration (FDA) approved	Evidence-based, alternative (vaginal misoprostol)	Evidence-based, alternative (sublingual misoprostol)	Evidence-based, alternative (buccal misoprostol)
Mifepristone dose 200 mg/tab	600 mg (3 tabs)	200 mg (1 tab)	200 mg (1 tab)	200 mg (1tab)
Misoprostol dose 200 ug/tab	400 µg (2 tabs)	800 µg (4 tabs)	800 µg (4 tabs)	800 µg (4 tabs)
Where misoprostol is taken	Office	Home	Home	Home
When misoprostol is taken after mifepristone	48 h	6–24 h	48 h	24–48 h
Estimated cost	$90/mifepristone × 3 tabs=$270 $1/ miso tab × 2 tabs=$2 Cost of three office visits	$90/mifepristone × 1 tab=$90 $1/miso pills × 4 tabs=$4 Cost of two office visits	$90/mifepristone × 1 tab=$90 $1/miso pills × 4 tabs=$4 Cost of two office visits	$90/mifepristone × 1 tab=$90 $1/miso pills × 4 tabs=$4 Cost of two office visits
Gestational age limit	≤49 days gestation	≤63 days gestation	≤63 days gestation	≤63 days gestation
Efficacy (%)	92–97	95–98	98	96
Timing of follow-up visit	Approximately day 14	Within 14 days	Within 14 days	Within 14 days

Case Study

A 23-year-old nulliparous female presents to your office after missing her menses. Her last menstrual period was 6 weeks ago. She and her partner experienced a condom break a couple of months ago, but she did not know about emergency contraception. She is a young graduate student and does not feel ready to be a parent at this time. After pregnancy options and abortion options counseling, she decides to proceed with a medication termination. Her examination today reveals a 6-week-size, anteverted uterus with no adenexal masses or tenderness. A transvaginal ultrasound reveals an intrauterine pregnancy approximately 6.2 weeks by crown-rump length.

Diagnosis (Algorithm 26-1)

- 6.2-week intrauterine pregnancy
- Desire for elective termination

Differential Diagnosis

- Normal, intrauterine pregnancy
- Ectopic pregnancy
- Heterotopic pregnancy: concomitant presence of an intrauterine and ectopic pregnancy
- Early pregnancy failure: threatened, incomplete, or complete spontaneous abortion

Indications (Algorithm 26-1)

- Elective procedure
- May also be medically necessary for women with comorbidities in which carrying pregnancy to term poses a threat to health and/or life

Contraindications (Algorithm 26-1)

- Confirmed or suspected ectopic pregnancy or undiagnosed adnexal mass
- Intrauterine device in place (remove prior to treatment)
- Chronic adrenal failure

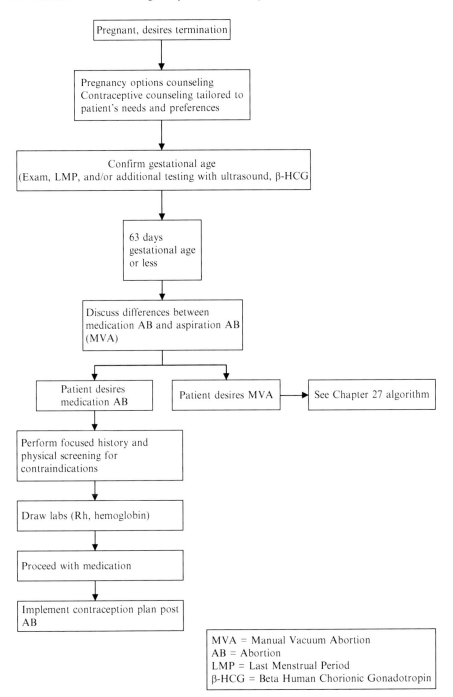

Algorithm 26-1 Decision tree for abortion options

- Current long-term, systemic corticosteroid therapy
- Allergy to mifepristone, misoprostol, or other prostaglandins
- Inherited porphyria
- Hemorrhagic disorder or current anticoagulant therapy

Special Considerations

- Patients with severe anemia (hemoglobin <10 mg/dl, hematocrit <30%) should be evaluated individually for symptoms and presence of current bleeding in order to determine the safest method of pregnancy termination.
- Any patient with chronic medical conditions (e.g., cardiac disease, hepatic disease, uncontrolled diabetes, uncontrolled seizure disorder, inflammatory bowel disease, renal disease, pulmonary disease) should be evaluated individually to determine the safest method of pregnancy termination.
- Breastfeeding mothers: There is no evidence that mifepristone is harmful to breastfeeding infants. Women should be warned that misoprostol can cause mild side effects such as diarrhea in infants, but they do not necessarily need to stop breastfeeding during this time.

Equipment (Fig. 26-2)

- Evidence-based medication abortion consent form (Fig. 26-3)
- Danco® Patient Agreement Form and the Mifeprex® Medication Guide (download from website www.earlyoptionpill.com)
- Patient Instructions for Medication Abortion Form (Fig. 26-4)

Fig. 26-2 Mifepristone 200 mg pills

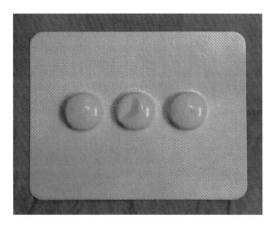

EVIDENCE-BASED MEDICATION ABORTION
CONSENT FORM

The following consent form should be modified accordingly based upon the specific regimen being used (e.g., vaginal misoprostol, buccal, sublingual, oral misoprostol).

Initial each line indicating that you understand and agree with each statement.

_____ I have been appropriately informed about all pregnancy options and abortion options.

_____ "Medication abortion" means using drugs to cause an abortion. A suction abortion uses instruments to empty the uterus or womb. I know that I should not begin a medication abortion unless I am sure I want to end my pregnancy. I am willing to have a suction abortion if the medication abortion fails.

_____ I have received the **Mifeprex® Patient Agreement** and **Mifeprex® Medication Guide**.

_____ I understand that this consent differs from the **Mifeprex® Patient Agreement**.

_____ I understand that the medication abortion must be done within the **first 9 weeks of pregnancy**.

_____ The first medication I will take is **mifepristone** (also known as "Mifeprex®" or "RU486"), which blocks a hormone needed to continue a pregnancy. I will take a 1 pill (200 mg) because research shows this dose is effective. The second drug I will take is **misoprostol** (also known as "Cytotec®"). It causes bleeding and cramping, which pushes the pregnancy tissue out of the womb.

_____ Before I take these medications, I will have a blood tests done as recommended by my clinicians, such as a check for anemia (low blood level). I will have my Rh type confirmed by a donor card, prior blood test or a new blood test. If I am "Rh negative," I will get a shot of MICRhoGAM® as a precaution to prevent any problems with future pregnancies.

_____ I will swallow the **mifepristone** tablet before I leave today. I know that mifepristone can cause bleeding and cramps, or I may feel nothing at all.

_____ I will take **4 misoprostol** tablets home with me. **I will take the misoprostol tablets as directed [INSERT YOUR PROTOCOL HERE]** because research shows this method is effective. I will take the misoprostol even if I have already started bleeding.

_____ I understand that 1-6 hours after I take the **misoprostol**, I will have cramping and bleeding. If I soak more than two maxi pads each hour for two hours in a row, I will call my provider. I will also call if I do **NOT** bleed within 24 hours of inserting the misoprostol.

_____ I have been given prescriptions for pain and nausea. To the best of my knowledge, I am not allergic to mifepristone or misoprostol or any prescription medications given me.

_____ I understand that possible complications from a medical abortion can include: incomplete emptying of my uterus, infection, sepsis (severe infection), bleeding that may (rarely) require a blood transfusion or emergency surgery, allergic reaction, requiring another procedure or surgery.

_____ If I start to feel very ill, I will call my provider. Very rarely, women have had serious "toxic shock" illness after a medication abortion.

_____ I will return for a check-up in 1-2 weeks to be sure that the abortion is complete. At this visit, an ultrasound or a blood test may be done. If the abortion is not complete, I may need a suction procedure to end the pregnancy.

_____ I understand that the abortion must be complete because misoprostol can cause serious birth defects.

Fig. 26-3 Evidence-based medication abortion consent form (source: Reproductive Health Access Project http://www.reproductiveaccess.org/)

____ I have read this form and have had time to think about it. I have had all of my questions answered.

____ If a complication occurs, I request and allow the physician to do whatever is necessary to protect my health.

____ I hereby consent that Dr. _____ give me mifepristone and misoprostol for an early medication abortion.

Patient name (print): _____

Patient Signature: _____   Date: _____

Witness: _____   Date: _____

Provider: _____   Date: _____

Mifeprex®, Danco Laboratories, New York, NY;
Cytotec®, Pfizer, New York, NY;
MICRhoGAM®, Ortho Clinical Diagnostics, Raritan, NJ

Fig. 26-3 (continued)

- Ultrasound (not mandatory per FDA protocol)
- Ultrasound documentation form (if applicable)
- Mifepristone 200 mg pills (must be a registered provider with Danco® http://www.earlyoptionpill.com) (Fig. 26-2)
- Misoprostol 200 mcg tablets (order in bulk)
- Urine pregnancy test
- Ability to document Rh status, hemoglobin, or hematocrit

Procedure (Algorithm 26-1)

1. Perform pregnancy options counseling. Important points to consider:
   - Ask open-ended questions in a nonjudgmental manner (e.g., "How do you feel about being pregnant?").
   - Inquire about the woman's support network (partner, family, friends, etc.).
   - Discuss all options as necessary: continuing the pregnancy and becoming a parent; continuing the pregnancy and opting for an adoption; ending the pregnancy.
   - Assess that the woman's decision, whatever it may be, has not been coerced.
2. Confirm pregnancy diagnosis and gestational age:
   - Assess Last Menstrual Period (LMP) and perform a bimanual to check for consistency between history and examination.
   - Obtain a urine pregnancy test or serum β-HCG, as indicated.
   - Obtain or perform an ultrasound, as indicated.

A Note about Ultrasound: While ultrasonography is widely used for gestational age dating, it is not mandatory to perform in an ultrasound for medication abortion

Medication Abortion Patient Instructions

1. Today, (*date*:_____ , *time*: _____ am/pm) you took 1 pill of **Mifepristone** (RU-486 or Mifeprex®, Danco Laboratories, New York, NY) to end your pregnancy. You may have some vaginal bleeding after taking this pill or you may feel nothing at all.

2. At (*date*:_____ *time*____am/pm) you will take another medicine, **Misoprostol** (Cytotec®,Pfizer, New York, NY). Be sure to get a good meal and plenty of rest beforehand. Take the pain medications prescribed to you (such as 2 pills of Ibuprofen) one hour before you take the Misoprostol – this will help decrease your cramps. You must take the Misoprostol even if you have already started to bleed.

3. Taking misoprostol: You and your provider have already discussed which protocol you are using. Wash your hands prior to handling the misoprostol.

☐ If you are doing the **buccal protocol**: Place **2 misoprostol pills in each cheek** (for a total of 4 pills). Leave the pills there for 30 minutes, and then swallow the rest of the pills with water. The pills may taste chalky and dry.

☐ If you are doing the **sublingual protocol**: Place **4 misoprostol pills under the tongue**. Leave the pills there for 30 minutes, and then swallow them with something to drink

☐ If you are doing the **vaginal protocol**: Your provider may have given you gloves. If so, put on the gloves and lie down on a bed. Push **4 misoprostol pills high into your vagina**, one by one. The pills do not have to be put in a special spot, just push them as far back as you can. Rest on your back for thirty minutes. After you get up, it is OK if you see a few partly dissolved pills come out if you go to the bathroom.

4. **Symptoms to Expect: Misoprostol** (the second medicine) causes cramping within 2-4 hours after taken for most women. The cramping can be very strong for a few hours, but usually not for more than 24 hours. You will also have bleeding that can be quite heavy with clots for a few hours. You may see some pregnancy tissue (usually white or gray). After the abortion is complete, you may have light to moderate bleeding that lasts 1-4 weeks, on and off.

You may have bad cramps. If so, take pain medicine as instructed by your health care provider. You can also use a heating pad. Some women get nausea, diarrhea, or chills soon after taking the second medicine. This should get better in a few hours. If it does not, call your provider.

5. **IMPORTANT: Call if any of the following happens:**
-Your bleeding soaks through **more than 2 maxi pads per hour for 2 hours**, OR
-You do **not** bleed within 24 hours after inserting the misoprostol, OR
-You have a **fever**, OR
-You start to **feel very ill** 24 hours after you have taken misoprostol

6. **To contact us:** Call the 24-hour number: _____. If you have any questions, think something is wrong, or think you have an emergency, PLEASE CALL and we will call you back. Feel free to call, no question is too small.

7. **Follow-up:** You have an appointment on _____ at _____ am/pm. At this visit, we will make sure that the abortion is complete. **This is an important appointment**, as you can have bleeding and cramping and still not have completed the abortion.

8. **Birth Control:** We have already talked about your birth control plan:_____. Remember that **you can get pregnant even right after an abortion**. You should start your birth control on _____ even if you are still bleeding.

Fig. 26-4 Patient instructions for medication abortion (adapted from: Reproductive Health Access Project http://www.reproductiveaccess.org/)

per FDA protocol. According to the Mifeprex® Prescribing Information, "the duration of pregnancy may be determined from menstrual history and by clinical examination. Ultrasonographic scan should be used if the duration of pregnancy is uncertain, or if ectopic pregnancy is suspected" [11]. It has been shown that women seeking abortions can accurately estimate their gestational age [12] and that clinician assessment of gestational age (based on exam and LMP) had a high correlation with sonography [13]. Based upon this evidence, some providers have advocated for an "ultrasound as needed" protocol, such that an ultrasound is performed only under certain circumstances [14,15]. This approach can greatly improve access to abortion services, particularly in sites where the cost of an ultrasound machine is prohibitive and/or there are no trained ultrasonographers. Indications for ultrasonography premedication abortion:

- Discrepancy between gestational age as assessed by uterine size and LMP
- Uncertain LMP
- Adnexal mass or pain
- LMP at the end of a course of hormonal contraception
- Provider uncertainty with exam
- History of previous ectopic pregnancy
- Confirm eligibility criteria and conduct other medical screening as indicated (e.g., Pap smear, sexually transmitted infection (STI) testing). The performance of such screening tests in otherwise asymptomatic patients is not mandatory prior to providing medication abortion.
- Help the woman choose a birth control method. Discuss emergency contraception and provide advance prescriptions if necessary.
- Confirm Rh type: review blood donor cards and/or old prenatal labs, or send for testing.
- If the woman is Rh negative, a dose of MICRhoGAM® (50 μg) (Ortho Clinical Diagnostics, Raritan, NJ) should be given just prior to using misoprostol or within 72 h of bleeding.
- Testing for hemoglobin or hematocrit is not mandatory per the Mifeprex® Medication Guide. Providers may choose to routinely screen for anemia depending on the local prevalence on anemia and/or by individual risk factors and clinical history [16].
- Review your *Evidence-Based Medication Abortion Consent Form* (Fig. 26-3) and the *Patient Agreement Form* ® (required by Danco®, the manufacturer of mifepristone). The patient should also be given the *Mifeprex® Medication Guide*. Document that you reviewed the differences between the FDA-approved regimen and any alternative regimen(s) you offered the patient.
- Counsel the patient on what to do and expect (Fig. 26-4).
- The patient should pick a convenient time to administer the misoprostol, after mifepristone ingestion. Review *how and when* to administer the misoprostol, depending on which route has been chosen.
- Advise on the use of pain and/or nausea medications prior to misoprostol administration (e.g., ibuprofen, Phenergan® [Wyeth, Madison, NJ]).
- Review when to call: if no bleeding occurs within 24 h, if soaking through two pads an hour for two consecutive hours, if sustained fever >100.4°F.
- Advise that cramping and bleeding may occur a couple of hours (h) after taking the misoprostol, which may peak in 3–5 h. The cramping ranges from mild to intense. Approximately two-thirds of women will complete the abortion process within 4 h. By 24 h, 90% of women will have successfully completed the abortion.

- The bleeding is similar to a heavy period with or without clots. The woman should be told that she will see blood and tissue (like a wet facial tissue), and it would be unusual to recognize fetal parts, even at 63 days gestation.
- Have the woman take the mifepristone in your office under direct observation. Document the time and date and the lot number of the mifepristone.
- Prior to leaving, the woman should have:
- Misoprostol tablets (record the lot number and expiration date) to self- administer at home
- Prescriptions for pain and/or nausea
- Prescriptions for birth control and, if necessary, emergency contraception
- A follow-up appointment in 12 weeks
- A 24-h provider contact number
- The Patient Instruction Form (Fig. 26-4)

At Follow-Up Visit

1. Confirmation of pregnancy termination can be confirmed by:
   - Patient history (a description of cramping and bleeding, passage of pregnancy tissue) *and*
   - Physical examination *or* ultrasound *or* documentation of declining serum β-HCG level (at least 80% decline from baseline) [16]; Postabortion indications for ultrasonography:
     - History not consistent with successful abortion
     - Woman still feels pregnant
     - Serum b-HCG not declining
     - Provider uncertainty with history
2. If the abortion is incomplete (persistent sac, no evidence of fetal cardiac activity), the patient can be offered repeat misoprostol or an aspiration abortion. An aspiration abortion may need to be involved for problematic bleeding and/or ongoing pregnancy (presence of fetal cardiac activity).
3. Clinicians should inquire about the woman's reactions to the abortion process and provide support and reassurance as appropriate. It is not unusual for women to feel a wide range of emotions following an elective abortion, including relief, sadness, anxiety, and guilt.
4. Review the contraceptive plan and initiate the method that day, if possible.

Complications and Risks

Less than 1% of all US abortion patients experience a major complication. The risk of death associated with abortion in the United States is less than 0.6 per 100,000 procedures, which is less than one-tenth the risk associated with childbirth. Complications and risks are:

- Significant bleeding requiring intervention: <1%
- Infection: <1%
- Sepsis: <0.01%
- Incomplete abortion, requiring a uterine aspiration procedure: 0.16–5%

A Note about Sepsis: On July 15, 2005, the US Food and Drug Association (FDA) issued a public health advisory regarding four deaths in the United States (all in California) that occurred following vaginal administration of misoprostol and oral mifepristone for medication abortion. *Clostrium sordelli*, a virulent gram-positive bacteria, was identified as the causative agent in all cases. Other cases of *Clostrium sordelli*-related deaths have involved cases of spontaneous abortion and childbirth. After an extensive investigation, the Centers for Disease Control and Prevention, the FDA, and the National Institute of Allergy and Infectious Diseases concluded that there is no definitive causal relationship between mifepristone and the deaths [17]. Clinicians should be familiar with the signs and symptoms of sepsis and initiate prompt evaluation of women who present with sustained fever, severe abdominal pain, prolonged heavy bleeding, syncope, or abdominal pain or general malaise that occurs more than 24 h after taking misoprostol [11]. For more information on this topic, please visit the CDCwebsite (http://www.cdc.gov/ncidod/dhqp/id_Csordellii.html).

Tricks and Helpful Hints

- Some women who otherwise meet medical eligibility may not be appropriate candidates for medication abortion for psychosocial reasons.
- Clinicians should consider the following questions to identify patients who may be unable to carry out instructions or follow up: Does the patient have a phone, a car, childcare? How far does she live from your office? Is there a language barrier?

Procedure Note

See Fig. 26-5 for the Medication Abortion Charting Form.
   (Provider to fill in blanks/circle applicable choice when given multiple choices and customize as needed.)

Patient Name : _____
Chart Number: _____

MEDICATION ABORTION CHARTING FORM

		Yes	No	N/A
Options counseling documented				
Protocol explained:	Timing of medications, adverse effects			
	Need for follow-up visit			
	On-call system			
Contraindications ruled out:	No IUD in place			
	No allergy to prostaglandins/mifepristone			
	No chronic adrenal failure			
	No long-term systemic corticosteroid tx			
	No concurrent anticoagulant therapy			
	No ectopic pregnancy			
	No hemorrhagic disorder			
Mifeprex medication guide given				
Mifeprex provider/patient agreement signed				
Informed, evidence-based consent form signed				
Rh status (circle one): Positive Negative				
Rhogam given (if indicated)				
Initial beta-HCG level: (if indicated)				
Hemoglobin level (if indicated):				
Ultrasound dating done (if indicated):				
Pain medication prescribed:				
Mifeprex lot #: Exp date: Date administered:				
Misoprostol lot #: Exp date: # of pills dispensed:				
Follow-up visit completed on:				
Abortion completion assessed by: History /Exam				
	Beta-HCG level			
	Sonogram			
Contraception plan: _____ Date initiated:				

Fig. 26-5 Medication abortion procedure note/charting form (adapted from: Reproductive Health Access Project http://www.reproductiveaccess.org/)

Coding

CPT® Codes (Current Procedural Terminology, AMA, Chicago, IL)

For the visit	99204 or 99214	level 4 new or established patient E/M visit
For the ultrasound	76817	transvaginal ultrasound, pregnant uterus
	76815	limited ultrasound, pregnant uterus
For medication(s)	J8499	prescription drug, oral, nonchemo, not otherwise specified
	J3490	unclassified drug
	90385	MICRhoGAM®, if given in office

ICD 9-CM-Diagnostic Codes (International Classification of Diseases, 9th Revision, Clinical Modification, Center for Disease Control and Prevention) [non-comprehensive]

Legally induced abortion, without mention of complication, complete	635.92

If J codes not accepted by insurance carrier, use 99070 (a cost of materials CPT code) for Mifeprex® or S0190 for Mifeprex®. Note: Each insurance carrier may reimburse for Mifeprex® using a different code. The name of the drug (Mifeprex®), the dosage (200 mg), and the 11-digit National Drug Code (NDC) from the drug package must accompany this claim. In addition, submit a copy of the drug invoice to show the cost of the drug.

Patient Instructions

See Fig. 26-4.

(Provider to fill in blanks/circle applicable choice when given multiple choices and to customize as needed.)

Case Study Outcome

The patient took 200 mg of mifepristone the day of the office visit in your office. She self-administered 800 µg of misoprostol vaginally at home approximately 24 h later and experienced bleeding similar to a heavy period 3–4 h later. She also had cramping that eventually subsided with ibuprofen and a heating pad. At her follow-up visit, an ultrasound revealed a thick endometrial stripe but no intrauterine pregnancy. She was bleeding lightly and pain free, and reported relief that the process was over. You advised her to start her birth control pills that day.

References

1. Finer L, Henshaw K. Disparities in rates of unintended pregnancy in the United States, 1994 and 2001. *Perspect Sex Reprod Health* 2006;38(2):90–96.
2. Henshaw SK. Unintended pregnancy in the United States. *Fam Plann Perspect* 1998;30(1):24–29, 46.
3. Finer LB, Henshaw SK. Abortion incidence and services in the United States in 2000. *Perspect Sex Reprod Health* 2003;35(1):6–15.
4. Schaff EA, Fielding SL, Westhoff C, Ellertson C, Eisinger SH, Stadalius LS, Fuller L. Vaginal misoprostol administered 1, 2, or 3 days after mifepristone for early medical abortion: a randomized trial. *JAMA* 2000;284(15):1948–1953.
5. World Health Organisation Task Force on Post-ovulatory Methods of Fertility Regulation. Comparison of two doses of mifepristone in combination with misoprostol for early medical abortion: a randomised trial. *BJOG* 2000;107(4):524–530.
6. Bartley J, Brown A, Elton R, Baird DT. Double-blind randomized trial of mifepristone in combination with vaginal gemeprost or misoprostol for induction of abortion up to 63 days gestation. *Hum Reprod* 2001;16(10):2098–2102.
7. Hamoda H, Ashok PW, Flett GM, Templeton A. A randomised controlled trial of mifepristone in combination with misoprostol administered sublingually or vaginally for medical abortion up to 13 weeks of gestation. *BJOG* 2005;112(8):1102-1108.
8. Middleton T, Schaff E, Fielding S, Scahill M, Shannon C, Westheimer E, Wilkinson T, Winikoffet B. Randomized trial of mifepristone and buccal or vaginal misoprostol for abortion through 56 days of last menstrual period. *Contraception* 2005;72:328–332.
9. Creinin M, Fox M, Teal S, Chen A, Schaff E, Meyn L, for the MOD Study Trial. A randomized comparison of misoprostol 6 to 8 hours versus 24 hours after mifepristone for abortion. *Obstet Gynecol* 2004;103(5):851–859.
10. Tang OS, Chan C, Ng E, Lee S, Ho PC. A prospective, randomized, placebo-controlled trial on the use of mifepristone with sublingual or vaginal misoprostol for medical abortions of less than 9 weeks gestation. *Hum Reprod* 2003;18(11):2315–2318.
11. Danco Laboratories, LLC. Mifeprex® Medication Guide. NY, NY: [updated 7/19/05, cited 10/30/07]. Available from: http://www.earlyoptionpill.com/pdfs/medication071905.pdf
12. Ellertson C, Elul B, Ambardekar S, Wood L, Carroll J, Coyaji K. Accuracy of assessment of pregnancy duration by women seeking early abortions. *Lancet* 2000;355:877–881.
13. Fielding SL, Schaff EA, Nam NY. Clinicians' perception of sonogram indication for mifepristone abortion up to 63 days. *Contraception* 2002;66:27–31.
14. Clark WH, Gold M, Grossman D, Winikoff B. Can mifepristone abortion be simplified? A review of the evidence and questions for future research. *Contraception* 2007;75:245–250.
15. Clark WH, Panton T, Hann L, Gold M. Medication abortion employing routine sequential measurement of serum hCG and sonography only when indicated. *Contraception* 2007;75(2):131–135.
16. World Health Organization. Safe abortion: technical and policy guidance for health systems. Geneva: WHO, 2003.
17. Aldape MJ, Bryant AE, Stevens DL. Clostridium sordelli infection: epidemiology, clinical findings, and current perspectives on diagnosis and treatment. *Clin Infect Dis* 2006;43:1436–1446.

Additional Resources

Websites

To obtain the Mifeprex® Medication Guide and Patient Agreement Form, visit: www.earlyoption-pill.com

For patient and clinician resources regarding early abortion care (including the methotrexate/misoprostol regimen), visit The Reproductive Health Access Project: http://www.reproductive-access.org/

For information regarding abortion training in family medicine residencies, visit The Center for Reproductive Health Education in Family Medicine: www.rhedi.org

For educational resources and a clinical curriculum regarding medication abortion, visit The National Abortion Federation: http://www.prochoice.org/education/resources/index.html

For information regarding state laws on abortion, visit The Center for Reproductive Rights: http://www.reproductiverights.org/

Chapter 27
Manual Vacuum Aspiration (MVA) Abortion

Justine Wu

Introduction

Traditionally, "surgical" abortions referred to dilation and curettage (D&C), or to sharp curettage performed in the operating room under general or regional anesthesia or moderate sedation. Surgical abortion can also occur via vacuum aspiration with an electric pump machine or manually with a 60 cc handheld syringe (a manual vacuum aspirator). These methods are commonly referred to as "aspiration abortion" and can be performed safely and effectively in the outpatient setting [1], with local anesthesia alone or combined with light to moderate sedation. Aspiration abortion is associated with lower rates of complications, including infection and perforation, compared to sharp curettage. According to the World Health Organization [2], aspiration abortion and medication abortion are preferred over sharp curettage whenever possible.

Aspiration abortion performed with a Manual Vacuum Aspirator (MVA) is a safe, simple procedure particularly adaptable for use in the primary care setting because of several features of the MVA: (1) low cost and ability to reuse the manual aspirator; (2) small size and portability of the manual aspirator; (3) its ability to aspirate tissue without extensive fragmentation, allowing for easier identification of early pregnancy tissue; and (4) its ability to work without an electrical source. The MVA is also a quieter machine than the electric vacuum, which may reduce patient anxiety. Use of the MVA is clinically indicated for elective abortions up to 12 weeks by uterine size or Last Menstrual Period (LMP). Other uses of the MVA technique include treatment of early pregnancy failure and endometrial biopsy.

After the United States (US) Food and Drug Administration's (FDA) approval of mifepristone for medication abortion in 2001, the number of medication abortions

J. Wu (✉)

Department of Family Medicine, University of Medicine and Dentistry of New Jersey, Robert Wood Johnson Medical School, 1 Robert Wood Johnson Place, MEB 2nd Floor, CN19, New Brunswick, NJ, 08903-0019, USA
e-mail: drwuju@yahoo.com

S.M. Sulik and C.B. Heath (eds.), *Primary Care Procedures in Women's Health*, DOI 10.1007/978-0-387-76604-1_27, © Springer Science+Business Media, LLC 2010

performed in the US has steadily increased. Medication abortion offers an important alternative for women seeking early abortion services (see Chap. 26). In order to provide comprehensive abortion options counseling, clinicians should be familiar with the advantages and disadvantages of medication abortion versus aspiration abortion from a patient perspective (Table 27-1 see patient handout).

Clinicians should be familiar with state regulations for first trimester abortion provision prior to introducing MVA in their practice. Regulations may include mandatory waiting periods, parental consent for minors, and/or mandatory health department reporting. Advanced practice clinicians (nurse practitioners, physician assistants) should specifically check if "physician-only" laws apply for abortion provision in their state.

Less than 1% of all US abortion patients experience a major complication. The risk of death associated with abortion in the United States is less than 0.6 per 100,000 procedures, which is less than one-tenth the risk associated with childbirth [3].

The routine use of antibiotics just prior to or following induced abortions <16 weeks is associated with a 42% reduction in the incidence of postabortal upper genital tract infection, regardless of the woman's preprocedure risk status [4]. It is not clear which antibiotic regimen has the greatest preventive effect. In the US, doxycycline (100 mg orally twice a day) is used widely, with durations ranging from 1 to 7 days.

Case Study

A 42-year-old G3P2002 female presents to your office with complaints of nausea. Her last menstrual period was 8 weeks ago. She stopped using birth control pills a year ago, citing that "I was too old to be on the pill." She and her husband already have two teenagers. She is shocked when her pregnancy test is positive and feels overwhelmed about the thought of having another child. After pregnancy options counseling, she goes home to talk with her husband. The couple returns the next week, having decided to proceed with an aspiration abortion. Her examination reveals an 8-week-size, anteverted uterus. A transvaginal ultrasound reveals an intrauterine pregnancy approximately 8.6 weeks by crown-rump length.

Diagnosis (Algorithm 27-1)

- 8.6-week intrauterine pregnancy
- Desire for elective termination

Differential Diagnosis

- Normal, intrauterine pregnancy
- Ectopic pregnancy

- Heterotopic pregnancy (concomitant presence of an intrauterine and ectopic pregnancy)
- Early pregnancy failure (threatened, incomplete, or complete spontaneous abortion)

Indications (Algorithm 27-1)

- Elective abortion up to 12 weeks
- Treatment for early pregnancy failure up to 12 weeks
- Medical necessity for women with comorbidities in which carrying a pregnancy to term poses a threat to health and/or life
- Endometrial biopsy (instead of using endometrial pipelle)

Contraindications (Algorithm 27-1)

- Gestational age is greater than the limit set by the clinical site
- Inability to tolerate MVA under local anesthesia and available analgesia
- Known hydatidiform mole
- Hemodynamic instability
- Severe medical illness (e.g., suspected diabetic ketoacidosis, uncontrolled seizure disorder, acute asthmatic attack) for which surgery would be life-threatening

Special Considerations/Contraindications

- Active intrauterine infection: Clinicians should decide whether or not to proceed with the procedure depending on the patient's clinical status. Treatment should be initiated promptly per the Centers for Disease Control (CDC) Sexually Transmitted Diseases Treatment Guidelines [5].
- Mucopurulent cervicitis: The patient should be treated per CDC guidelines for presumptive gonorrhea and chlamydia cervicitis [5]. The patient can still undergo the procedure that day but should complete treatment postprocedure.
- Significant medical comorbidities: Examples include uncontrolled diabetes, cardiovascular or pulmonary disease, seizure disorder, and blood-clotting disorders. Patients should be medically stable prior to the procedure and/or referred to a facility that is able to treat women with such conditions.
- Cervical stenosis: May require cervical ripening agents, special dilation techniques.
- Severe anemia: Defined as hemoglobin <8 mg/dl, hematocrit <24%, and/or symptomatic. Clinicians need to determine whether to proceed or delay the procedure.
- Suspected and/or known ectopic pregnancy: Evaluate, treat, and refer according to local protocol.

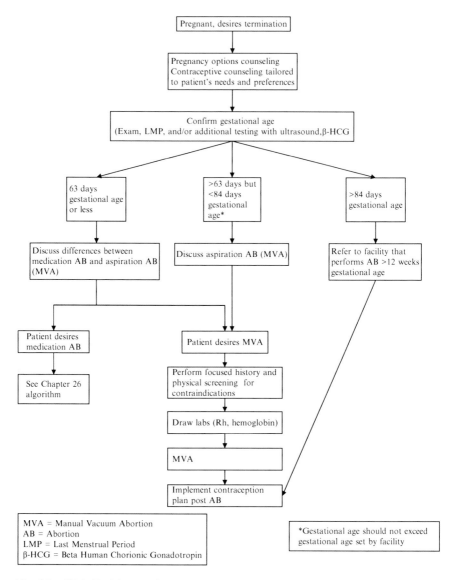

Algorithm 27-1 Decision tree for women desiring elective termination

Equipment (Fig. 27-1)

Sterile instrument trays containing the following:

- Specula (various sizes)
- Ringed forceps (sponge stick)
- Iodine cups

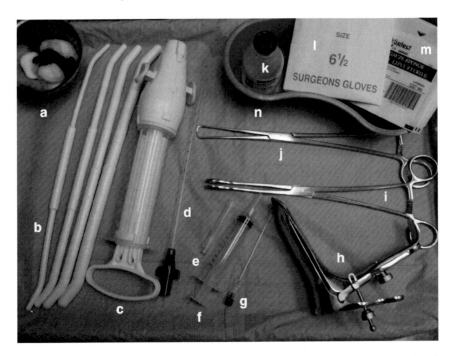

Fig. 27-1 Equipment set-up (sterile) for MVA. (a) Antiseptic soaked cotton balls in basin; (b) Cervical dilator set; (c) Manual vacuum aspirator; (d) Flexible cannula; (e) Needle; (f) Syringe; (g) Long needle; (h) Speculum; (i) Rings forceps; (j) Tenaculum; (k) Lidocaine; (l) Sterile gloves; (m) Gauze sponge (Select Medical Products); (n) Kidney-shaped basin

- Tenaculums
- Vaginal dilators (e.g., Denniston or Pratt)

For viewing and processing Products of Conception (POC):

- Light box (available at a photography or craft store)
- Glass pyrex dish (traditional pie size)
- Strainer (kitchen supply)
- Long forceps (to move and pickup POC)
- Pathology specimen jars or disposal cups

Additional supplies:

- 10–12 cc syringes
- 22 gauge 1½ in. spinal needles/18 gauge needles, needle extenders
- Sharps containers
- 60 cc aspiration syringe (e.g., IPAS MVA Plus®, IPAS, Chapel Hill, NC)
- Flexible cannulas in sizes 5–12 (e.g., IPAS Karman® [IPAS, Chapel Hill, NC], MedGyn® [Medgyn, Lombard, IL], Berkeley® [Berkeley Medevices, Richmond, CA])

- Nonsterile gloves/Sterile gloves
- Sterile gauze
- Betadine
- Kidney basins
- Autoclave and supplies for cleaning and wrapping equipment

Medications:

- Lidocaine 1% (may dilute 50/50 with Normal Saline)
- RhoGAM® (Ortho Clinical Diagnostics, Raritan, NJ)
- For emergency use:
  - Methergine® (Novartis, Basil, Switzerland) (for excessive bleeding)
  - Misoprostol (for cervical ripening, excessive bleeding)
  - Atropine
  - IV tubing, IV fluid, IVs in various gauges, tape
  - Albuterol inhaler
  - Epinephrine 1:1,000

Ultrasound and Supplies (if an ultrasound is on-site):

- Probe covers
- Probe disinfectant
- Ultrasound gel
- Printer paper (if printer available)

Patient items:

- Drape
- Gown
- Sanitary napkins

Documents:

- MVA Consent Form (Fig. 27-2)
- MVA Preprocedure Form (Fig. 27-3)
- MVA After-Care Instructions and Information (Fig. 27-4)
- Relevant birth control education

Procedure (Algorithm 27-1)

Pre-procedure Steps

1. Perform pregnancy options counseling. Important points to consider:
   - Ask open-ended questions in a nonjudgmental manner, e.g., "How do you feel about being pregnant?"
   - Inquire about the woman's support network (partner, family, friends).
   - Discuss all options as necessary: (1) continuing the pregnancy and becoming a parent; (2) continuing the pregnancy and opting for an adoption; or (3) ending the pregnancy.
   - Assess that the woman's decision, whatever it may be, has not been coerced.
2. Confirm pregnancy diagnosis and gestational age by assessing LMP, performing a bimanual examination, and obtaining an ultrasound. Obtain a urine pregnancy test or serum β-HCG, if indicated.
3. Confirm eligibility criteria and conduct other medical screening as indicated (e.g., Pap smear, STI testing). The performance of such screening tests in otherwise asymptomatic patients is not mandatory prior to performing MVA.
4. Help the woman select an appropriate birth control method. Discuss Emergency Contraception (EC) and provide advance prescriptions of EC if necessary.
5. Providers may choose to routinely screen for anemia depending on the local prevalence of anemia and/or by individual risk factors and clinical history [6].
6. Confirm Rh type (review blood donor cards, old prenatal labs, or send for testing).
7. Review consent form and obtain the patient's signature (Fig. 27-2).

Performing MVA

Throughout the procedure, the *"no-touch"* technique should be followed such that instrument parts that enter the vagina or cervical os are never touched.

Step 1: Prepare the Woman and Prep the Cervix (Fig. -27-5)

- Have the woman empty her bladder.
- Explain the procedure steps to the woman and answer all her remaining questions.
- Help the woman into dorsal lithotomy position on the table.
- Wash hands, put on appropriate barrier equipment; gloves can be sterile or nonsterile.
- Perform a bimanual examination, noting the size, shape, and position of the uterus.
- Insert the speculum so that the entire cervix is well visualized.
- Clean the cervix with an antiseptic soaked sponge.

MVA CONSENT FORM

Initial each line, indicating you understand and agree with each statement.

_____ I request a Manual Vacuum Aspiration (MVA), a procedure that will empty my uterus. This procedure may be used as an aspiration abortion or as treatment for a miscarriage or a failed medication abortion.

_____ I understand that if I am pregnant, the MVA will end my pregnancy. I have been appropriately informed about all pregnancy options and abortion options.

_____ I understand that before the MVA, I may have a blood test done to check for anemia. I will document my Rh type by donor card, prior blood test or a new blood test. If I am Rh negative, I will get a shot of MICRhoGAM® (Ortho Clinical Diagnostics, Raritan, NJ) as a precaution to prevent any potential problems with future pregnancies.

_____ I understand that I might be offered medications before the MVA, such as ibuprofen to lessen the cramping and misoprostol to help open my cervix. I will have local anesthesia with lidocaine solution injected. To the best of my knowledge, I am not allergic to ibuprofen, misoprostol, or lidocaine.

_____ I understand that the possible complications from MVA include: incomplete emptying of my uterus, infection, bleeding that may (rarely) require a blood transfusion or emergency surgery, allergic reaction, perforation (poking a hole in the uterus), injury to the cervix, uterus, vagina or nearby organs, requiring another procedure or surgery.

_____ I have read this form and have had time to think about it. I have had all of my questions answered.

_____ I have been given an information sheet explaining how and when to get help should a question or problem arise after the procedure.

_____ In the event of an unexpected complication during the MVA, I request and authorize the physician to do whatever is needed to protect my health and welfare.

_____ I hereby consent that _____ do the procedure "manual vacuum aspiration" for me.

Signature of patient: _____   **Date:** _____

Provider signature: _____   **Date:** _____

Witness: _____   **Date:** _____

Fig. 27-2 MVA consent form (adapted from Reproductive Health Access Project: http://www. reproductiveaccess.org/)

Step 2: Administer a Paracervical Block (Fig. 27-6)

- Inject 1–2 cc of local anesthetic at the planned tenaculum site (12:00 for an anterverted uterus, 6:00 for a retroverted uterus).

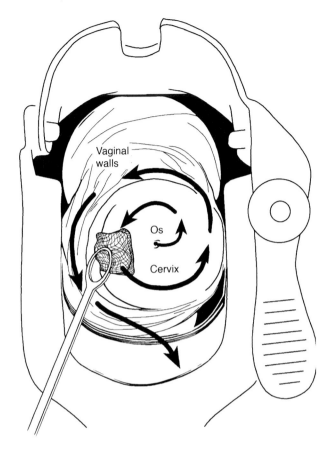

Fig. 27-5 Prepping the cervix (courtesy of IPAS, Stephen C. Edgerton, illustrator)

- Place the tenaculum at the anesthetized site by opening the tenaculum and closing the "teeth" around a generous amount of cervical tissue, which allows gentle counter traction to be applied to straighten the uterus.
- Using the tenaculum, move the cervix to the side to visualize the "reflection," the site at which smooth cervical tissue meets vaginal tissue.
- Inject half of the remaining amount of anesthetic at the "reflection," first at 4:00 and then at 8:00 (or vice versa), burying the needle to a depth of 1–1.5 in. and taking care to pull back on the plunger first to avoid injecting in a blood vessel.

Step 3: Dilate the Cervix (Table 27-2)

Table 27-2 displays the recommended dilation and cannula size needed for corresponding gestational age. During dilation, maintain gentle traction on the tenaculum to pull the uterine axis as straight as possible.

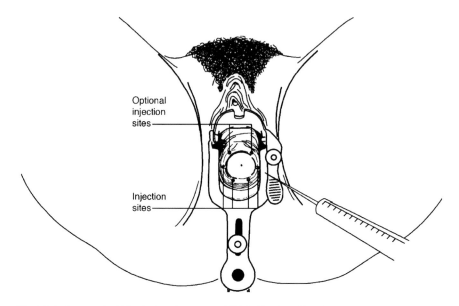

Fig. 27-6 Paracervical block sites (courtesy of IPAS, Stephen C. Edgerton, illustrator)

Table 27-2 Suggested dilation and cannula by gestational age

Gestational age (weeks) by ultrasound	Pratt dilator (measured in circumference; French)	Denniston dilator (measured in diameter; mm)	Flexible Karman Cannula size (mm)
5.0–5.4	19	6	6
5.5–6.4	19	6	6
6.5–7.4	21	7	7
7.5–8.4	25	8	8
8.5–9.4	27	9	9
9.5–10.4	31	10	10
10.5–11.4	31 or 37	10 or 12 (no 11 cannula)	10 or 12
11.5–12.0	37	12	12

1. Gently insert the first dilator into the cervix so that it is introduced just beyond the internal os. A slight "give" may be felt as the dilator slides from the wider external os past the internal os.
2. Take the dilator out and turn it over to dilate with the other side of the dilator (which is the next size up). Progressively dilate to the appropriate size.

Step 4: Insert the Cannula and Attach the Syringe (Fig. 27-7)

1. Insert the cannula into the cervix, past the cervical os and into the uterine cavity.
2. Attach a "primed" MVA syringe to the cannula, holding the tenaculum and the end of the cannula in one hand and the aspirator in the other.

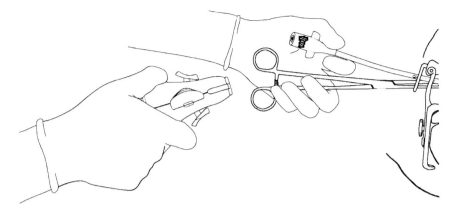

Fig. 27-7 Cannula inserted and attaching aspirator (courtesy of IPAS, Stephen C. Edgerton, illustrator)

Step 5: Evacuate the Uterus

- Release the valve buttons of the MVA aspirator, which will start the suction (Fig. 27-8).
- Gently and slowly rotate the syringe 360°, using an in-and-out motion at the same time. There should be a return of blood and tissue through the cannula and into the syringe (Fig. 27-9).
- Once the aspirator is filled or once no further return of tissue occurs, withdraw the cannula beyond the cervical os until the vacuum is lost (a soft "whoosh" will be heard as the seal is broken).
- Reinsert the cannula just beyond the os at this time. Detach the aspirator from the cannula (Fig. 27-10). Empty the aspirator contents into a kidney basin.
- "Prime" the aspirator and attach it to the cannula. Repeat steps 4 and 5 until evacuation is complete.

Step 6: Assess for Complete Uterine Evacuation

The following signs indicate the uterus is completely evacuated:

- A "gritty" sensation is felt as the cannula passes over the uterine wall.
- The uterus "tightens" around the cannula.
- Red or pink foam appears and no more tissue passes through the cannula.
- The woman complains of uterine cramping in response to uterine contractions.

Step 7: Complete the Procedure

- Take the cannula and aspirator out of the cervix.
- Take the tenaculum off. This can be facilitated by releasing the clamp and then gently rotating the entire tenaculum clockwise 360°, effectively lifting the "teeth" out of the cervical tissue.

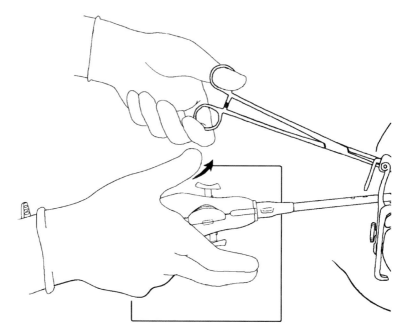

Fig. 27-8 Release the valve buttons of the MVA aspirator, which will start the suction (courtesy of IPAS, Stephen C. Edgerton, illustrator)

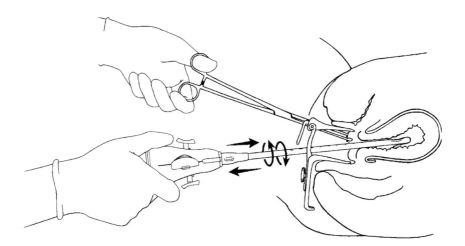

Fig. 27-9 Evacuating uterine contents (Courtesy of IPAS, Stephen C. Edgerton, illustrator)

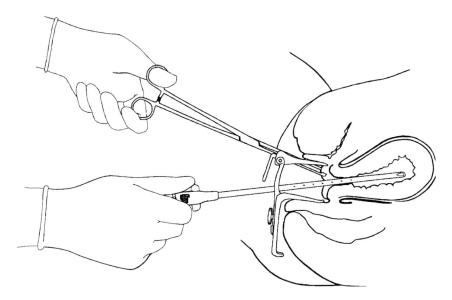

Fig. 27-10 Aspirator detached from cannula. (Courtesy of IPAS, Stephen C. Edgerton, illustrator)

- Use a sponge stick to gently swab any remaining blood out of the vaginal vault.
- Observe for any active bleeding, particularly from the tenaculum site. Apply pressure to any sites of bleeding.
- If an intrauterine device is desired, it can be safely inserted at this time, although patients should be warned of slightly higher expulsion rates [7].
- Remove the speculum.
- Remove barriers and gloves, and wash hands.
- Help the woman into a comfortable position on the table.

Step 8: Inspect the Products of Conception (POC)

- The tissue should be rinsed in a strainer and placed in a clear, glass dish with water to help "float" the tissue.
- For best visualization, the dish should be placed on a light box.
- Identify villi, gestational sac, and decidual tissue (Fig. 27-11). As early as 8.5 weeks, fetal parts may be visible. Fetal parts must be positively identified in pregnancies 10–13 weeks LMP.
- If no POC are visible or are less than expected for gestation age, an ultrasound and/or reaspiration should be considered, as well as reevaluation of the diagnosis. The differential for absent POC or POC less than expected includes: (1) incomplete abortion; (2) spontaneous abortion that already completed; (3) a uterine anomaly that precluded complete aspiration; (4) a failed abortion; or (5) ectopic pregnancy.

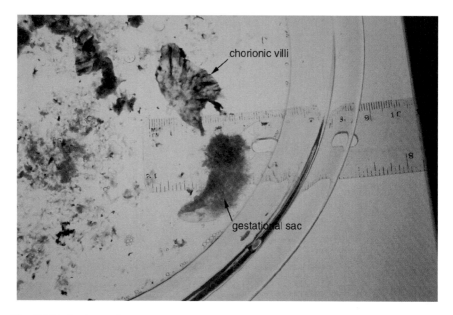

Fig. 27-11 Products of conception: villi and gestational sac (courtesy of Deborah Oyer, MD, Aurora Medical Services, Seattle, WA)

- After satisfactory inspection, the POC should be discarded per medical waste guidelines or sent to a pathology laboratory if required by institutional/state regulations.

Complications and Risks

- Significant bleeding (first-trimester rate): 0.1%
- Infection: 0.1–0.5% (with the use of prophylactic antibiotics)
- Hematometra (retained uterine clots): 0.2%
- Need to reaspirate (retained tissue or continuing pregnancy): 0.3–2%
- Perforation: 0.1%

Tricks and Helpful Hints

- Cervical preparation: Cervical priming with misoprostol (a prostaglandin) for first trimester abortion has been shown to increase initial cervical dilatation, decrease blood loss, and require less dilation force [6]. The benefits of cervical priming must be weighed against the disadvantages of increased side effects, such as nausea, vomiting, diarrhea, bleeding, and cramping that can occur prior to the procedure. Common protocols for cervical priming include 400 μg (two tablets) of misoprostol taken 3 hours (h) prior to the procedure via oral or vaginal administration [8,9]. Potential indications for preprocedure misoprostol cervical preparation may include:

- Pregnancies over 9 weeks in nulliparous women
- Any situation in which the risk of perforation is increased (e.g., stenotic os)
- Pregnancies over 12 weeks
- Performing the paracervical block: To reduce patient anxiety and pain, some clinicians like to ask the patient to cough just as the needle is inserted into the cervix. The cough serves to push the cervix forward towards the needle and most importantly, it is a pain distracter. This technique can also be used when placing the tenaculum.
- Difficult dilation of an extremely anteverted or retroverted uterus: Changing to a shorter blade speculum (e.g., Klopfer, Weisman-Graves, Moore-Graves) allows the provider to pull the cervix closer. It also provides more anterior and posterior space to accommodate the dilators and cannula at a steeper angle to follow the uterine axis.

Procedures

Name:
MR#:

MVA PRE-PROCEDURE NOTE

Date: _____

Vitals: BP ____/____ Pulse_____ Temp ____

☐ Patient was counseled regarding her pregnancy options.
☐ Procedure explained, alternatives discussed, side effects, adverse events reviewed.
☐ Informed consent obtained, filed in chart.

History:

Age: ____ G ____ P: ___ # of C/S: ___ Prev abs: ___ Surg ___ Med___ SAB

Hb: ___/dl. **Rh Type:** ☐ Negative ☐ Positive Confirmed by:_____

Relevant gyn history:

LMP:

Last PAP:

Allergies: ☐ NKDA ☐ Yes Indicate med and reaction:_____

Ultrasound Exam: (see Ultrasound documentation form)
Gestational Age _____ determined by ☐ CRL ☐ GS
WNL/Notes:

Assessment:

☐ Patient is a candidate for aspiration abortion
☐ Post procedure contraception:_____
☐ 800 mg Ibuprofen dispensed for oral administration. Time: ____
☐ If Misoprostol given: ____ dose _____ route

Clinician Signature: _____

1

Fig. 27-3 MVA preprocedure note and procedure note (adapted from Reproductive Health Access Project: http://www.reproductiveaccess.org/)

MVA PROCEDURE NOTE:

Name:

MR#:

Physical Examination:

Uterus: Size in weeks (bimanual): _____ AV/Mid / RV

Cervix: WNL / CMT, parous/nullip

Vagina: WNL / discharge noted: _____

Procedure:

☐ Cervix and vagina swabbed with Betadine.

☐ Lidocaine 1%, _____cc total injected.

☐ Tenaculum applied _____ o'clock.

☐ Cervix progressively dilated to: _____.

☐ Cannula inserted, size _____.

Estimated blood loss: _____ cc.

Additional comments:_____

Additional procedures:

☐ Pap done

☐ GC, Chlamydia done

☐ Wet prep done Results: _____

Tissue Exam:

☐ Decidual tissue

☐ Villi

☐ Gestational sac

☐ Tissue appropriate for gestational age

Post-Op Ultrasound if done:

☐ No IUP visualized   Other: _____

Assessment:

☐ Patient stable, AB complete

☐ Post-procedure vital signs:

B/P____   P____

☐ Other notes: _____

Plan:

☐ Expected symptoms discussed; post-procedure instructions given.

☐ Rh negative? Yes/No   If yes, RhoGAM® (Ortho Clinical Diagnostics, Raritan, NJ) given? Yes/No

☐ Doxycycline 100 mg tabs BID x ____ days

☐ Contraception: _____

☐ Follow up appointment given for_____

Clinician Signature: _____

2

Fig. 27-3 (continued)

Coding

CPT® Codes (Current Procedural Terminology, AMA, Chicago, IL)

For the visit	99204 or 99214 (level 4 new or established patient E/M visit)
For the ultrasound	76817 (transvaginal ultrasound, pregnant uterus) or 76815 (limited ultrasound, pregnant uterus)

For the procedure and medications

59840	Induced abortion, by dilation and curettage
J2000	Lidocaine
64450	Injection, nerve block
A4550	Surgical tray
99000	Specimen handling
J2210	Methergine®
90385	MICRhoGAM®
90782	Therapeutic injection

ICD 9-CM-Diagnostic Codes (International Classification of Diseases, 9th Revision, Clinical Modification, Center for Disease Control and Prevention)

635.92	Legally induced abortion, without mention of complication, complete

Postprocedure Patient Instructions

- The woman should be allowed to rest and recover for at least 30 min.
- Continue to monitor her vitals and symptoms. Uterine cramping and bleeding should continue to subside. Prolonged cramping and excessive bleeding are not normal.
- Rh negative patients should be given a dose of MICRhoGAM® (50 μg) (Ortho Clinical Diagnostics, Raritan, NJ).
- The following items should be reviewed carefully with the patient (Fig. 27-4):
  - Postprocedure self-care
  - Signs and symptoms requiring medical attention
  - How to "QuickStart" birth control (begin that day), review correct use, possible side effects
  - The woman should be discharged home with the following:
  - A follow-up appointment in 1–2 weeks
  - Prescriptions or supplies for ibuprofen or analgesic of choice
  - Prescriptions or supplies of birth control to start as soon as possible

- Prescriptions or supplies of a postabortion antibiotic regimen
- A 24-h provider contact number
- The Patient After-Care Instructions and Information Form (Fig. 27-4).

(Provider to fill in blanks/circle applicable choice when given multiple choices.)

Case Study Outcome

The patient underwent an uncomplicated MVA in the office. She had a copper intrauterine device placed immediately after the procedure. The products of conception were consistent with 8.5-week pregnancy. She was discharged home in good condition.

Patient Handout

Pre Procedure Handout

Table 27-1 Comparison of early abortion options: a patient resource

Abortion pill/medication abortion (mifepristone and misoprostol)	Aspiration abortion (suction or vacuum aspiration)
1. How far along in the pregnancy can I be?	
Up to 9 weeks into the pregnancy (some offices may have an 8-week limit)	Up to 12 weeks into the pregnancy
2. What will happen?	
The actual abortion takes place at home	The abortion takes place in the office
In the office, you will swallow the abortion pill (mifepristone)	The actual abortion procedure takes 5–10 min
At home, 24–48 h later, you take the misoprostol pills	The doctor will put instruments in your vagina and uterus to remove the pregnancy
The abortion usually starts 1–4 h after you take the misoprostol. You will probably have heavy bleeding and cramps for a couple of hours	You will have cramps for about 1–2 min during this time
You will come back to the office about 1 week later	You will come back to the office about 1 week vlater
3. How painful is it?	
Women have mild to very strong cramps off and on. Pain pills help. Each woman is different in how she experiences pain	Women have mild to very strong cramps during the abortion. Pain pills help. Each woman is different in how she experiences pain

(continued)

Table 27-1 (continued)

Abortion pill/medication abortion (mifepristone and misoprostol)	Aspiration abortion (suction or vacuum aspiration)
4. How much will I bleed?	
Heavy bleeding with clots is common during the abortion. After that, lighter bleeding with clots lasts 1–2 weeks or more. The amount of bleeding is similar to that of an aspiration abortion, although it takes longer	Most women have light bleeding for 1–7 days. Bleeding may continue off and on for a few weeks
5. How much does it cost?	
$350 and up. Your insurance company may cover some of that cost	$350 and up. Your insurance company may cover some of that cost
6. Can the abortion fail?	
The pills work 95–98% of the time. If they fail, you must have an aspiration abortion	It works 99% of the time. If it fails, you must have a repeat aspiration
7. Can I still have children afterwards?	
A safe, legal abortion does *not* change your baseline fertility (your chance of getting pregnant based on your own body)	A safe, legal abortion does *not* change your baseline fertility (your chance of getting pregnant based on your own body)
8. Is it safe?	
Both pills have been used safely for over 10 years. Big problems are rare. Your doctor will review the risks with you (bleeding, infection, incomplete abortion)	Aspiration abortion has been done safely for over 25 years. Abortion in the first 12 weeks leads to very few problems. Your doctor will review the risks with you (bleeding, uterus perforation, infection, incomplete abortion)
9. What are the advantages?	
To some, it feels more natural, like a miscarriage	It is over in a few minutes
You will not have shots, anesthesia, or instruments in your body, unless the pills do not work	You see less bleeding than you would with a medication abortion
Being at home instead of in an office may be more private and comfortable for you	Medical staff are there
	It can be done later in the pregnancy than with a medication abortion
10. What are the disadvantages?	
It is a 2-day process at minimum	A clinician must insert instruments inside the uterus
Bleeding can be very heavy and lasts longer than with an aspiration abortion	Pain medicines may cause side effects
Cramping can be severe and lasts longer than with an aspiration abortion	The woman has less control over the abortion procedure
It fails more often than an aspiration procedure	

Adapted from the Reproductive Health Access Project: www.reproductiveaccess.org

Post Procedure Handout

ASPIRATION ABORTION
PATIENT AFTER-CARE INSTRUCTIONS AND INFORMATION

Today _____ you had a procedure called an "aspiration abortion." You will probably feel fine when you go home. You can go back to your regular activities as soon as you want to. You can take a shower and wash your hair as soon as you want to. You can eat normally, although you may still feel nauseated for another few days.

Follow-up visit: You have an appointment _____ at _____am/pm.

Are there things you should not do? Until you come back next week, do not put anything in your vagina. To be safe, do not use tampons, do not douche, and do not have sex.

WHAT TO EXPECT

Vaginal Bleeding: You can expect to have bleeding for up to 2 weeks. It is common for the bleeding to stop and start for several weeks after the abortion. Some women have no bleeding for 2-3 days and then begin to have bleeding like a period. Other women have only spotting for a few days and then no more bleeding at all. If you exercise or have a lot of activity, you may notice the bleeding increases; this is not dangerous.

Cramping: Some women have cramps off and on during the week following an abortion. You can use pain medication like Tylenol®, Ibuprofen (Motrin® or Advil®), or Naproxen (Aleve® or Naprosyn®). You can also use a heating pad.

Sadness or very emotional: Most women feel relieved when the abortion is over. Some women also feel sad and feel like crying. These feelings are partly from the changes in hormones, now that you are no longer pregnant. Feeling emotional at this time is normal. If you think your emotions are not what they should be, please talk to us.

When will your period come back? You can expect a period in 4-8 weeks. It is not the same for all women.

WHAT ARE DANGER SIGNS?

Heavy bleeding: If you are soaking through more than 2 maxi pads an hour for more than 2 hours.

Severe cramps: Cramps that are getting stronger and are not helped by pain medication.

Fever: If your temperature is higher than 101 degrees.

EMERGENCY CONTACT: Call the 24-hour number: _____. If you have any questions, think something is wrong, or think you have an emergency, PLEASE CALL and we will call you back. It may take us 10-15 minutes to return your call. Feel free to call, no question is too small.

PREGNANCY PREVENTION: You can get pregnant right after an abortion even BEFORE YOUR PERIOD COMES BACK. We have already talked about your birth control plan:_____. You should start this (date:_____) even if you are still bleeding. If you have sex without protection, you can use Emergency Contraception (EC) to prevent another pregnancy.

Tylenol®, McNeil, New Brunswick, NJ
Advil®, Wyeth, Madison, NJ
Motrin®, McNeil, New Brunswick, NJ
Aleve®, Bayer, Pittsburgh, PA
Naprosyn®, Hoffmann-La Roche, Nutley, NJ

Fig. 27-4 MVA patient instructions (adapted from: Reproductive Health Access Project: http://www.reproductiveaccess.org/)

References

1. Westfall JM, Sophocles A, Burggraf H, Ellis S. Manual vacuum aspiration for first trimester abortion. *Arch Fam Med* 1998;7(6):559–562.
2. World Health Organization (WHO). *Safe abortion: technical and policy guidelines for health systems.* Geneva: WHO, 2003.
3. Henshaw SK. Unintended pregnancy and abortion: a public health perspective. In Paul M, Lichtenberg ES, Borgatta L, Grimes DA, Stubblefield PG (eds) *A clinician's guide to medical and surgical abortion.* New York: Churchill Livingstone, 1999, pp 11–22.
4. Sawaya GF, Grady D, Kerlikowske K, Grimes DA. Antibiotics at the time of induced abortion: the case for universal prophylaxis based on a meta-analysis. *Obstet Gynecol* 1996;87:884–890.
5. Centers for Disease Control and Prevention. Sexually transmitted diseases treatment guidelines. *MMWR* 2006;51(RR-6):7-61.
6. World Health Organization. *Safe abortion: technical and policy guidance for health systems.* Geneva: WHO, 2003.
7. Grimes D, Lopez LM, Schulz K, Stanwood N. Immediate postabortal insertion of intrauterine devices. *Cochrane Database Syst Rev* 2004(4):CD001777
8. Ngai SW, Chan YM, Tang OS, Ho PC. The use of misoprostol for pre-operative cervical dilatation prior to vacuum aspiration: a randomized trial. *Hum Reprod* 1999;14(8):2139–2142.
9. Singh K, Fong YF, Prasad RN, Dong F. Evacuation interval after vaginal misoprostol for pre-abortion cervical priming: a randomized trial. *Obstet Gynecol* 1999;94(3):431–434.

Additional Resources

Websites

For patient and clinician resources regarding early abortion care, visit The Reproductive Health Access Project: http://www.reproductiveaccess.org/

For information regarding abortion training in family medicine residencies, visit The Center for Reproductive Health Education in Family Medicine www.rhedi.org

For educational resources and a clinical curriculum regarding medication abortion, visit The National Abortion Federation: http://www.prochoice.org/education/resources/index.html

For information regarding state laws on abortion, visit The Center for Reproductive Rights: http://www.reproductiverights.org/

For information regarding MVA aspirators and supplies: www.ipas.org

Chapter 28
Botulinum Toxin A Injections for Reduction of Facial Rhytids

Sharon D. Gertzman

Introduction

Botulinum Toxin A, commonly known as Botox® or Botox® Cosmetic (both: Allergan, Irvine, CA) or Dysport (Medicis, USA), is a neurotransmitter blocker that is used in aesthetic procedures to erase the fine lines of the face known as active lines. The mechanism of action of this drug is to block neurotransmitters in the facial muscles by binding the muscle receptor site on the muscles necessary to make the muscle fire. Botox® or Botox® cosmetic take approximately 2–7 days to work their way into the muscle and remain tightly bound to the muscles for approximately 3–5 months, whereas Dysport takes effect in 1.5 days and remains effective for 4–6 months. Botox has been available for use in the US since the early 70s. Dysport was approved for cosmetic use by the FDA in 2009. It has however, been in use for cosmetic purposes in Europe under the trade name Reloxin for approximately 20 years.

When injecting patients with Botulinum Toxin A, it is imperative to distinguish the difference between an active and a passive line. Active lines are those wrinkles on the face that are caused by expression. They primarily appear when the face is in motion and disappear or become remarkably softer when the facial muscles are at rest. When an active line has been present for years or even decades, it will often leave a line in the skin when the muscles are at rest. The most common active lines treated with Botulinum Toxin A are the horizontal forehead lines caused by the frontalis muscle, the vertical lines at the glabella caused by the corrugator and procerus muscles, and the horizontal lines lateral to the eyes, commonly known as "crow's feet" caused by the orbicularis oculi muscles. In fact, at the time of this publication, the vertical lines at the glabella are the only FDA-approved cosmetic use for Botulin Toxin A. Any other use of Botulinum Toxin A is considered off-label and must be presented to the patient for informed consent as such (see section on Patient Handout.).

S.D. Gertzman (✉)
Serenity Medical Spa, 2425 Pennington Road, Suite 100, Pennington, NJ 08534, USA
e-mail: sgertzman@yahoo.com

S.M. Sulik and C.B. Heath (eds.), *Primary Care Procedures in Women's Health*,   385
DOI 10.1007/978-0-387-76604-1_28, © Springer Science+Business Media, LLC 2010

Passive lines are those lines that are present regardless of movement. They primarily appear as a result of facial lipoatrophy that comes with age, combined with the forces of gravity. Passive lines are generally seen along the nasolabial fold as well as along the labial–mental lines (lateral edges of the mouth to the lateral edges of the chin). These are commonly known as "marionette lines."

As a general rule for those new to injecting Botulinum Toxin A, it is a safe generalization to treat those areas above the nose with Botulinum Toxin A, whereas those areas below the nose are reserved for dermal fillers. It is not to say that Botulinum Toxin A is not used in areas below the nose, but these injections should be done only by experienced clinicians. These risks include facial asymmetry and loss of ability to pronounce some letter sounds.

Choosing the right individual for optimal success is important. An individual whose forehead moves more than approximately ½ in. with superior or inferior traction is not a candidate for Botulinum Toxin A in that area, as relaxing those muscles would result in his/her brow dropping significantly. This result is not aesthetically pleasing. The best recommendation for such an individual would be a brow lift.

Studies show that 20–40 units per area of Botox cosmetic, or 50–60 units of Dysport is the appropriate amount of botulinum toxin A to achieve an aesthetic result that should last approximately 4 months [1]. At the time of this publication, the FDA-approved manner for botulinum toxin A preparation is with nonpreserved saline solution. The toxin must be used within 4 h of reconstitution and stored in the refrigerator between uses by patients. In 2003, a study was conducted that showed the toxin could be stored in the freezer and used as many as 4–6 weeks later with equal outcomes [2].

Case Study

A 40-year-old woman presents to your office with the complaint that, while she feels fine, she is frequently asked if she is tired, angry, or upset. She states that she frequently finds herself furrowing her brow when she is concentrating or stressed. Her medical history is completely benign, including her annual check-up and blood work done within 30 days.

On physical exam, she appears fatigued with moderate rhytids horizontally in her forehead as well as deeper "frown lines" vertically between her eyebrows at her glabella. When she smiles, horizontal rhytids radiate away from her eyes laterally and infralaterally. Upon palpating her relaxed forehead and putting traction superiorly and inferiorly on her brow, it does not appear that she uses her forehead musculature to hold her brow up.

Diagnosis (Algorithm 28-1)

Active rhytids of the forehead, glabella, and orbicularis oculi.

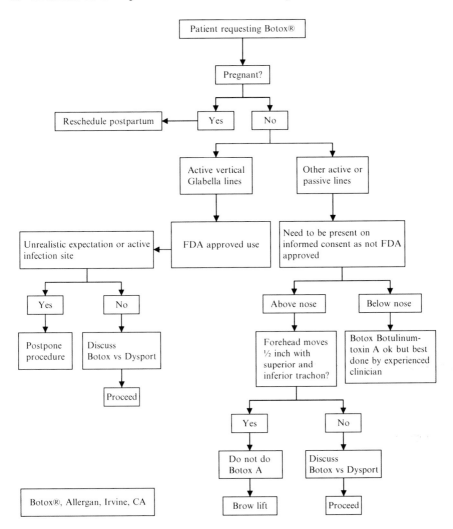

Algorithm 28-1   Botox® (Allergan, Irvine, CA) indications and contraindications

Indications (Algorithm 28-1)

Active rhytid of the facial musculature that affects the patient's sense of well-being and his/her interaction with others.

Contraindications

- Pregnancy
- History of adverse reaction to botulinum toxin A

- Unrealistic expectation
- Active infection at the injection site

Equipment

- 1 vial Botox® Cosmetic with 100 unit of Botulinum Toxin A or 1 vial Dysport with 300 units Botulinum Toxin A
- 2.5 cc nonpreserved sterile saline for injection for Botox 1.5 cc for Dysport
- 22 gauge, ½ in. sterile needle
- 3 cc sterile syringe
- 30 gauge ½ in. sterile needle
- Two 1 cc tuberculin type sterile syringes
- Alcohol wipes
- Bowl with ice
- Surgical marker with disposable ruler
- Nonsterile gloves
- Digital camera

Procedure

1. Patient preparation:
   (a) Review and sign informed consent with patient (See Patient Handout section.).
   (b) Give copy to patient, and keep original in patient records.
   (c) Photograph patient with treatment areas at rest and with muscles contracted.
2. Clean treatment areas with alcohol swab.
3. Mark each injection site with surgical marker as follows:

   Orbicularis Oculi
   (a) Palpate the lateral border of the orbit at the level of the outer canthus.
   (b) Measure ¼ in. lateral to that border, in the body of the orbicularis oculi.
   (c) Mark two subsequent points in ¼ in. increments paralleling the line of the inferior orbit (Fig. 28-1).
   (d) Repeat for the other side.

   Forehead
   (a) Have patient raise eyebrows to determine levels of furrowing.
   (b) At the level of the mid-pupillary line on each side, mark two areas within the frontalis muscle.
   (c) Mark two more areas at the mid-glabellar line (total of 6 points).
   (d) See Fig. 28-1.

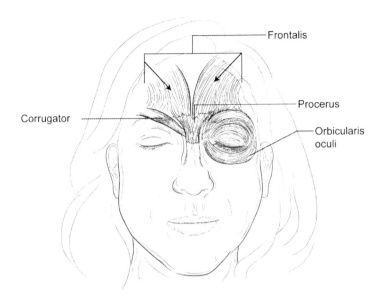

Fig. 28-1 Facial musculature and injection sites

Glabella
(a) Have the patient frown to furrow his/her glabella.
(b) Palpate and mark two points in the body of the glabella.
(c) Palpate and mark two points on each side of the glabella along the eyebrow line to affect the corrugator muscles and some fibers of the procerus muscles. On most patients, it is quite easy to visualize the musculature by making them repeatedly contract and relax their brow. Care should be taken to avoid the distal fibers of the frontalis muscle as this will cause a "V" shape to the eye brows or a quizzical look, which is not aesthetically pleasing (Fig. 28-1).

4. Prepare the Botulinum Toxin solution (to be done immediately prior to use):
(a) Botulinum Toxin prep: Wipe the Botox® or Dysport vial and the saline vials with alcohol.
(b) Using the 22 gauge needle and 3 cc syringe, draw up 2.0 cc of sterile saline for Botox, 1.5 cc sterile saline for Dysport.
(c) Separate the 22 gauge needle from the syringe.
(d) Insert the 22 gauge needle in to the Botox® or Dysport vial, listening for the vacuum release. (If there is no vacuum release, do not use the vial and report it to the manufacturer.) This method prevents the injected saline from traumatizing the botulinum toxin, which helps maintain its efficacy.
(e) Reattach the needle, and add the saline to the vial of Botox® or Dysport.
(f) Swirl gently.
(g) Discard the 3 cc syringe, leaving the 22 gauge needle in the vial.

(h) Attach the tuberculin syringe, and draw up 0.6 cc of fluid (30 units) of Botox or 0.3 cc of Dysport for each area.

(i) Remove the tuberculin syringe from the 22 gauge needle, attach a clean tuberculin syringe, and place the vial with needle into the bowl with ice; store in refrigerator for next case. This method minimizes needle punctures into the botox vial, ensuring sterility of the vial.

(j) Attach the 30 gauge needle to the full tuberculin syringe.

5. Inject 0.1 cc of concentrated Botox or 0.05 cc Dysport subcutaneously to each of your previously marked areas. Using this dilution, 0.1 cc deposits 5.0 units per injection of Botox or 0.05 cc injects 10 units of Dysport, which is sufficient for the average facial muscle. Other dilutions are acceptable; however, this constitution allows for a small amount of fluid at each injection site. This minimizes trauma to the site and discomfort. It also lessens the amount of migration of the toxin.

6. Massage up and away from the eyes. Direct pressure to any bleeding areas.

7. Review postprocedure instructions with patient.

8. Return botulinum toxin A to refrigerator or freezer.

Complications and Risks

- Paralysis of a nearby muscle that could interfere with opening the eye(s) (Ptosis-presents as a 1–2 mm droop of upper eyelid; generally lasts for 2–10 weeks.)
- Local numbness
- Headache, nausea, or flu like symptoms
- Swallowing, speech, or respiratory disorders
- Swelling, bruising, or redness at injection site
- Disorientation or double vision
- Temporary asymmetrical appearance
- Abnormal or lack of facial expression
- Inability to smile when injected in the lower face
- Facial pain
- Product ineffectiveness

Tricks and Helpful Hints

- Advise patients to avoid all aspirin, nonsteroidal antiinflammatories, Vitamin E, and Gingko for 1 week prior to procedure to minimize risk of bruising.
- If patient is prone to bruising, he/she should begin taking *Arnica Montana* (available in any health food store or full service pharmacy) 3 days prior to and 3 days postprocedure.
- Try to visualize and subsequently avoid any subcutaneous vessels during injection, especially in the orbicularis oculi where they are prevalent.
- Use ice packs pre and postinjection to minimize discomfort and bruising.

Procedure Note

(Provider to fill in blanks/circle applicable choice when given multiple choices and customize as needed.)

After informed consent and preprocedure photos, the patient's skin is cleansed with alcohol and marked with a surgical marker as needed. 0.1 cc of botulinum toxin A or 0.05 cc of Dysport of lot_____ with expiration date_____ reconstituted with _____ cc sterile nonpreserved saline is injected into each marked area. Written and verbal postprocedure instructions were reviewed with the patient. Follow up was scheduled in 1 week.

Coding

CPT® Codes (Current Procedural Terminology, AMA, Chicago, IL)
J0585   Botulinum Toxin Type A, per unit

ICD 9-CM-Diagnostic Codes (International Classification of Diseases, 9th Revision, Clinical Modification, Center for Disease Control and Prevention)
701.8   Atrophic conditions of skin/Rhytidosis Facialis

Suggest cash payment at the time of service; insurance companies do not reimburse for this procedure.

Some physicians bill per unit medication used, plus a small mark-up for medication wasted, which is inevitable due to medication in the syringe and the difficulty with storage. $10–$15 per unit results in: Botox horizontal frown line treatment at $300–450. Alternatively $5–8/unit of Dysport results in a cost per area treated price of $300–480. Other physicians charge per site, with discount for multiple sites.

Postprocedure Patient Instructions

The patient should be notified that for the next 3–6 hours (h) she should try to maintain her head in a neutral position. The patient should not look down, lie down, or lie on her side for the next 3–6 h. The patient should avoid manipulation of the area for 4 h. The patient should try to use the muscles involved as much as possible for the next 2–3 days, as the more the muscle is used, the faster the botulinum toxin A will take effect. Facial exercise in the area of treatment is recommended: frown/smile every hour. These measures *should minimize* the possibility of *ptosis* to almost 100%.

The patient should expect to begin seeing relaxation of the muscles later the same day w/Dysport w/full effect in 3–4 days. Patients treated w/Botox will see the effect begin approximately 2 days after treatment with full effect expected approximately 7–10 days after treatment. The benefits may last 3–6 months; on average, they last

4 months with Botox, and a slightly longer duration with Dysport. A touch-up may be necessary in 1–2 weeks. The patient should contact the provider after 8 days if the desired effect is not received.

Case Study Outcome

After extensive consultation, review of risks, benefits, and complications, the patient elected to have her horizontal rhytids of her forehead injected with Botulinum Toxin A. She returned to the office 3 months later, requesting to have her glabella injected after having received numerous comments from a variety of people that she looked much more relaxed and happy.

Patient Handouts

(Provider to fill in blanks/circle applicable choice when given multiple choices and customize as needed.)

Patient Informed Consent for Administration of Botulinum Toxin A

Botox and Dysport are made from Botulinum Toxin A, a protein produced by the bacterium Clostridium botulinum. For the purpose of improving the appearance of wrinkles, small doses of the toxin are injected into the affected muscles blocking the release of a chemical that would otherwise signal the muscle to contract. The toxin thus paralyzes or weakens the injected muscle. The Food and Drug Administration (FDA) approved the cosmetic use of Botulinum Toxin Type A for the temporary relief of moderate to severe frown lines between the brow and recommends that the procedure be performed no more frequently than once every 3 months.

It is not known whether Botulinum A Toxin can cause fetal harm when administered to pregnant women or can affect reproductive capabilities. It is also not known if Botulinum A Toxin is excreted in human milk. For these reason, Botulinum A Toxin should not be used on pregnant or lactating women.

I authorize and direct_____, with associates or assistants of her choice, to perform the following procedure of Botulinum A Toxin injections on _____ (patient name) for the treatment of _____ (e.g., brow, forehead, crow's feet).

___The details of the procedure have been explained to me in terms I understand.

___Alternative methods and their benefits and disadvantages have been explained to me.

___I understand the FDA has only approved the cosmetic use of Botulinum A Toxin for frown lines between the brow. Any other cosmetic use is considered off label.

___I understand and accept the most likely risks and complications of Botulinum A Toxin injection(s) include but are not limited to:

- Paralysis of a nearby muscle that could interfere with opening the eye(s)
- Local numbness
- Headache, nausea, or flu-like symptoms
- Swallowing, speech, or respiratory disorders
- Swelling, bruising, or redness at injection site
- Disorientation or double vision
- Temporary asymmetrical appearance
- Abnormal or lack of facial expression
- Inability to smile when injected in the lower face
- Facial pain
- Product ineffectiveness

___I understand and accept that the long-term effects of repeated use of Botox Cosmetic are as yet unknown. Possible risks and complications that have been identified include but are not limited to:

- Muscle atrophy (weakness)
- Nerve irritability
- Production of antibodies with unknown effect to general health

___I understand and accept the less common complications, including remote risk of death or serious disability, that exist with this procedure.

___I am aware that smoking during the pre- and postoperative periods could increase chances of complications.

___I have informed the doctor of all my known allergies.

___I have informed the doctor of all medications I am currently taking, including prescriptions, over-the-counter remedies, herbal therapies, and any others.

___I have been advised whether I should take any or all of these medications on the days surrounding the procedure.

___I am aware and accept that no guarantees about the results of the procedure have been made or applied.

___I have been informed of what to expect posttreatment, including but not limited to: estimated recovery time, anticipated activity level, and the necessity of additional procedures if I wish to maintain the appearance this procedure provides me.

___I am not currently pregnant or nursing, and I understand that should I become pregnant while using this drug there are potential risks, including fetal malformation.

___If pre- and postoperative photos and/or videos are taken of the treatment for record purposes, I understand that these photos will be the property of the attending physician.

___I understand that these photos may only be used for scientific or record keeping purposes.

___The doctor has answered all of my questions regarding this procedure.

___I have been advised to seek immediate medical attention if swallowing, speech, or respiratory disorders arise.

Patient Consent

I certify that I have read and understand this treatment agreement and that all blanks were filled in prior to my signature.

_____   _____
Patient's Signature/Date   *Witness' Signature/Date*

_____   _____
Print Patient Name   *Print Witness Name*

References

1. Carruthers A, Carruthers J, Said S. Dose-ranging study of botulinum toxin A in the treatment of glabellar rhytids in females. *Dermatol Surg* 2005;31:414–422.
2. Hexsel DM, Trinidad De Almeida A, Rutowitsch M, Alencar De Castro I, Silveria VLB, Gobatto DO, Zechmeister M, Mazzuco R, Zechmeister D. Multicenter, double-blind study of the efficacy of injections with botulinum toxin A reconstituted up to six consecutive weeks before application. *Dermatol Surg* 2003;29:523–529.
3. Brandt F, Swanson N, Baumann L, A phase III, randomized double blind, Placebo-Controlled study to assess the efficacy and safety of reloxin® in the treatment of glabellar lines. Presented at the 31st Hawaii dermatology seminar March 3–9, 2007 Maui, HI.
4. Moy R, Maas C, Monheit G, Huber B, Reloxin investigational group. Long-term safety and efficacy of a new botulinum toxin type A in treating glabellar lines. *Arch Facial Plast Surg.* 2009;11:77–83.

Chapter 29
The Use of Cosmetic Lasers in Clinical Practice

Donald J. Brideau

Introduction

As the baby boomer generation ages, many want to remain active and maintain their youthful appearance. The growth of this segment of our population continues to fuel the cosmetic procedures industry. Clinical uses of lasers include hair removal, acne treatment, skin rejuvenation, vascular lesions and a variety of pigmented lesions, and skin tightening [1]. Additionally, as lasers and other light therapies become less complicated, safer to use, and have more applications, more physicians are providing the services that their patients previously received elsewhere.

As routine health care reimbursement remains stagnant, physicians are also looking for ways to improve their bottom line while they provide high-quality comprehensive services to their patients. This chapter will serve as an introduction for those not providing these services yet. Many procedures performed in family medicine can be more efficiently performed with a laser, such as treating a large number of seborrheic keratoses at one visit.

Unlike many of the chapters in this book, laser procedures and the settings used are quite specific to the particular wavelength of the laser medium and the particular brand of laser used. Therefore, this chapter will discuss techniques, clinical applications, and pearls, since specific settings might not be applicable to the laser used in each practice.

Laser is an acronym for Light Amplification by Spontaneous Emissions of Radiation. The target or chromophores vary in their ability to absorb light of various wavelengths. Rox Anderson in the early 1980s developed the concept of selective thermolysis [2]. The targeted chromophore will be selectively damaged if it can be heated by the specific wavelength faster than the thermal relaxation time of the target chromophore and slower than the thermal relaxation time of the surrounding

D.J. Brideau (✉)
Georgetown University Medical School and George Washington School of Medicine
and Health Science, and President, Cosmetic Laser and Skin Services, Alexandria, VA, USA
e-mail: dbrideau@vacoxmail.com

S.M. Sulik and C.B. Heath (eds.), *Primary Care Procedures in Women's Health*,
DOI 10.1007/978-0-387-76604-1_29, © Springer Science+Business Media, LLC 2010

structures. Simply put, the targeted tissue is damaged while the surrounding tissue remains unharmed.

In general, no limit exists to the number of pulses used for a treatment. Therefore, individuals may have multiple treatment areas treated on the same day. However, if a topical anesthetic is used, the surface area may be the limiting factor, thus necessitating multiple visits. Cost may be the other limiting factor for the patient. Some treatments, such as those of vascular and pigmented lesions, may be priced by the number of pulses used. Patients may choose to treat a certain number of their lesions based on their budget and return for additional treatments later.

Case Study

A patient presents to your office complaining of unwanted facial hair. She has been waxing her upper lip and chin for many years, and has decided she would like to pursue a more permanent method of hair removal. She presents for initial consultation and requests information about frequency of visits and costs.

Indications (Algorithm 29-1)

There are numerous clinical indications for lasers in primary care. While many are truly cosmetic in nature, other procedures can replace current techniques already being used in practice.

Laser Hair Removal

* Unwanted hair on almost any area of the body
* Pseudofolliculitis Barbae

Acne Treatment for New Lesions and Reduction of Acne Scars

* Adjunct to typical medical therapies [3]
* Improvement in scar appearance

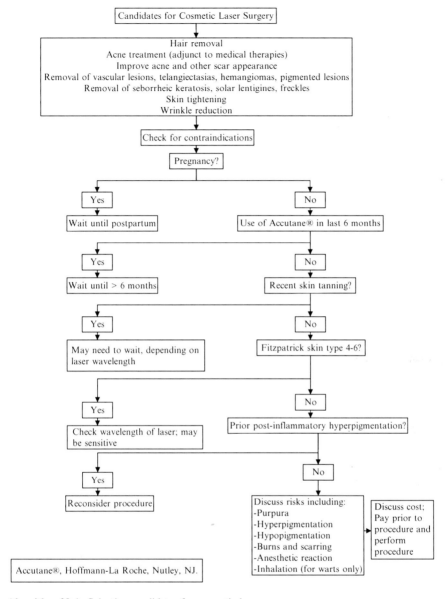

Algorithm 29-1 Selecting candidates for cosmetic laser surgery

Vascular Lesions

- Telangiectasias of legs and face
- Hemangiomas

Wrinkle Reduction and Skin Tightening

Pigmented Lesions

- Seborrheic Keratosis
- Solar Lentigines
- Freckles

Contraindications

- Pregnancy
- Prior postinflammatory hyperpigmentation

Relative Contraindications

- Fitzpatrick Skin Types 4–6 (darker skinned individuals) may be more sensitive to pigment changes depending on the wavelength
- Use of Isotretinoin (Accutane®, Hoffmann-La Roche, Nutley, NJ) in last 6 months (increased sensitivity of skin to complications)
- Presence of tan (dependent on wavelength of laser) or recent tan

Equipment

- Correct protective eye wear for patient and operator (Each wavelength has specific types of goggles.)
- Laser (Fig. 29-1 shows an example.)
- Premoistened towelettes (used to cool skin during certain procedures)
- Ice pack (used during and after certain procedures)
- Topical Anesthetic (used for some procedures and may be dependent on the type/brand of laser)
- Digital Camera for before and after procedure photographs

Procedure

1. Consultation: Individuals must be evaluated as to their specific desires for cosmetic treatment and goals.
2. Setting and Appropriate Expectations: It is important not to oversell the results; setting appropriate expectations up front will ensure that your patients are satisfied

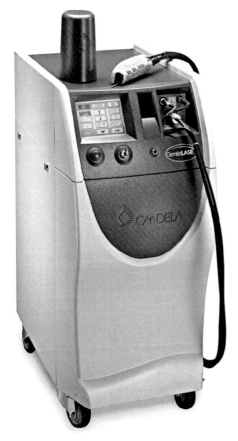

Fig. 29-1 GentleLASE® Candela laser (used with permission from Candela Corporation, Wayland, MA)

and pleased with the results. Failure to do so will most likely lead to unhappy patients. Use photographs to show before and after results. Also, when performing wrinkle reduction or skin tightening procedures, one can show a patient what is expected at the end of treatment by touching and moving the skin.

3. Consent:
   - Individuals should have the procedure explained in depth.
   - Number of treatments for a particular condition and cost per treatment should be discussed.
   - Risks of procedures should be reviewed.

4. Photographs: Individuals should have pictures of the area to be treated prior to any procedures.

5. Choosing Settings for Laser: There are multiple lasers, each with various settings that control the energy levels of the laser, the time for each pulse, and the spot

size that will be used. Additionally, some lasers must also set coolant levels. Laser manufacturers provide a set of guidelines that will list the type of procedure with a range of settings. Please refer to these guidelines.

Hair Removal

- Perform test dose on the patient in an area near the area to be treated. Hair removal areas should not be double pulsed. Watch for erythema of the skin as the dose is increased. Most blisters will show up in 15–30 seconds if too much energy is used.
- Several minutes after treating with adequate energy, one may notice peri-follicular edema, like a small mosquito bite. This means that adequate damage has been done to the base of the hair follicle.
- Individuals usually need 4–6 treatments spaced at various intervals depending on the area of the body being treated:
- Facial Hair: every 4–6 weeks
- Axillary and Bikini: every 6–8 weeks
- Chest and legs: 8–12 weeks
- For individuals with Fitzpatrick Skin Types 4–6, perform a test dose of various levels and wait 2 weeks to determine if any unexpected hyper- or hypopigmentation develops. A 1064 nm Nd:YAG is considered the safest laser wavelength in these classes of skin type.
- To decrease discomfort during procedures, especially when treating sensitive areas like the face and neck, touching the skin immediately after treatment relieves some of the discomfort felt. This may be done with your fingers or may be with an aloe or a premoistened towelette to soothe the skin. Additionally, one can apply an ice pack for brief periods of time.

Vascular Lesions: Telangiectasias

- Measure size of the vessel to be treated. Smaller lesions need higher energy levels since the energy is delivered in Joules/cm^2 and thus fills a smaller area of the laser spot.
- If your laser allows you to vary the pulse width, start at the lower range of the energy level and at longer pulse widths. The longer the pulse width, the less likely purpura will occur.
- Watch for vascular spasm.
- If this does not occur, decrease the pulse width before increasing the energy dose. (Follow the specific guidelines for your laser.)
- After treating, advise the patient that they may feel a slight raised area along the vessel treated. Avoid sun exposure while it is raised.
- Advise that it may take 6–12 weeks for the vessel to completely disappear.

- If vessel still blanches at 8 weeks, it can be retreated.

Pigmented Lesions

Most lasers use some form of cooling to protect the epidermis. When treating superficial pigmented lesions, the skin must absorb the energy to produce the desired effect. Thus, one must turn off or minimize the cooling used by the laser.

- Darker lesions may need lower energies since they will absorb more.
- Start at the lowest energy level for a specific spot size based on your laser's guidelines.
- Listen for a snapping sound and/or changing of color of the pigmented lesion.
- Retreat if necessary in 4 weeks.

Complications and Risks

With current lasers, improved safety has decreased the likelihood of serious complications. Most clinicians in primary care will be using nonablative lasers: those designed not to burn the skin to achieve the therapeutic effect. However, individual lasers as well as individual responses to light therapies can result in similar complications. The most common would include [4]:

- Purpura (bruising, especially when performing vascular treatments)
- Hyperpigmentation
- Hypopigmentation
- Burns and scarring
- Eye damage (incorrect wearing of protective eye wear or not wearing protective eye wear)

- Anesthetic reaction (too much used and/or occlusion)
- Inhalation (plume from viral particles when treating warts)

Procedure Note

(Provider to fill in blanks/circle applicable choice when given multiple choices and customize as needed.)

The patient was counseled to the risks and benefits of the elective procedure for (insert type: hair removal, vascular treatment, wrinkle reduction, etc.). The (specific laser type) laser was used with test dosing based on established guidelines. The settings were used as indicated in the consent document. The patient tolerated the procedure well and was advised to avoid any tanning during the next few days. Skin care was discussed.

Coding

Most procedures require no coding since these are generally cosmetic in nature and not covered by insurance. Determining payment method prior to performing the procedure must occur

Several procedures may be coded although they may not be covered or their reimbursement may not justify the use of the laser

17110	Wart Treatment (up to 14 lesions)
17110	Destruction of lesions – benign up to 14 lesions
17111	for more than 14 lesions
7106	Treatment of vascular lesions 1 for <10 sq cm

Patient Instructions

Prior to your appointment, please avoid sun exposure as this can increase the likelihood of side effects. If you were advised to apply anesthetic such as topical lidocaine 4%, begin applying 1 hour prior to the procedure and repeat every 20 min. Follow the instructions of the clinician for appropriate dosage of the anesthetic.

After the procedure, you should again avoid sun exposure to the area treated, as this skin may be more sensitive to burning.

Case Study Outcome

The patient opted to have the laser hair treatments done and presented every 4 weeks for six total treatments. She has had good resolution of the hair and is very pleased with the outcome. She will follow up if she has any new hair growth and any problems.

References

1. Kauvar A, Hruza G (eds). *Principles and practices in cutaneous laser surgery.* Boca Raton: Taylor and Francis Group, 2005.
2. Anderson RR, Parrish JA. Selective photothermolysis: precise microsurgery by selected absorption of pulsed radiation. *Science* 1983;220(4596):524–527.
3. Mariwalla K, Rohrer T. Use of lasers and light-based therapies for treatment of acne vulgaris. *Lasers Surg Med* 2005;38:1–15.
4. Wiley A, Anderson RR, Azpiazu JL, et al. Complications of laser dermatologic surgery. *Lasers Surg Med* 2006;37:333–342.

Chapter 30
Glycolic Peels

Kathleen M. O'Hanlon

Introduction

Chemical peeling describes a treatment using chemical substances that cause a controlled reaction in the skin and provide both a superficial and deep stimulus for dermal structure renewal [1]. Various wounding agents are used, and peels are typically classified as superficial, medium, or deep. The chemicals used for superficial peels, in which the injury extends through the stratum corneum to the basal cell layer of the epidermis, include alpha hydroxyl acids such as glycolic acid, salicylic acid, low-strength trichloroacetic acid, and the 5-fluorouracil products [2].

In the case of the glycolic peel, concentrated glycolic acids, which are fruit acids found naturally in sugarcane, are applied to the skin for a short period of time and then neutralized to end the treatment [3]. This promotes removal of the outer layer of surface skin cells and stimulates cell rebuilding and restructuring of deeper layers. Healing time depends on the depth of the injury, which depends on the pH or strength of the acid and the duration of time the acid contacts the skin. A series of peels done at 3–4 week intervals can promote the desired changes over 4–6 months.

Case Study

A 49-year-old woman presents to your office for a skin consultation. She has an extensive history of sun exposure, and, on exam, she exhibits significant photodamage of the face including abnormal pigmentation, scattered roughened areas suggestive of actinic keratoses, and a tough, leathery texture.

K.M. O'Hanlon (✉)
Department of Family Practice, Joan C. Edwards Marshall University School of Medicine,
1600 Medical Center Drive, Suite 1500, Huntington, WV, 25701, USA
e-mail: kohanlon@marshall.edu

S.M. Sulik and C.B. Heath (eds.), *Primary Care Procedures in Women's Health*,
DOI 10.1007/978-0-387-76604-1_30, © Springer Science+Business Media, LLC 2010

Diagnosis (Algorithm 30-1)

Actinic Damage

Differential Diagnosis

- Actinic keratoses
- Lentigo
- Melasma
- Dyschromia

Indications [3] (Algorithm 30-1)

- Reverse solar elastosis
- Reverse basal cell atypia
- Reverse abnormal deposition of melanin
- Decrease comedones and papulopustular lesions
- Normalize keratinization and promote normal cell turnover
- Provide the skin with smoothness

Contraindications

- Pregnancy/Lactation
- Active herpetic or varicella lesions in area
- Open wounds in area
- History of Isotretinoin use in previous 6 months
- Genetic syndromes causing skin fragility (i.e., Ehlers–Danlos)

Equipment (Fig. 30-1)

- Surgical bonnet or shower cap
- Cotton balls and mild skin cleanser/prepeel cleanser
- Cotton-tipped swabs/petroleum jelly
- Brushes (to apply wounding agent)
- Dispensing cup and various strengths of glycolic acid (Fig. 30-2)
- Eye protection/ocular wash
- Timer or watch
- Neutralizer spray
- Hand towels
- Postpeel products (sunscreen and moisturizer)

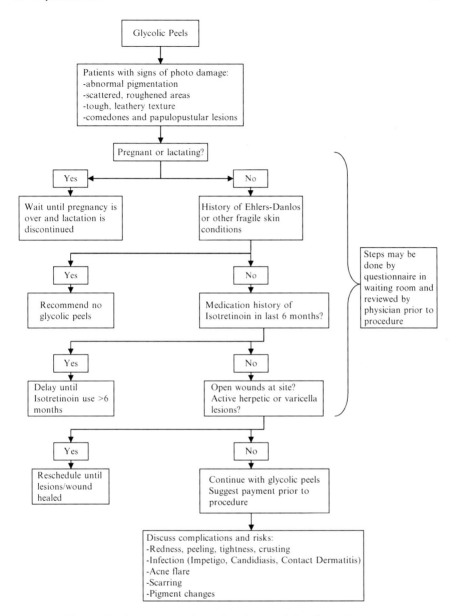

Algorithm 30-1   Indications and contraindications for use of glycolic peels

Optional Equipment

- Small fan (for patient comfort)
- Topical anesthetic (EMLA®, [AstraZeneca, Wilmington, DE], ELA-Max® [Ferndale Laboratories, Ferndale, MI], or betacaine/lidocaine/tetracaine cream from compounding pharmacy)

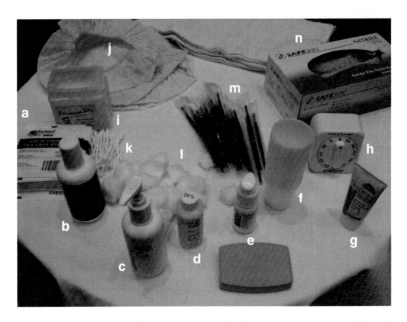

Fig. 30-1 Equipment for glycolic peel treatment. (a) 4×4 cm gauze sponge (Select Medical Products); (b) Neostrata® Optimal PrePeel Cleanser; (c) NeoStrata® Facial Cleanser; (d) Neostrata® Glycolic Acid Skin Peel; (e) Neostrata® Bionic Face Serum; (f) Dispensing cups; (g) Postpeel cream: Neostrata® Daytime Protection Cream; (h) Timer; (i) Petroleum jelly (CVS, Woonsocket, RI); (j) Surgical cap; (k) Cotton tipped applicators; (l) Cotton balls; (m) Brushes for peel; (n) Gloves (Safeskin® Nitrile Gloves, Kimberly–Clark, Roswell, GA). (Not pictured: Peel Neutralizer) (NeoStrata® is a trademark of The NeoStrata Company, Princeton, NJ)

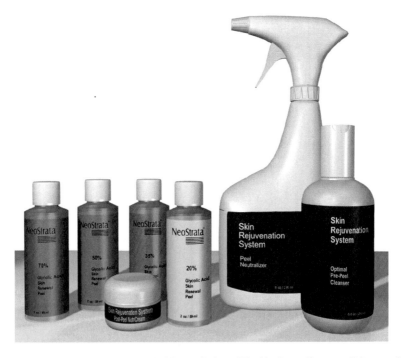

Fig. 30-2 Glycolic acid strengths (used with permission of The NeoStrata Company, Princeton, NJ)

Procedure

1. Cleanse face with gentle cleanser to remove makeup and sebum.
2. Lie patient supine, protect hair with bonnet, and drape with towels.
3. With cotton swab, apply petroleum jelly sparingly to areas of pooling (lateral canthae of eyes, nasolabial folds, and lips).
4. Begin timer and rapidly brush chemical on skin, beginning with forehead, cheeks, and then lower face.
5. Apply carefully around eyes, nose, and lips and sparingly to areas of potential pooling (if solution enters eyes, flush immediately).
6. Complete initial application within 45 seconds; continuous reapplication can be done until neutralization to ensure even skin coverage without fear of over-applying due to layering.
7. Observe for erythema, and query patient about stinging/burning/pain. Pain, vesiculation, blanching, and frosting are reasons to neutralize glycolic acid immediately.
8. If tolerated, allow the acid to contact the skin for 5 minutes (min). When the timer reaches 5 min, protect eyes with damp cotton balls and spray treated areas liberally with bicarbonated neutralizer.
9. Pat with towel and then reapply neutralizer. When foaming ceases, neutralization is complete. Pat dry.
10. Apply moisturizer and sunscreen.

Complications and Risks

- Redness, peeling, light scabbing, mild swelling
- Infection: impetigo, candidiasis, contact dermatitis, reactivation of latent herpes simplex virus
- Pigmentary changes
- Acne flare
- Scarring

Tricks and Helpful Hints

Cold 4×4 gauze sponges or ice packs may be applied to achieve comfort.

Interpretation of Results

Expect some redness and tightness. Fine crusting and peeling may occur over 4–5 days.

Procedure Note

(Provider to customize as needed.)

> The patient was placed in the supine position, and the hair/face appropriately draped. The skin was gently cleansed, and prepeel cleanser was applied using cotton balls. Petroleum jelly was sparingly applied to the lateral canthae of the eyes, nasolabial folds, and the commissures of the lips using a cotton-tipped swab. 20% glycolic acid was rapidly brushed onto the skin and allowed to sit for 5 min. Moist cotton balls were placed for eye protection, and the acid was spray-neutralized and pat-dried with towels twice. Moisturizer and sunscreen were applied. The patient tolerated the procedure without difficulty.

Coding

CPT® Codes (Current Procedural Terminology, AMA, Chicago, IL)

15788	Chemical Peel, facial; epidermal
15789	Chemical Peel, facial; dermal
15792	Chemical Peel, nonfacial; epidermal
15793	Chemical Peel, nonfacial; dermal

ICD 9-CM-Diagnostic Codes (International Classification of Diseases, 9th Revision, Clinical Modification, Center for Disease Control and Prevention)

706.1	Acne
695.3	Rosacea
702.0	Actinic keratosis
709.2	Disfigurement d/t scar
709.00	Dyschromia, unspec.
709.09	Lentigo, Melasma

Postprocedure Patient Instruction

The patient should use gentle cleansers, and apply moisturizer at least twice a day. Strict sun protection and tanning-booth avoidance should be practiced. Redness, tightness, fine peeling, and possibly crusting may be expected for 4–7 days. Unnecessary handling of the skin should be avoided: no rubbing or picking. The patient should return to the office if signs of secondary infection (extreme redness, pustules, vesiculation, purulent drainage, or fever) develop. The patient may also return for repeat peeling after 4–6-week intervals.

Case Study Outcome

Subtle but recognizable signs of skin improvement were achieved following a series of peels, beginning with the 20% strength and gradually advancing to the 70% strength as tolerated.

Patient Handout

(Provider to customize as needed.)

A chemical peel is a technique for skin renewal involving application of concentrated glycolic acids to the skin for a short period of time. This promotes removal of the outer "damaged" layer of surface skin cells and stimulates cell restructuring of deeper layers.

Glycolic acid is one of the Alpha-Hydroxyl Acids (AHAs), a group of naturally occurring substances found in fruits and foods such as sugarcane. Since their discovery in the 1970s, dermatologists worldwide have appreciated the skin results of AHA treatments.

To ensure that you are a candidate for chemical peeling, we will review your medical history, skin sensitivities, and expectations. Pregnancy, active cold sores, or open wounds, and acne treatment with isotretinoin (Accutane®, Hoffmann-La Roche, Inc, Nutley, NJ) are reasons to postpone peeling.

Improvements that may result from a series of peels include: softening of fine lines, evening of skin tone, diminution in size of enlarged skin pores, increased smoothness of skin texture, fewer blemishes in acne-prone skin, and improved glow and radiance.

After your glycolic peel, your skin may be a bit pink and puffy. For most, these changes are subtle, and you can return to your normal activities immediately. It may take up to a week for the renewal process to allow your skin texture and appearance to completely return to normal. During this time, you may experience: stinging, itching, burning, tightness, sun sensitivity, and superficial peeling. Intermittent use of cool compresses and analgesics such as acetaminophen or ibuprofen can be used to treat mild pain and swelling if needed. The skin should be allowed to heal naturally: do not peel, pick, or scratch, and avoid sun or tanning booth exposure.

Rare side effects of the glycolic peel can include: (1) an acne flare up due to deep pore cleansing; (2) a cold sore flare up in those who are prone to these (preventive treatment should be used); (3) infection around the mouth (peri-oral dermatitis); (4) transient skin discoloration (hyper- or hypopigmentation). Please inform your doctor if any of these conditions occur so that proper treatment can be rendered.

After your peel:

- Wash the treated areas gently with soap-free cleansers and apply moisturizer twice daily. Make-up may be applied as usual when tolerated.
- Avoid use of irritants (i.e., retinoids) until the skin has fully healed.
- Strictly avoid sun exposure or tanning booths. Use a broad spectrum sunscreen (SPF at least 30).

Follow up every 3–4 weeks or as advised by your physician.

References

1. Bernstein EF. Chemical peels. In Kaminer MS, Dover JS, Arndt KA (eds) *Atlas of cosmetic surgery*. Philadelphia: WB Saunders, 2002.
2. Fulton, JE, Porumb S. Chemical peels: their place within the range of resurfacing techniques. *Am J Clin Dermatol* 2004;4(3):179–187.
3. Ditre CM, Nini KT, Vagley RT. *Introduction: practical use of glycolic acid as a chemical peeling agent*. From the Department of Dermatology, Hahnemann University, Philadelphia, PA. Private Practice, Princeton and East Brunswick, NJ, and The Pittsburgh Institute of Plastic Surgery, Pittsburgh, PA.

Additional Resources

Books

Brody HJ. *Chemical peeling and resurfacing*, 2nd Ed. St. Louis, MO: Mosby, 1997.
Coleman III WP, Coleman KM. Techniques for peeling of the face. In Merli GJ (ed): *The clinical atlas of office procedures: basic cosmetic procedures*. Philadelphia: WB Saunders, 2000.

Index